Yves Keravel Marc Sindou

Giant Intracranial Aneurysms

Therapeutic Approaches

In Collaboration with
G. Debrun · Ph. Decq · F.G. Diaz · V. Dolenc
J. Duquesnel · A. Gaston · Y. Guegan · J. Huppert
C. Marsault · Ph. Mercier · J. Moret · F.R. Nelson
J.P. Nguyen · G. Perrin · J. Pialat

Foreword by M.G. Yaşargil

With 123 Figures

Springer-Verlag
Berlin Heidelberg NewYork
London Paris Tokyo

Professor Dr. Yves Keravel
Service de Neurochirurgie de l'Hôpital Henri-Mondor
51, Ave. du Maréchal-de-Lattre-de-Tassigny
F-94000 Créteil, France

Professor Dr. Marc Sindou
Hôpital Neurologique et Neurochirurgical Pierre Wertheimer
59, Bld. Pinel, F-69003 Lyon, France

Originally published in French under the title
"Les anévrysmes géants intracrâniens. Approches thérapeutiques"

Revised and enlarged edition translated by S. Rao

ISBN-13: 978-3-642-83173-7 e-ISBN-13: 978-3-642-83171-3
DOI: 10.1007/978-3-642-83171-3

Library of Congress Cataloging-in-Publication Data. Anévrysmes géants intracrâniens. English. Giant intracranial aneurysms. Translation of: Les anévrysmes géants intracrânien. Bibliography: p. Includes index. 1. Intracranial aneurysms – Surgery. I. Keravel, Y. (Yves), 1944– . II. Sindou, M. (Marc), 1943– . III. Debrun, G. IV. Title. [DNLM: 1. Carotid Artery Diseases – complications. 2. Cerebral Aneurysm – surgery. WL 355 A5799] RD594.2.A5413 1987 617'.481 87-26321
ISBN-13: 978-3-642-83173-7 (U.S.)

Softcover reprint of the hardcover 1st edition 1988

2122/3130-543210

Foreword

The first aneurysms explored by such pioneers of neurosurgery as Cushing and Dandy were the giant intracranial aneurysms. These giant aneurysms present many therapeutic difficulties and, because of their unique anatomical features and size, may present in a multitude of ways. With the advent of specialized imaging techniques such as computed tomography (CT), magnetic resonance imaging (MRI) and selective angiography, preoperative diagnosis today is most often accomplished without difficulty. However, completely thrombosed giant aneurysms may mimic other lesions with mass effect (such as basilar meningiomas, chordomas or chondromas) and their true anatomical shapes and relations to other cranial structures can only be ascertained by direct operative inspection.

Due to their morphological features (thrombosed, nonthrombosed, partially thrombosed, fusiform), anatomical variations and difficult locations, giant aneurysms present new challenges for the modern neurosurgeon. Although microsurgical techniques have rendered direct surgical treatment of giant intracranial aneurysms safer, elimination of the aneurysm without disturbing the hemodynamics continues to be problematic. Some of these lesions have relatively small necks and can therefore be clipped fairly easily. Others have large necks, are fusiform, or contain perforators; how best to treat these lesions is a question still unresolved by presentday neurosurgery.

The authors have presented and discussed the pathology and hemodynamics as related to the mechanism of formation of giant intracranial aneurysms. They have included neuroradiological techniques (especially CT, MRI and arteriography) as pertinent in the management of these difficult vascular lesions. They have carefully reviewed the various clinical approaches for treatment of giant intracranial aneurysms. Finally they have summarized guidelines for management of treatment according to clinical and anatomical considerations.

The authors have provided a work of superior all-round quality which should be considered a valuable reference for the serious neurosurgeon.

M.G. Yaşargil

Preface

This work, devoted to the difficult problem of the management of giant intracranial aneurysms, is based on the combined experience of the authors, the cooperative study of the French-Speaking Neurosurgical Society, and a review of the world literature published during the last 12 years.

The study was previously published in a French monograph entitled "Les anévrysmes géants intracrâniens: approches thérapeutiques", published by the French-Speaking Neurosurgical Society in 1984 in *Neurochirurgie* [30 (Suppl 1) 1–128]. In the present book, new cases have been added from the authors' personal experience, the literature review has been updated to 1985, and several chapters have been enriched with new, up-to-date additions.

The authors are grateful to S. Rao for the translation and Heidrun Herion and Ursula Davis of Springer-Verlag for their useful advice during preparation of this edition.

Y. Keravel
M. Sindou

Foreword to the French Edition*

Through Louis Mansuy's good offices, Yves Keravel and Marc Sindou have asked me to write a brief introduction to their report. This tactful manner of approach, at a time when my name has begun to fade away from the public memory, is most touching. No less moving is the thought that, from beyond the grave, Mr. Wertheimer, one of the founders of the French-Speaking Society of Neurosurgery, is to witness a gathering of some of his students and myself at a Congress chaired by Jacques de Rougemont, who was also a student of his. And yet, what has a man still to say whose career in neurosurgery was cut short by superannuation 6 years ago? First and foremost, he would be remiss – and in this particular case, it is not just a matter of politeness – if he did not emphasize the rare quality of this work, its thoroughness, and the authors' obvious efforts to understand each problem as it arose.

Going beyond the usual pathologic, clinical, diagnostic and therapeutic issues, the authors devote two pithy chapters to the role of anatomical and hemodynamic features in the formation and growth of giant aneurysms. Not content with making deductions from the laws of fluid mechanics, they resort to firsthand experimentation to enrich our knowledge of the modes of flow, of blood turbulence within the aneurysmal sac, and, as a result, of the organization of thrombi or the risks of rupture. Equally laudable are the pains they have taken some chapters later, to give their colleagues an exact picture of the technology of clips, taking care not to overlook the risks attending most of them (except austenic clips) during follow-up by magnetic resonance imagery. Here I should perhaps mention that throughout their report the authors have not neglected silk ligatures, the enormous possibilities of which I personally have always valued.

One final comment, so as not to overstep the limit fixed for me by the editor. I find altogether praiseworthy the lucid descriptions of recent technical advances (Vinko Dolenc's, for instance, concerning intracavernous aneurysms). So, also, on the therapeutic plane, is the rigorous analysis of the results of occlusion of the arterial pedicles or their intravascular obliteration with balloons, both of which can be used as a last resort.

The latter technique, introduced by Serbinenko, has been improved upon by G. Debrun so radically that C. Drake himself has not hesitated to use it – which goes to show how very difficult it is to manage giant aneurysms in a not inconsiderable proportion of cases.

The handful of neurosurgeons in Europe and elsewhere in the world who, since the latter half of the 1940s, have avoided systematic ligature of the arteries at the cervical level cannot help mentioning the headway made. They used to operate under local anesthesia, that is to say, without tracheal intubation and – at least initially – without the option of controlled hypotension, and with a poorly lit operative field. Only the grim spontaneous

* Presented at a meeting of the French-Speaking Neurosurgical Society held in Grenoble June 28–30, 1984.

course of aneurysms of any size can account for their courage, not to say their rashness. Their faith has now found its reward, and their approach its vindication, in the more numerous safer options that are available to us today. But what will perhaps prove most satisfying to those of us who have reached the end of their careers is to find, in the final chapter setting out the general conclusions of the report, that Sindou and Keravel harbor the same burning faith which drove their predecessors to "forge ahead towards a safer and more efficacious" mode of treating giant intracranial aneurysms.

We who are on our way out can draw comfort from them. For my own part, I owe them my warmest and most sincere thanks.

EMILE LAINE
Honorary Professor of Neurosourgery

Contents

Introduction

Giant intracranial aneurysms, owing to their volume and anatomical features, have always been considered as lesions presenting great therapeutic difficulties, such that in the past they were most often approached by indirect methods. A generation of neurosurgeons, represented by Norlen and Laine in Europe and Drake in North America, showed that it was possible to manage giant aneurysms of some types and in certain localizations by direct surgical approach without undue risk. More recently, several neurosurgeons such as Sundt and Hosobuchi in the United States, Pertuiset and Yasargil in Europe, and Suzuki, Ishii, and Sugita in Japan, have proceeded further along this path. Besides direct surgical management, which has been rendered safer by microsurgical techniques, methods of occlusion of the parent artery, where the attendant risks of ischemia can be reduced by prior extra-intracranial bypass, also play an interesting role. Finally, progress in management by the intravascular methods developed by Serbinenko in the USSR, and Debrun in Europe and later on in the United States has made it possible to achieve occlusion in aneurysms until then considered difficult of access.

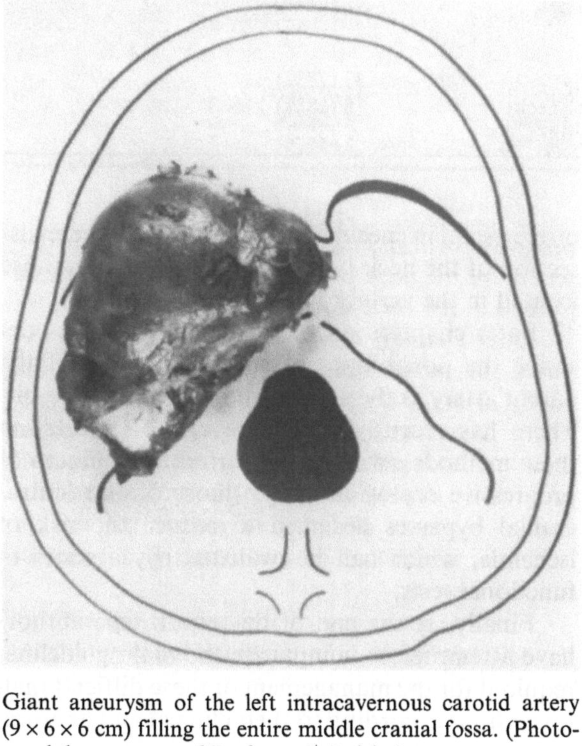

Giant aneurysm of the left intracavernous carotid artery (9 × 6 × 6 cm) filling the entire middle cranial fossa. (Photograph by courtesy of Professor J. Poirier)

Entrusted by the French-speaking Neurosurgical Society with the preparation of this monograph, we have endeavored to synthesize the current therapeutic approaches for the management of these malformations. This topic has gained particular interest owing to the technological advances of the past 10 years and the spate of papers which have appeared recently.

The present report has been based on three sources of information: (a) 80 personal cases treated by the authors at the Neurological Hospital of Lyon and Henri-Mondor Hospital of Créteil; (b) 309 observations collected from replies to a questionnaire sent to the members of the French-speaking Neurosurgical Society with a view to the preparation of this report (see table below); and (c) a detailed review of the literature over the past 12 years.

As is emphasized in its title, this report focuses on the numerous therapeutic approaches which have been proposed for the management of giant intracranial aneurysms. It also analyzes the anatomical, physiological, clinical, and neuroradiological data which have been found useful for these approaches.

The first chapters, devoted to the pathology and hemodynamics at the level of the parent artery and aneurysmal sac, stress the mechanisms of formation and forms of development of this type of aneurysm. An understanding of these phenomena is of paramount importance for determination of the management to be adopted.

The clinical study is presented briefly, as a detailed paper on the topic has recently been published by P. Creissard et al. in the journal *Neurochirurgie* (reference 19 in the bibliography to the chapter entitled "Clinical Study").

The chapter concerning the neuroradiological features mainly deals with computed tomography

A cooperative study by the French-speaking Society of Neurosurgery involving 309 cases from 1973 to 1983
The numbers of cases are different in the various headings, due to a lack of information in some series. In the following tables dealing with localizations or treatment we have only considered cases in which complete data concerning mortality, morbidity and good results were available.

Sex distribution		Clinical presentation		Pathological types	
Male	126 cases (40%)	Hemorrhagic:	142 (48%)	Nonthrombosed:	164 (60.5%)
Female	183 cases (60%)	Pseudotumoral:	140 (47%)	Thrombosed:	23 (8.5%)
		Thromboembolic:	14 (5%)	Partly thrombosed:	75 (28%)
				Serpentine:	8 (3%)

Topographical types		Management		
		Direct surgical approach (%)	Parent artery ligation (%)	Intravascular occlusion (%)
Cavernous sinus	66 (23.5%)	1.5	58.5	19
Carotid ophthalmic	46 (16.5%)	48	46	6
Posterior communicating	54 (19%)	78	19	3
Carotid bifurcation	25 (9%)	58	26	16
Middle cerebral	56 (20%)	96	4	
Anterior communicating	28 (10%)	87.5	12.5	
Vertebral	3 (1%)	25	50	25
Basilar trunk	13 (4.5%)	33.3	66.3	
Basilar trunk bifurcation	1 (0.3%)			
Other sites	7 (2.5%)	25	50	25

Results:

1. Direct surgical management: 155 cases (54%)

Mortality:	41 cases (26.5%)	by neck occlusion:	133 (87%)
Morbidity:	38 cases (24.5%)	by wrapping:	20 (13%)
Good results:	76 cases (49%)		

2. Occlusion of parent artery: 90 cases (31%)

Mortality:	8 cases (8.8%)	proximally:	71 (86.5%)
Morbidity:	9 cases (10%)	by trapping:	11 (13.5%)
Good results:	73 cases (81.2%)		

3. Intravascular occlusion: 43 cases (15%)

Mortality:	7 cases (16%)	proximally:	33 (77%)
Morbidity:	8 cases (18.5%)	in front of neck:	8 (18%)
Good results:	28 cases (65.5%)	in aneurysm:	2 (5%)

(CT), which is essential for the diagnosis, surgical indications, and follow-up of these malformations.

The first chapter devoted to therapeutic approaches deals with direct surgical approaches for selective occlusion of the neck, which whenever feasible is the treatment of choice.

Although beyond the limits of the topic, we have found it useful to include chapters on subjects of more general interest such as those relating to clip technology and extracorporeal circulation. As a matter of fact, recent advances in these fields have made some of these giant malformations more accessible to direct surgical management. Special attention is paid to other interesting direct methods, like intraluminal thrombosis, which only requires minimal exposure of the sac and may prove useful in specific anatomical types where dissection of the neck is very difficult (notably, those located in the vertebrobasilar circulation).

Later chapters on therapeutic approaches describe the possibilities of surgical ligation of the parent artery at the cervical and intracranial levels. There has recently been a revival of interest in these methods owing to the current techniques of progressive occlusion and to those of extra-intracranial bypasses designed to reduce the risk of ischemia, which can be evaluated by a series of functional tests.

Finally, at the end of this report, the authors have attempted to summarize the main guidelines required for the management of these difficult malformations according to their clinical and anatomical characteristics.

Anatomical Definition

Giant aneurysms are classically defined by their size; an outer diameter equal to or greater than 25 mm is the criterion accepted by most authors. Even more than their size, their anatomical peculiarities – responsible for technical difficulties – make them a distinct entity (Fig. 1).

The neck, which is usually wide, can be either fragile or rigid because of atheromatous plaques or mural thrombi, which makes clipping difficult.

The sac, a frequent site of partial thrombosis, often adheres to collaterals of the parent artery. Moreover, collateral branches may arise directly from the neck.

The aneurysmal mass is often difficult to separate from the anatomical site from which it develops and to dissect from the adjacent cerebral tissue and the surrounding cranial nerves.

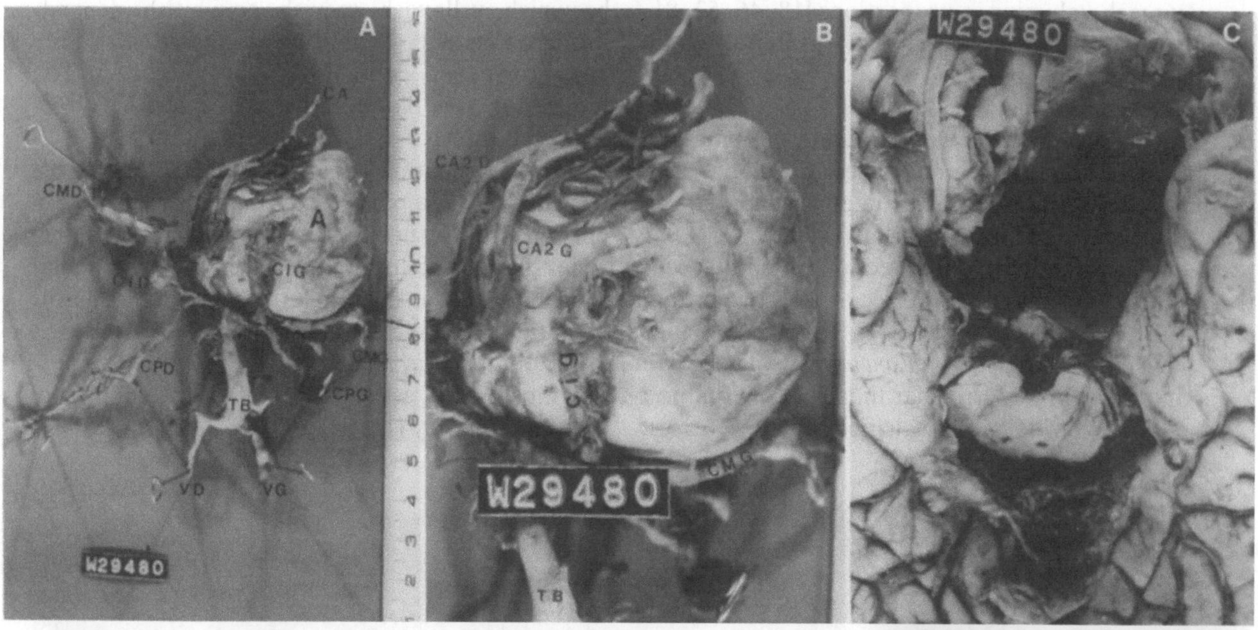

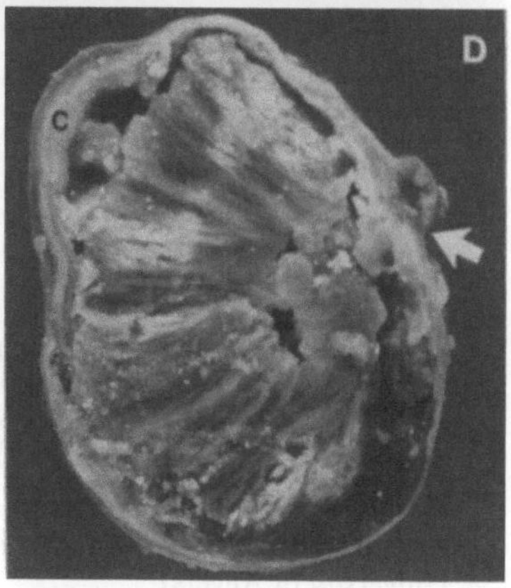

Fig. 1 A–D. Anatomical definition. **A** Left carotid ophthalmic aneurysm on circle of Willis (∅45 mm). **B** The aneurysm is attached to the left juxtaclinoid carotid with a large neck. The carotid is rooted in the base of the aneurysm. Note displacement of vessels adjacent to the aneurysm, especially the two anterior cerebral arteries and middle cerebral artery. **C** Cavity corresponding to the site of the aneurysm at the base of the left frontal lobe. Note upward displacement of diencephalon and backward displacement of cerebral peduncles. **D** Transverse cut of aneurysmal sac which is totally thrombosed and calcified after proximal carotid ligation. Note attachment site of sac on carotid (*arrow*) and thickness of calcified aneurysm wall (*C*). *A*, aneurysm; *CA*, anterior cerebral artery; *CA2D*, right anterior cerebral artery (ACA2); *CA2G*, left anterior cerebral artery (ACA2); *CID*, right internal carotid artery; *CIG*, left internal carotid artery; *CMD*, right middle cerebral artery; *CMG*, left middle cerebral artery; *CPD*, right posterior cerebral artery; *CPG*, left posterior cerebral artery; *VD*, right vertebral artery; *VG*, left vertebral artery; *TB*, basilar trunk

Mechanisms of Formation: Pathologic Features

This chapter will describe successively the macroscopic and microscopic features of giant intracranial aneurysms and the neuropathologic factors involved in their formation.

Macroscopic Findings

Most giant aneurysms are saccular. They are located on arterial bifurcations of the circle of Willis or on its main branching arteries. They may be unique or multiple in number [21, 26, 28], and may reach voluminous proportions [18, 46, 52, 81, 93], up to $12 \times 8 \times 6$ cm in size, as reported by Pianetti et al. [74].

The aneurysmal sac (Fig. 2) is most often whitish and hard. Its neck may contain atheromatous plaques. The neck is more or less developed and most often large. Leptomeninges around the sac are thickened and may be yellowish (see Fig. 1).

After formalin fixation, section of giant saccular aneurysms may reveal three aspects, according to the extent of thrombosis:

1. *Nonthrombosed giant aneurysms:* Their wall is thicker and more irregular than that of common aneurysms but is rarely calcified. In these cases, considered nonthrombosed by the clinician, the internal wall of the sac is covered by a laminated mural thrombus. This has led Stehbens [94] to consider such aneurysms as almost always partly thrombosed.

2. *Partly thrombosed giant aneurysms:* The thrombus accounts for a noticeable reduction of the sac. The fibrous and irregular wall contains areas of nodular thickening, which give a multilobulated external appearance to the pouch [97]. It often contains small, laminated calcifications. The thrombus lining the internal surface of the sac is brownish, yellowish, greyish, or whitish, depending upon its age. It may be laminated with grey and brown concentric layers (see Fig. 7A). The lumen contains blood and is off-centered with irregular borders.

The "serpentine" aneurysm [23, 27, 53, 73, 85, 97, 101, 104] is a partly thrombosed sacciform aneurysm with tortuous, off-centered channels sometimes giving rise to blind recesses. This particular morphological entity is mostly found in the middle cerebral, internal carotid, and vertebral arteries.

3. *Totally thrombosed giant aneurysms.* These are most often associated with a thrombosis of the parent artery [12, 89, 108].

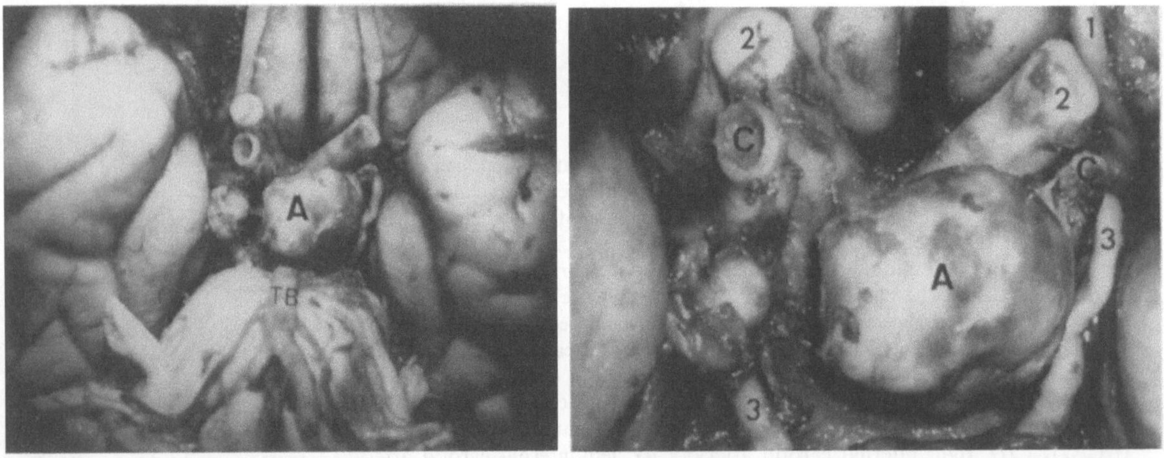

Fig. 2. Left carotid-ophthalmic aneurysm (*A*) of the infraoptochiasmatic type (inferior view). *TB*, basilar artery; *C*, carotid artery; *1*, olfactory nerve; *2*, optic nerve; *3*, oculomotor nerve. (Photographs by courtesy of Professor G. Guy, University of Angers)

Figure 1 gives a macroscopic view of a thrombosed aneurysm after carotid ligation. The thrombus within the sac is homogeneous, greyish-white, and with fine calcifications arranged linearly from its base.

Giant saccular aneurysms unrelated to arterial forks are more rare. They are usually encountered in older patients in a highly atheromatous circle of Willis, especially in the vertebrobasilar system. The sac is very atheromatous and calcified. The adjacent leptomeninge contains a rich capillary network. Sometimes multiple aneurysms are present.

Giant fusiform aneurysms are very similar to megadolichoarteries as Little et al. [57] have suggested, though with a greater diameter. Their arterial trunk presents a concentric dilatation which, by definition, is 25 mm large or more. Their elective location is the basilar artery (three cases out of 9000 post-mortem examinations [80]) and, more rarely, the supraclinoid segment of the carotid or the middle cerebral artery [68]. As saccular aneurysms unrelated to arterial forks, their walls are calcified and severely atherosclerotic, but they do not tend to develop a true sac. Giant fusiform aneurysms are also observed in children [100], and may be calcified [55].

In giant aneurysms, *the parent artery and its branches* are often incorporated in the sac [29, 101], or are at least closely attached by fibrous, meningeal, and/or glial tracts (see Fig. 1). At bifurcations, the parent artery is only slightly atheromatous, except in the neck of saccular aneurysms. Giant aneurysms unrelated to bifurcations as well as giant fusiform aneurysms show marked atheromatous deposits, except in children.

Examination of the *circle of Willis* often shows other aneurysmal sacs with small, thin-walled ectasic, parietal changes which may correspond to aneurysmal sacs in formation and which are referred to as "preaneurysms." Developmental abnormalities are frequently present in the circle of Willis. They may be implicated in the formation of aneurysms through the hemodynamic changes they cause. Examples are: hypoplasia of anterior cerebral artery segment A1, arterial agenesis [51], azygos anterior cerebral artery [44] and fenestrations of the vertebrobasilar system [87], or other vestigial vessels such as trigeminal arteries [64] (Fig. 3). According to Sonntag et al. [88] and other authors, such abnormalities are present in about one third of cases.

An association between angiomas (arteriovenous shunts) and giant aneurysms has been reported [1, 11, 66, 100, 103]. The consequent increase in blood flow is considered a precipitating factor in the formation of such aneurysms.

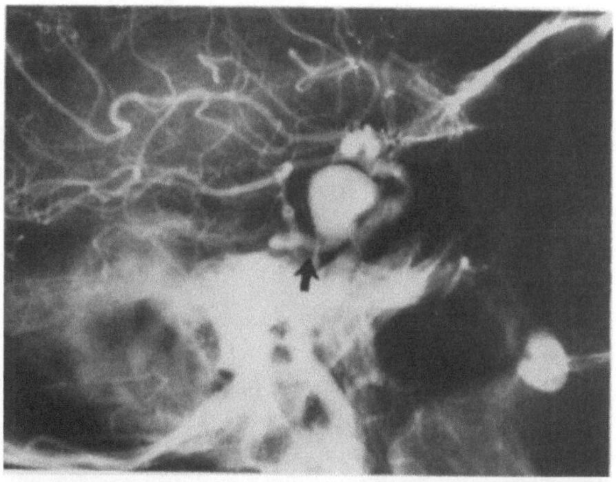

Fig. 3. M.G., a 69-year-old female. Aneurysm of the origin of a right trigeminal artery (*arrow*), opposite the superior orbital fissure, revealed by abducens palsy (lateral view)

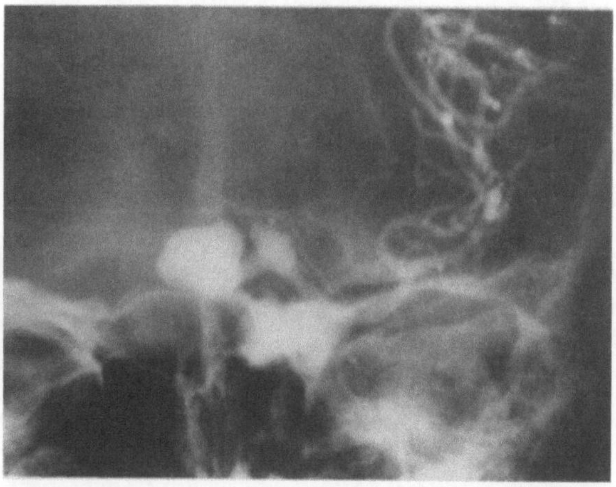

Fig. 4. Multiple aneurysms. G.L., a 40-year-old female with four aneurysms: giant left intracavernous aneurysm (anteroposterior diameter of 25 mm); left carotid-ophthalmic aneurysm; left carotid artery bifurcation aneurysm; anterior communicating artery aneurysm fed by right carotid artery (not seen in this photograph)

The presence of a giant aneurysm, especially if associated with aneurysms, *should prompt examination for blood-vessel dysplasia:* fibromuscular dysplasia of the media [45, 50, 76], connective tissue disorders such as Ehlers–Danlos syndrome [61], elastic pseudo-xanthoma, or Marfan's disease [22, 61, 62, 79] (Fig. 4). Associated malformations such as polycystic kidney disease or aorta coarctation should also be investigated [41, 47]. Such associations have only been rarely described; however, it must be stressed with giant aneurysms that post-

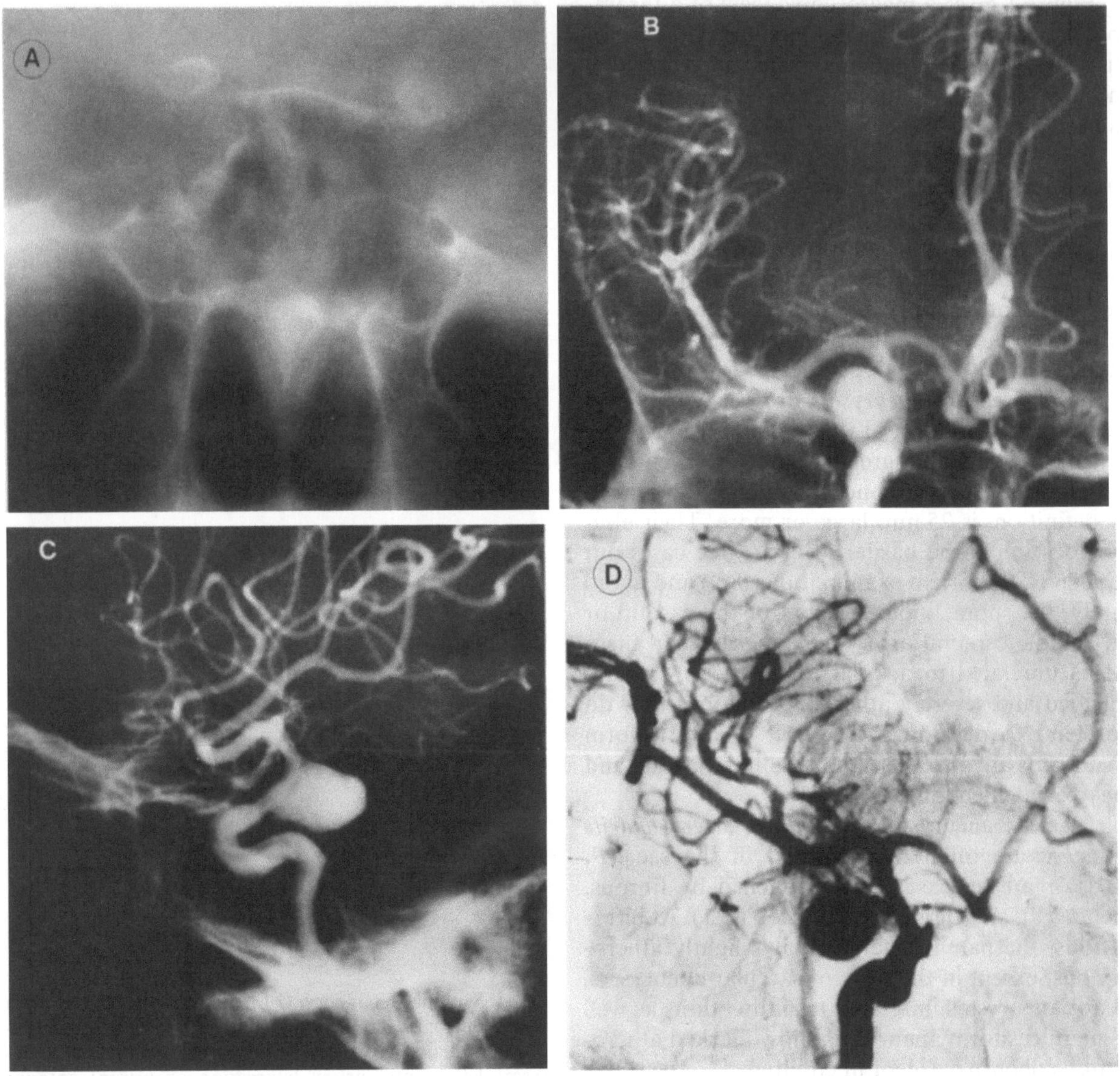

Fig. 5A–D. P.L., a 24-year-old male, was referred in December 1985, after a cranial traumatism with a third nerve palsy, for an osteodural fistula responsible for three successive bouts of meningitis. As the CT scan and the basal skull tomogram revealed important fractures of the sphenoid on the right side (**A**), a right carotid angiogram was obtained to check the integrity of the carotid artery. It demonstrated a large vascular aneurysm (**B, C**), arising from the juxtaclinoid carotid segment through an apparently 3-mm-long channel (**D**). At the operation, the aneurysm walls and neck could not be clearly identified, so the internal carotid artery was exposed at the cervical neck in order to allow further dissection of the lesion with temporary proximal clamping. The dissection resulted in a rupture of the lesion which was actually a fibrinous reorganized pseudoaneurysm enclosed within a plastic arachnoiditis. It only could be controlled by undertaking an extra-intracranial trapping of the ICA. The operation was completed by doing an immediate superficial temporal-middle cerebral artery bypass, the superficial temporal artery having been preserved for that eventuality

mortem examinations have not systematically involved peripheral arteries (for example, carotid, renal, and splenic arteries).

Occasional associations of giant aneurysms with tuberous sclerosis were reported by two authors; once in a 53-year-old man [34] and once in a child [8]. Giant aneurysms were also reported ipsilaterally to congenital hemihypertrophy in association with capillary hemangioma and arteriovenous malformation [25]. Some other associations have been described: with facial nevus flammens, for instance [78].

Post-traumatic lesions of the arterial wall, though very unusual, can lead to aneurysmal formations. Some of these aneurysms may become giant, especially in the juxtaclinoid part of the carotid artery [82]. Their sac results from a fibrinous organization inside a subarachnoid cistern compartmented by a plastic arachnoiditis (Fig. 5).

Post-mortem examination of the brain and of cranial nerves adjacent to the aneurysm, especially in the case of pseudotumoral aneurysms, may allow an evaluation of compressive, ischemic, or embolic lesions linked with the presence of giant aneurysms and an assessment of the frequency of such associated lesions.

Microscopic and Ultrastructural Findings

A review of the past 12 years' literature shows a relative lack of histological studies dealing with giant aneurysms. Examination of five cases known to the authors has shown that the appearance of the aneurysmal wall was roughly similar to that described by Thauvoy et al. [102].

Light Microscopy

The wall thickness is variable, ranging from 0.2 to 2 mm, sometimes more. The wall of the aneurysm is contiguous to that of the parent artery, the internal elastic lamina and tunica media of which are usually completely interrupted beyond the neck.

In thinner zones, the wall is composed of dense, paucicellular collagenous tissue. This tissue may contain in its innermost part blood pigments, free or within macrophages, and vascular slits with some hemorrhages (Fig. 7B).

In thicker zones, the wall is often composed of two layers. The outer layer, exclusively fibrous, is difficult to distinguish from common scar tissue. The inner layer is thicker and is composed of young connective tissue, which is cellular and rich in blood vessels, with old or recent small hemorrhages more numerous in the neck. Between the two layers, fatty deposits rich in cholesterol crystals are frequently observed, containing lipid-laden macrophages and occasional multinucleate giant cells. Linear or clustered calcifications are seen in the fibrous outer layer and in the atheromatous plaques which can undergo ossification. Sometimes the inner layer is lined by organized mural thrombi appearing as more or less extensive fibrovascular proliferation covering the inner face of the sac (Fig. 8A, B). The aneurysm is surrounded

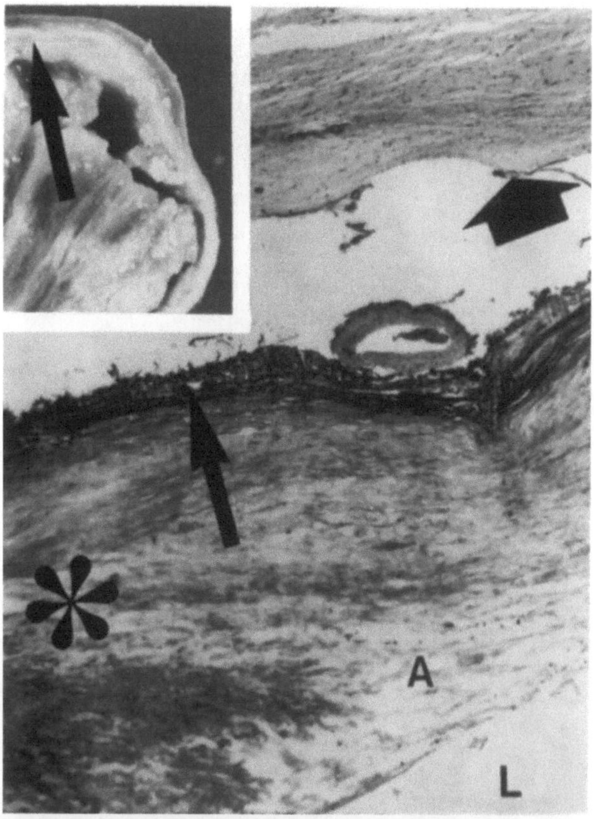

Fig. 6. Patient W.E. 29480 HPS (GI ×63). *Upper left:* macroscopic aspect of aneurysmal sac and corresponding histological feature (*arrow*). The lumen of aneurysm (*L*) is at *lower right*. The wall (*asterisk*) is irregularly thickened by dense sclerous collagen. Atheromatous deposit (*A*) inside it. The wall is covered by a thickened leptomeninge (*long arrow*). Gliosis of aneurysmal bed (*short arrow*)

by thickened leptomeninges (Fig. 8C), exteriorly covered by a glial lamina (Fig. 6). The meninge is often the site of recent subacute inflammatory reaction with fibrosis of the arachnoid, abundant inflammatory infiltrate, and occasional hemosiderin pigment. In older cases, the fibrous leptomeninge tends to become incorporated into the wall of the aneurysm (Fig. 8A).

The surrounding cerebral parenchyma shows a dense, reactive, fibrillar, astrocytic gliosis (Fig. 6). Perls' stain for iron shows ferrous pigments within the aneurysmal wall and adjacent leptomeninges, suggestive of fissure formation, or old, scarred, microscopic parietal ruptures.

"Serpentine" aneurysms show a characteristic non-endothelialized channel within the intrasaccular thrombus [101]. Fusiform and saccular aneurysms unrelated to arterial bifurcations are highly atheromatous. Aneurysms in children [2, 10, 30, 33, 56, 71, 72, 94, 106], although occurring early

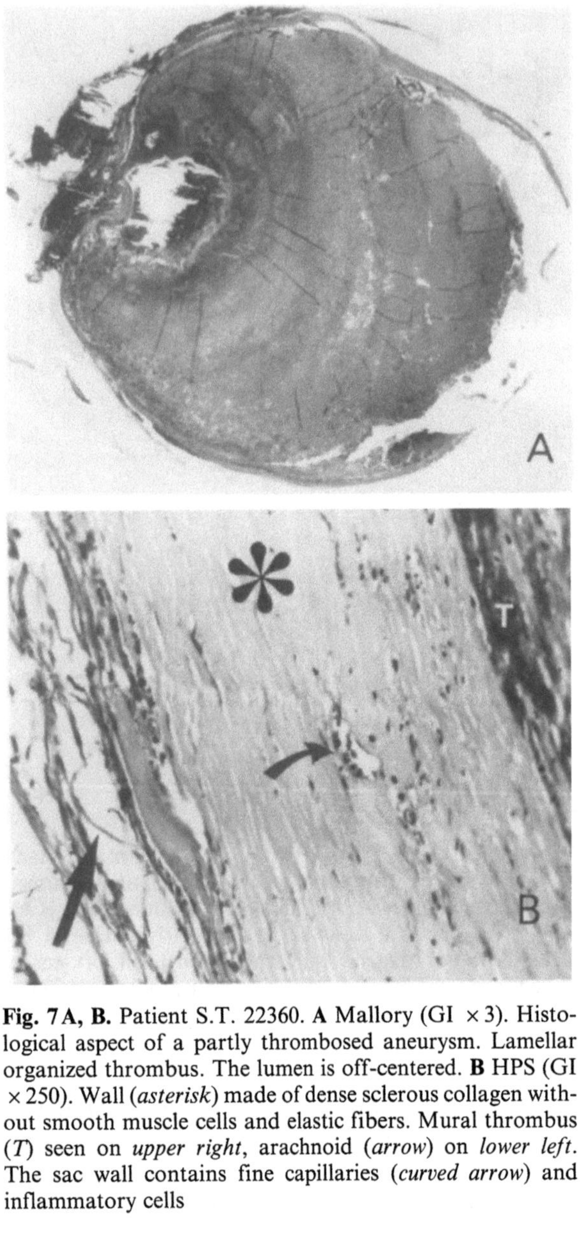

Fig. 7A, B. Patient S.T. 22360. **A** Mallory (GI ×3). Histological aspect of a partly thrombosed aneurysm. Lamellar organized thrombus. The lumen is off-centered. **B** HPS (GI ×250). Wall (*asterisk*) made of dense sclerous collagen without smooth muscle cells and elastic fibers. Mural thrombus (*T*) seen on *upper right*, arachnoid (*arrow*) on *lower left*. The sac wall contains fine capillaries (*curved arrow*) and inflammatory cells

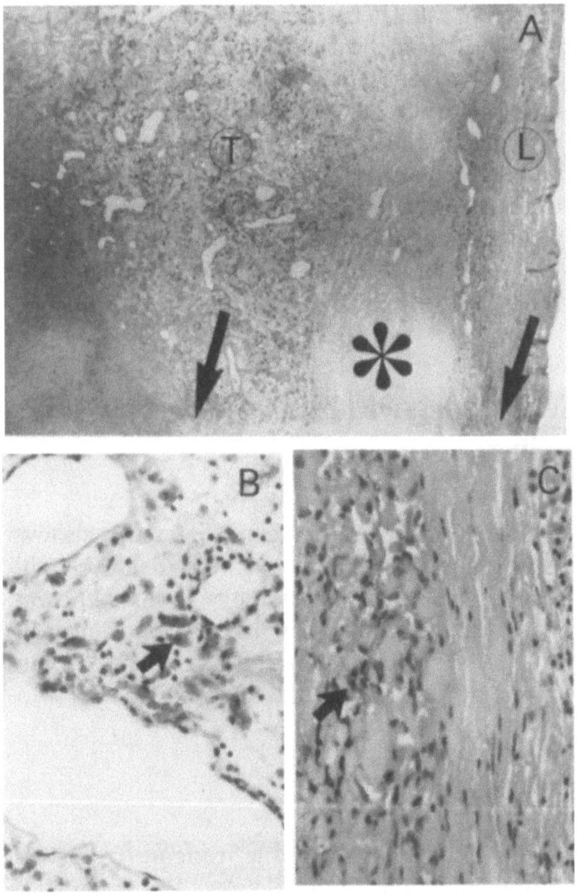

Fig. 8A–C. Patient F.X. 31273. **A** HE (GI ×63): Old aneurysmal wall (*asterisk*) with mural thrombus (*T*). A thickened leptomeninge (*L*). **B** HE (GI ×250): Details of organizing thrombus. Three newly formed capillaries within scleroedematous and inflammatory tissue. Note some hemosiderin-laden macrophages (*arrow*). **C** HE (GI ×250): Details of a thickened leptomeninge covered on the outside by wall of aneurysm (*arrow*). Fibrous thickening of the leptomeninges. Meningocyte proliferation with discrete inflammatory reaction. (Photograph by courtesy of Professor Pansini, University of Florence)

in life, are not necessarily related to blood vessel dysplasias. Some authors attribute them to a congenital focal abnormality of the arterial wall [56].

Finally, rare mycotic [15] or traumatic [19, 77] giant aneurysms have been reported.

Electron Microscopy

We have not found in the literature any mention of ultrastructural studies of giant aneurysmal walls. The ultrastructural studies of common aneurysmal sacs have given rise to various interpretations of the origin of aneurysms. Nyström [69] considers that they are secondary to developmental defects of the parietal wall. Lang and Kid [54] and Stehbens [96], as also Meyerman and Yasargil [63] more recently, believe that such vascular lesions correspond to a nonspecific degenerative reaction of the wall. Cajander and Hassler [9] think that the increasing fragility of the arterial wall is linked to a release of lysosomal particles from polymorphonuclear cells within the vessel's lumen. The degenerative arterial lesions are considered by Scanarini et al. [84] as ischemic and secondary to arteriosclerosis of the adventitial "vasa vasorum."

Scanning Electron Microscopy

Here again, accessible research has been found to deal with walls of aneurysms of ordinary dimensions [43, 83]. It describes crater-like lesions of the intima or findings closely resembling those seen in atherosclerosis.

Biochemical Study of Connective Tissue

The association of intracranial aneurysms with mitral valve prolapse was published by Jackson [48]. Although such lesions are quite common, this association may reflect a diffuse abnormality of the connective tissue. Neil Dwyer et al. [65] made a comparative study of the cutaneous and vascular collagens of patients with intracranial aneurysms and normal controls. Eight out of the 17 patients with an aneurysm had an abnormal type III collagen.

Experimental Data

Experimental aneurysms have been produced by various techniques [32, 60, 105]. In the most classic one, a vein graft is derived onto an artery [5, 6, 67, 95]. Using this technique, we attempted to reproduce giant aneurysms in the dog's cervical carotid artery. Most sacs formed by this technique have undergone thrombosis. This is not surprising if one considers the experimental findings of Black and German [6], who found that the bigger and thinner the sac, the greater its tendency to thrombosis. When experimental aneurysms undergo thrombosis, they show a complete organization and fibrosis, unlike human aneurysms, in which only part of the thrombus is organized.

The most elegant method of producing intracranial aneurysms in rats, described by Hashimoto et al. in 1978 [35, 36, 37], sometimes produces true giant aneurysms. The animals are given a lathyrism factor, β-aminoproprionitrile, which weakens the elastic and connective tissue of the arterial walls. Hypertension is induced by unilateral nephrectomy associated with a high salt diet and desoxycorticosterone administration. Unilateral ligature of the carotid artery produces hemodynamic disturbances which favor the appearance of intracranial aneurysms. This protocol produces the three factors apparently needed for aneurysm induction: weakening of the arterial wall, hemodynamic disorder, and arterial hypertension. In man, the last factor is still the subject of controversy. It must be stressed that rats with normal blood pressure which are submitted to the action of β-aminoproprionitrile do not form intracranial aneurysms [86], as found in an experiment carried out by the present authors on animals at the Institut National pour la Santé et la Recherche Médicale, Unit 37.

Natural History of Giant Intracranial Aneurysms

Pathogenetic hypotheses about the formation of aneurysms and their transformation into giant aneurysms are based on morphological findings. Giant aneurysms are formed in three stages: the first one leads to aneurysmal sac development through weakening of the internal wall; the second stage consists in the dilatation of the sac up to a "critical-sized" aneurysm; the third stage ends in a giant aneurysm.

The first two stages will be covered here briefly, since they are well known.

Weakening of the Arterial Wall and Induction of the Aneurysmal Pouch

Two groups of theories explain the remodellings of arterial walls which are necessary to the development of preaneurysmal lesions. The older so-called "congenital" theories [7, 20] have now been discarded. Forbus [24], Glynn [31], and Carmichael [13, 14] were the first to describe the parietal defects responsible for aneurysm formation. According to Forbus, the sites of least resistance of the arterial wall are in the bifurcation apex. Weakening of the wall is apparently due to a defect of the media. Glynn believes that elastic tissue and internal elastic lamina degeneration is the determining factor in aneurysm formation. Carmichael considers that concomitant lesions of the media and of the internal elastic lamina are necessary to the formation of aneurysms.

The theories of an "acquired" parietal defect leading to preaneurysmal lesions are defended by Stehbens [90, 91, 92, 93, 94], who believes that the defects of the media responsible for intracranial aneurysms are acquired and are different from those described by Forbus. Preaneurysms are apparently represented by funnel-shaped dilatations at bifurcation sites [39, 40, 41, 42], thinning parietal sites, and incipient aneurysms corresponding to parietal evaginations. According to Stehbens, such lesions have in common a disappearance of the media and of the internal elastic lamina of the parent vessels. The factors responsible are said to be hypertension (whose role is still contested), atherosclerosis [107], and hemodynamic stress.

From Formed Aneurysm to the "Critical" Phase

According to Suzuki and Ohara [99], the aneurysm first undergoes a phase of progressive expansion, explained by sac dilatation due to hemodynamic phenomena. Thus the volume of the sac can increase and its wall undergo modification. Initially, the wall is slender and regular over its entire length. Then, as a result of hemodynamic aggression, it thickens at the dome but its neck remains thin-walled. Finally, the aneurysmal walls become irregular with pronounced thinning zones contrasting with thickened zones. Parietal thinning is at the origin of "bullous" protrusions of the wall. Histologically, the aneurysmal sac becomes more and more sclerous in the course of its transformation. The "critical" phase for optimal weakening apparently depends upon its size. This is variously estimated by authors: a diameter of 4 mm according to Crompton [17], 5 mm according to McCormick and Acosta-Rua [59], 7 mm in the joint report by Locksley [58], and 6–15 mm according to Crawford [16].

From the "Critical"-Phase Aneurysm to the Giant Aneurysm

Progressive growing of intracranial saccular aneurysms has been proved occasionally by repeated angiography in cases treated conservatively or without decisive surgery. Artmann et al.'s review article [3] summarizes 131 such cases – including 23 cases of growing giant aneurysms – reported in the literature.

The progressive growth of giant aneurysms is usually attributed to a cyclic process of thrombosis and organization; however, phenomena exhibiting fissures and minimal ruptures of the sac are also implicated.

As its volume increases, the aneurysmal sac shows "bullous" expansions. Maximal parietal thinning zones apparently undergo thrombosis which organizes secondarily and accounts for a progressive increase in the size of the sac [16, 17, 38].

According to Thauvoy et al. [102] the wall of the giant aneurysm is fed internally by blood circulating in the lumen and peripherally by leptomeningeal vessels or by newly-formed vessels within the sac. When the thickness of the aneurysmal wall increases, mainly by apposition of mural thrombi, islands of lamellary ischemic necrosis have been said to occur in the wall. Under the effects of hemodynamic mechanisms these latter are penetrated and dissected by blood contained in the sac. The subsequent zones of hemorrhagic dissection secondarily undergo organization, stretching the sac and leading to its progressive growth.

The above pathogenetic mechanisms are not linked with the fissuring or rupture of the sac, unlike those discussed below.

Clinically, latent rupture or minimal or prodromal fissuring of the aneurysmal sac [70, 94, 99] would also explain the appearance of giant aneurysms. According to Stehbens [94], microscopic rupture of the aneurysm induces the formation of a thrombus which extends laterally to the walls of the sac. The thrombus produces a false sac which undergoes organization from the deep surface of the aneurysmal wall, which it tends to cover. Initially the false sac is rich in fibroblasts and newly formed vessels [98]. Then it is formed of a dense, scarring, sclerous collagen lamina which is difficult to distinguish from the fibrous wall of the initial sac.

Nyström [70] believes that the irritated arachnoid plays a role in sac repair and in parietal scar formation.

According to Suzuki and Ohara, following the appearance of a microscopic breach in zones of aneurysmal sac thinning, a fibrinous thrombus is formed at the rupture site under the coagulating effect of cerebrospinal fluid [4, 99]. The ability of cerebrospinal fluid to accelerate clot formation soon after the rupture of an aneurysm is an important factor in the formation of the protective layer of the ruptured aneurysmal wall. This newly formed protective layer is relatively weak in the first 3 weeks, during which the danger of recurrent bleeding is very high. It thus represents a weak point for recurrent hemorrhage with an inherent potential for further growth. After 3 weeks, the new wall is reinforced and thickened by capillary proliferation derived from the leptomeninges. These vessels will tend to fissure under the effect of intra-aneurysmal hemodynamic changes. This induces the formation of a new hematoma of the aneurysmal wall, which becomes fragile and progressively grows by incorporating successive new thrombi. Such episodes of blood leakage within and through the new aneurysmal wall, despite their latency, can be thought to lead to a progressive growth of the aneurysm. This mechanism was confirmed by recent electron microscopic studies of a large series of cerebral aneurysms obtained at operation. They demonstrate that microbleedings inside the aneurysm are more frequent than the clinical diagnosis of subarachnoid hemorrhage [63].

To summarize, the macroscopic, microscopic, and histogenetic *changes of the aneurysmal wall* together account for the progressive growth in size of aneurysms. However, they should not cover up a permanent potential risk of hemorrhagic rupture, whatever the size and degree of thrombosis and calcification of the sac. Moreover, there is some danger of distal embolism, especially in partly thrombosed and wide-necked giant aneurysms.

Mechanisms of Formation: Hemodynamic Features

This chapter is a summary of hemodynamic studies undertaken to elucidate further the mechanisms of growth, thrombosis, and rupture of giant intracranial aneurysms. The role of turbulent flow and intra-aneurysmal pressure is reviewed in the literature and studied with glass models of giant aneurysms.

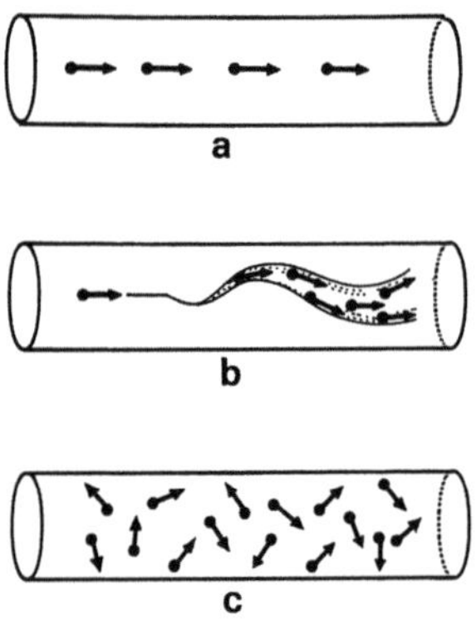

Fig. 9. a Laminar flow; **b** transition between laminar and turbulent flow; **c** turbulent flow

Review of the Literature

Turbulent Flow

There has been considerable speculation in the literature regarding the likelihood and possible significance of turbulence in human intracranial saccular aneurysms.

Turbulent Flow and Critical Reynolds Number

A low velocity fluid flow inside a cylindrical tube of constant diameter is defined by Poiseuille's law. Fluid particles move along streamlines parallel to the axis of the tube. The particles situated near the walls of the tube are immobile and their velocity progressively increases the nearer they are situated to its axis. This so-called laminar flow can be visualized by the injection of dye within the fluid (Fig. 9a). At higher velocity the movement of the particles is no longer linear. The dye stream becomes sinusoidal and progressively enlarges (Fig. 9b). At still higher velocity, the movement of the particles becomes completely random. This turbulent flow can be visualized by the injection of small particles of aluminium into the fluid (Fig. 9c). The factors that determine whether flow is laminar or turbulent are related by an experimentally determined, dimensionless constant given mathematical expression: R_e, i.e. as the Reynolds number. $R_e = D \cdot \frac{\rho}{\mu} \bar{V}$, where ρ is the fluid density, μ the fluid viscosity, $\bar{V}$ the mean flow velocity, and D the tube diameter. For small R_e values (low velocities) the flow is laminar. At high velocities, when R_e reaches a limit called the critical R_e number $(R_e)_c$, the flow becomes turbulent. For the case of a cylindrical tube and human blood at 37°, $(R_e)_c$ is in the range of 2000–2500. In models of circulation with pulsated flow, R_e numbers are lower. In cases of a tube of inconstant diameter, stenosis or bifurcation induces more complex fluid flow. At low velocities, fluid particles follow a regular curved trajectory which depends on the shape of the tube. As the velocity increases the flow becomes turbulent and the $(R_e)_c$ may also be determined. Figure 10 indicates the variations of the critical R_e numbers for different glass tube models [9] corresponding to various bifurcation angles. It can be seen that for a 90° bifurcation angle, the $(R_e)_c$ number is about half the number for a straight tube. Regarding the values of the arterial flow of the internal carotid artery, Ferguson considers that the R_e number at the level of the circle of Willis is about 600–750 [7].

Turbulent Flow in Saccular Aneurysms

Clinical evidence of turbulence has been suggested by cranial bruits associated with saccular aneurysms [16] and confirmed by direct visualization of the turbulent flow in serial angiography [23]. Experimentally in dogs, turbulence in side aneurysms was confirmed by the presence of a palpable thrill and audible bruit from the sac [12, 13].

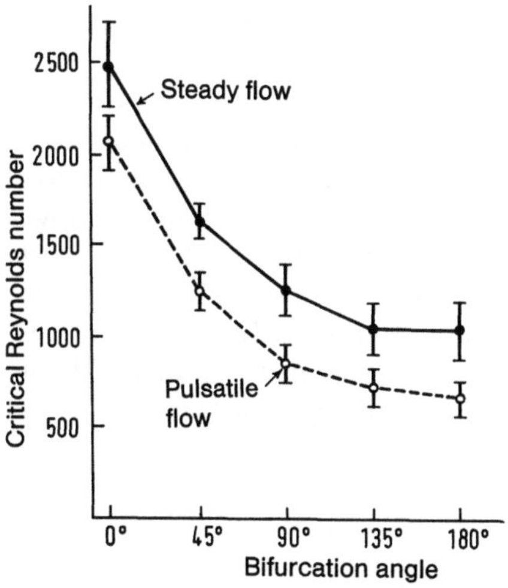

Fig. 10. Graph showing the critical Reynolds number corresponding to various bifurcation angles of glass models during steady and pulsatile flows. The bars represent ±1 SD. (Adapted from [9])

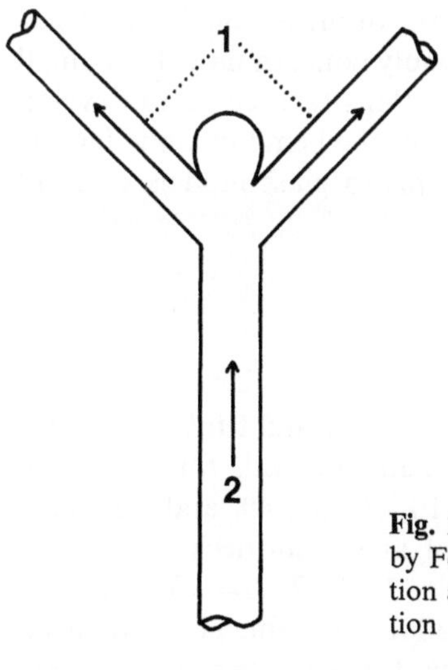

Fig. 11. Glass model used by Ferguson [6]. *1*, Bifurcation angle; *2*, flow direction

Ferguson [6] placed a glass model aneurysm at the level of a 90° bifurcation angle (Fig. 11) and used Evans blue-dye injections to demonstrate the turbulent flow. For a pulsatile flow, the $(R_e)_c$ number was 400, which is relatively low compared to the values obtained with a straight tube $[(R_e)_c = 2500)$. He concluded that turbulent flow pattern occurs in the sac of an aneurysm at a low flow rate. He suggested that the turbulent blood flow contributes to the degeneration of the elastica and the production of the atheromatous changes seen in the wall of aneurysms, which cause continuing enlargement and eventual rupture. Results obtained by two kinds of studies tend to confirm this hypothesis. On one hand, alteration of the structure of vessel's wall by turbulent flow has been well demonstrated in models of arterial stenosis [11, 31]. On the other hand, abnormally high blood flow and consequent turbulent flow induced by a cerebral arteriovenous malformation has been proved to be responsible for initiation and growth of cerebral aneurysms [16, 17, 18, 20, 24]. A similar phenomenon probably explains the following classic findings:

1. Aneurysms in connection with development of a collateral circulation after vascular occlusion.
2. High incidence of communicant artery aneurysms situated at the level of the dominant A_1 segment in cases of asymmetry of the circle of Willis [2, 15, 19, 29].

In contrast with these persuasive data concerning the role of turbulence, it is also important to mention that to some authors intra-aneurysmal flow appears mainly regular and not turbulent [14, 17].

Intra-aneurysmal Pressure

Since turbulent flow has been thought to be responsible for aneurysm enlargement, it was suggested that intra-aneurysmal pressure played the main role in aneurysm rupture [4]. Application of Laplace's law [5] to a sphere demonstrates this role: $T = PR/2_e$, where T represents the forces tending to disrupt the sphere along an equatorial circle, P is the pressure within the sphere, R the radius of an equatorial circle, and e the thickness of the wall (Fig. 12). It is thus apparent that the incidence of rupture is directly proportional to the increase in pressure. It is also apparent that the bigger an aneurysm, the higher the risk of rupture. Factors which influence intra-aneurysmal pressure have been studied by many authors. Black and Ferguson noted that intra-aneurysmal pressure is directly related to the systemic blood pressure. Black [1] measured this pressure by puncturing experimental aneurysms in dogs and Ferguson [8] in aneurysms surgically exposed in man. In other cases of human aneurysms, Wright [30] and Coll [3] found that the intra-aneurysmal pressure was lower than systemic pressure. These findings were considered to be due to a very narrow neck of the aneurysm in one case, and an intensive spasm of the middle cerebral artery proximal to the aneurysm in another case of Wright. For Coll, difference of pressure values is due to loss of energy along a certain length of the main artery whose

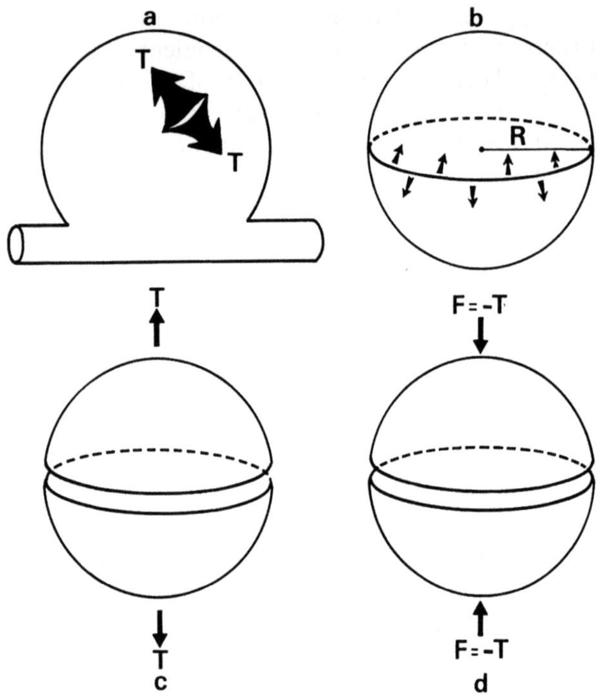

Fig. 12. At the level of any part of a sphere, the lateral force T may induce rupture (**a**). In case of rupture along an equatorial circle (**b, c**), $T=PR/2^{e}$, where P is the internal pressure, R the radius of the equatorial circle, and e the thickness of the wall. **d** F is the opposite force which could avoid rupture

cross-sectional area is progressively decreasing, and loss at the entrance to the aneurysm through the neck and in the expansion of the flow within the sac. Ozdamar [21] has confirmed these data in experimental aneurysms in cats. In this study aneurysm pressure was effectively found to be relatively low in cases of aneurysm having narrow necks and situated at 90° to the parent vessel blood flow.

Thrombosis

Black and German [1] have demonstrated in experimental aneurysms in dogs that a special anatomical configuration of aneurysms may be responsible of intra-aneurysmal thrombosis. They found that the intra-aneurysmal clotting tendency is high if the quotient of chamber volume to orifice area of the aneurysm is >28.3 mm. Such an anatomical configuration is compatible with low values of intra-aneurysmal pressure as seen in the preceding section. In addition, irregular repartition of intra-aneurysmal pressure in large, lobulated aneurysms [21] and the Coanda effect [22] may explain cases of irregular intra-aneurysmal repartition of clots and formation of serpentine aneurysms [10]. If a special anatomical configuration and low intra-aneurysmal pressure are the conditions which create a predisposition to thrombosis, clot initiation probably occurs in relation to turbulence flow. This relation has been demonstrated in animals with models of arterial stenosis [25, 26] and in human intracranial aneurysms [27]. It was suggested that turbulent flow causes endothelial damage which induces platelet aggregates.

Model Experiments

The review of the literature given above demonstrates the role and interaction of hemodynamic factors in the mechanism of initiation, growth, rupture, and thrombosis of intracranial aneurysms [7, 29]. These data mainly concern models or small aneurysms in humans. This fact led us to develop an experimental study of the hemodynamic factors in the same mechanisms in glass models of giant aneurysms.

Method

The models included long straight tubes of 4 mm and 6 mm internal diameter and, for each type of tube, aneurysms 10, 20, 30, 40, and 50 mm in diameter. The size of aneurysm neck is given by the following formula: $l=D_i/2$; $L=0.3\ \varnothing_a$; $\varnothing_a=h/0.4$, where L is the lateral diameter of the neck, l its frontal diameter, h the distance which separates the center point of the aneurysm from the axis of the tube, and $\varnothing_a$ the diameter of the aneurysm (Fig. 13). In each model the basic patterns of both steady and pulsatile flow were observed by Evans blue-dye injection, and the critical Reynold numbers $(R_e)_c$ were calculated. As shown above, the Reynold number (R_e) is given by the expression $R_e=D_i\frac{\rho}{\mu}\bar{V}$, where D_i is the internal diameter of the tube, $\frac{\rho}{\mu}$ the cinematic viscosity of the fluid $\left(\frac{\rho}{\mu}=1.10^{-6}\ \text{m}^2/\text{s}\right.$ for water at 20° C and 760 mmHg). The average fluid velocity V was calculated from the expression $\bar{V}=Q\pi r^2$, where Q is

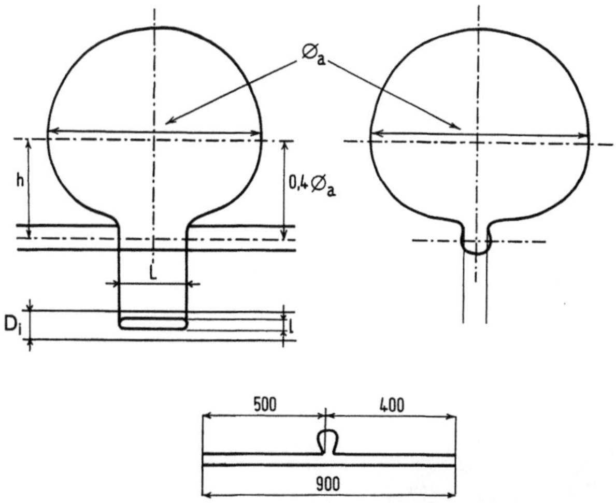

Fig. 13. Glass model aneurysms perpendicularly connected to the tube. *a*, aneurysm diameter; *L*, *l*, dimensions of the neck; D_i, internal diameter of the tube

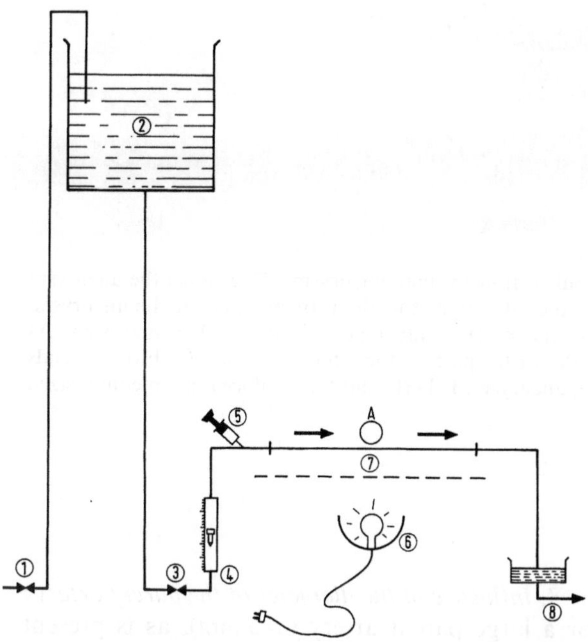

Fig. 14. Schema of the experiment. *1*, water supply; *2*, filling reservoir, which ensures a constant flow rate; *3*, precision sluice gate for regulation of flow rate; *4*, float spindle flowmeter; *5*, injection of Evans blue dye; *6*, light; *7*, diffusing screen; *8*, outflow; *A*, aneurysm

the flow rate through the tube. Variation of R_e was obtained by modification of Q or using tubes of different diameters (4 or 6 mm). Figure 14 gives a diagrammatic representation of the experimental apparatus.

Results

The dye never entered the aneurysm when flow within the tube was *laminar* ($R_e < 800$).

For $R_e > 1800$ (Q was about 330 ml/min for the 4-mm-diameter tube and about 580 ml/min for the 6-mm-diameter tube), flow within the tube was always *turbulent* and dye always entered the aneurysm. There were then two types of intra-aneurysmal flow:

No Turbulent Intra-aneurysmal Flow

In most cases, with a 4-mm tube, the fluid hits the distal edge of the neck and rebounds against the proximal wall of the aneurysm (Fig. 15A). Flow will then occur by layers in the proximal part of the aneurysm (Fig. 15B). This ascending flow begins to drop when the upper wall of the aneurysm has been reached (Fig. 15C). The bigger the aneurysm, the lower the values of R_e required to induce this type of intra-aneurysmal flow. For example, for an aneurysm 30 mm in diameter, this flow is obtained with R_e about 1500. For an aneurysm 10 mm in diameter, the same flow is obtained only if R_e is about 3500. By contrast, with the 6-mm tube, the size of the aneurysm does not influence its perfusion (R_e was the same for all sizes of aneurysm).

In some cases, particularly for the biggest aneurysm, the flow was different: the flow appeared to ascend in a straight, vertical line from the neck (Fig. 15D), with no difference between a 4-mm and a 6-mm tube.

Turbulent Intra-aneurysmal Flow

Intra-aneurysmal turbulent flow is demonstrated in Fig. 15E. The diameter of the tube influences the values of R_e required to obtain this type of flow. Thus, with the 6-mm-diameter tube, turbulent flow was obtained in all aneurysms, for R_e decreased as the size of aneurysm increased. For example, with a 10-mm-diameter aneurysm, R_e was about 5000. With a 50-mm-diameter aneurysm it was about 2500.

Pulsatile flow within the tube was obtained by simple rhythmic pressure on the soft part of the tube proximal to the aneurysm. The pulsatile flow contributes to decreasing the R_e values required for aneurysm supply. In all cases, the aneurysmal flow was turbulent (Fig. 15F).

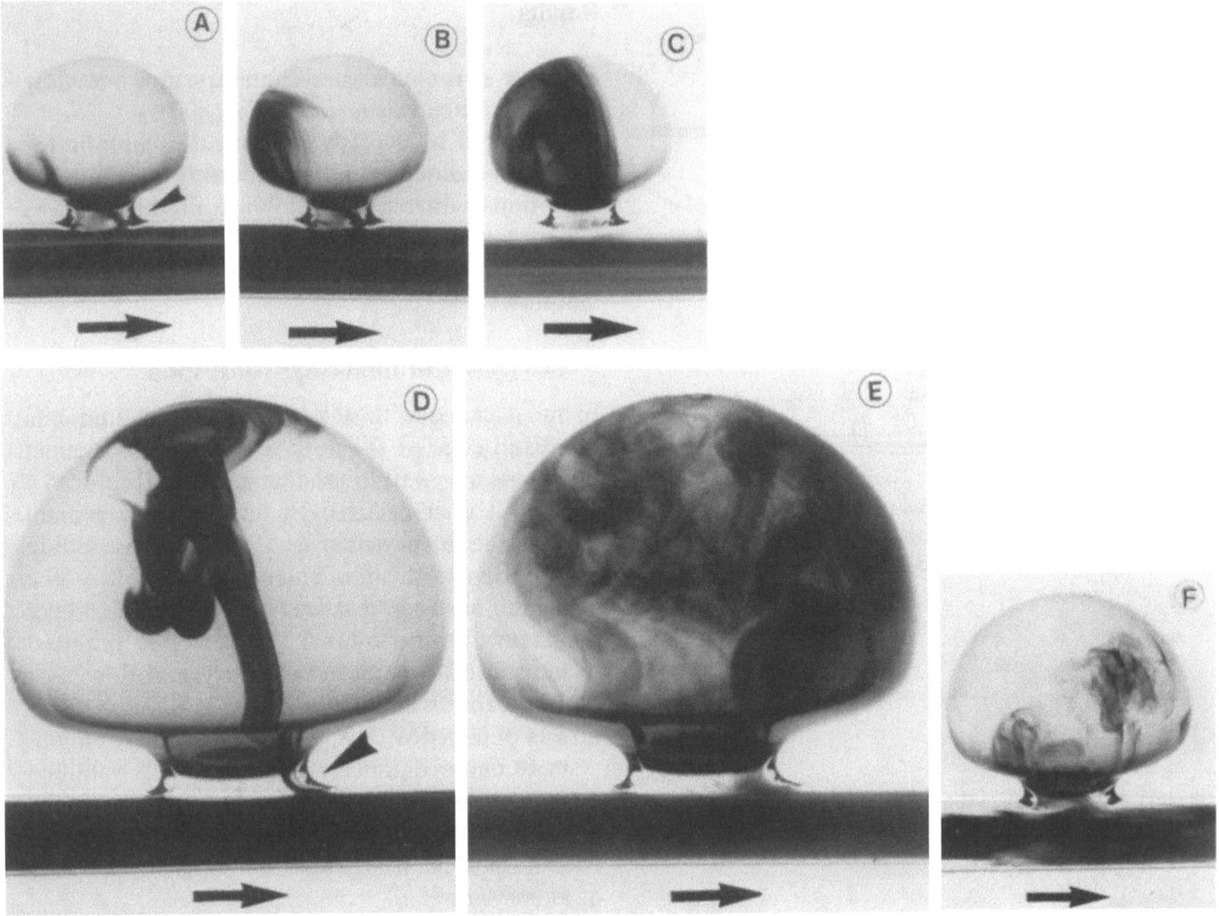

Fig. 15A–F. Intra-aneurysmal flow in glass models. **A–C** Nonturbulent flow in small aneurysms. Dye enters the aneurysm at the level of the distal part of the neck (**A**, *arrowhead*). Flow is then distributed to the proximal part of the aneurysm. There is a zone of less circulation in the distal part of the aneurysm. **D** Nonturbulent flow in a big aneurysm. As in the preceding case, dye enters the aneurysm at the level of the distal part of the neck *(arrowhead)*. Flow ascends in a straight, vertical line from the neck. **E** Turbulent flow in a big aneurysm. **F** Turbulent flow induced in a medium-sized aneurysm with a pulsatile flow in the tube

Comments

1. *Presence of turbulent flow in giant aneurysms:* in our study, turbulent flow was always demonstrated with pulsatile flow. The R_e values required were low and close to those suggested by Ferguson at the level of the circle of Willis. These data suggest that turbulent flow always occurs in giant aneurysms.

2. *Irregular distribution of the intra-aneurysmal flow:* injection of dye demonstrated clearly that both turbulent and nonturbulent intra-aneurysmal flow are irregularly distributed. In all types of aneurysms a zone of reduced circulation was visualized, which could explain partial thrombosis.

3. *Influence of the diameter of the parent artery:* for a large parent artery (>5 mm), as is present in most cases of human giant aneurysms (Fig. 16), supply of the aneurysm is easy to obtain with a relatively low R_e. By contrast, aneurysms attached to a smaller parent artery (<5 mm) are difficult to perfuse. These data may have therapeutic applications.

4. *Influence of flow rate in the parent artery:* like the diameter of the parent artery, a decrease in the flow rate decreases the values of R_e and reduces supply of all types of aneurysm.

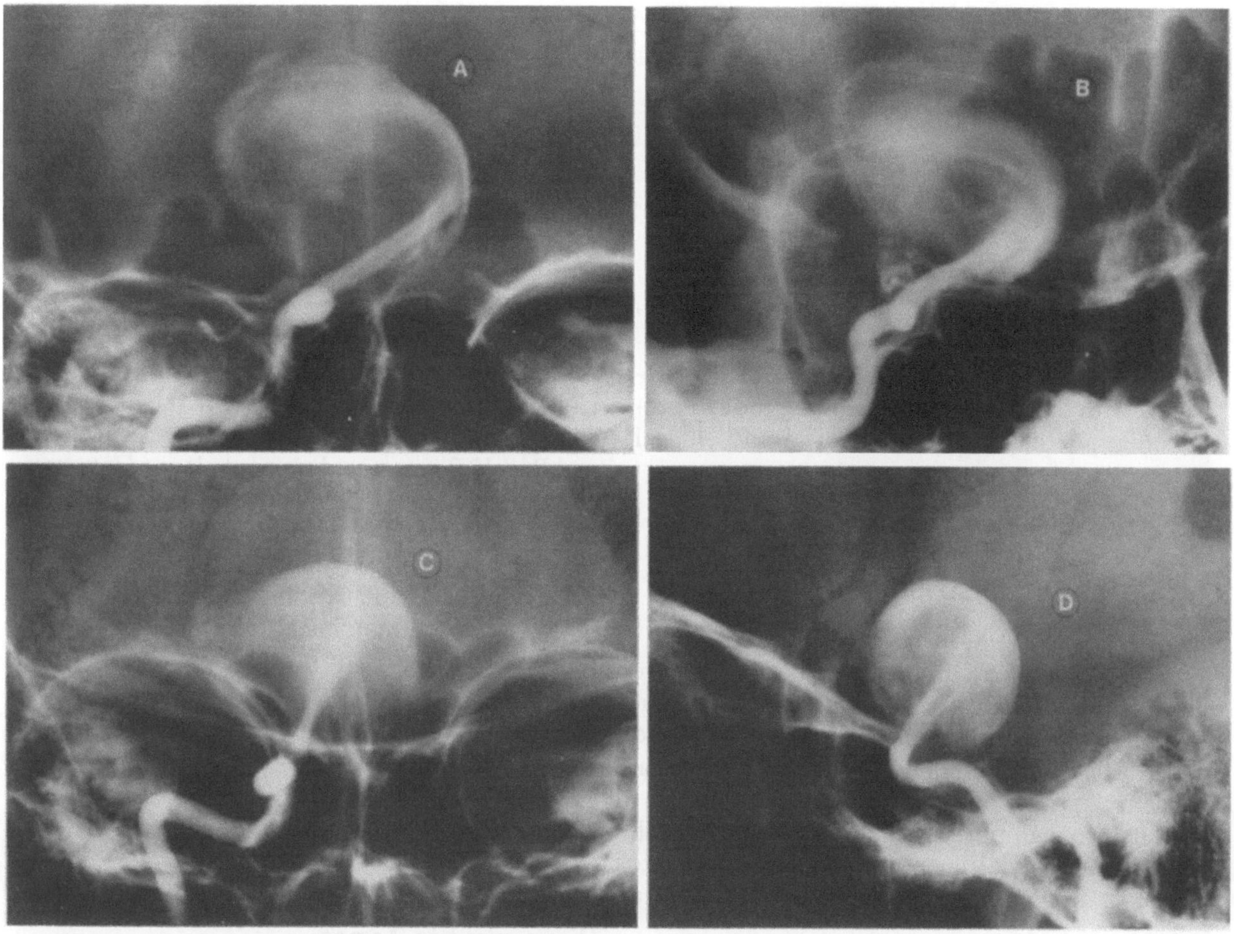

Fig. 16 A–D. Angiographic visualization of the intra-aneurysmal flow. In the first case (**A, B**) contrast medium is distributed in the superficial part of the aneurysm. In the second case (**C, D**), flow of contrast medium ascends straight from the neck. In both cases the parent artery is large

In conclusion, our results accord with the main data of the literature concerning turbulent flow in aneurysms. In our opinion, turbulence always occurs in giant aneurysms. Decreasing the flow rate in the parent artery and/or its diameter could reduce intra-aneurysmal turbulent flow. This could be probably obtained by an endovascular procedure when direct approach of the aneurysm is contraindicated, and may then reduce the risk of growth and rupture.

Clinical Study

Since a clinical study of giant aneurysms has recently been published in the French journal *Neurochirurgie* by Creissard [19], this chapter will merely deal with the main points regarding the symptomatology of the various anatomical and clinical types.

Incidence and Distribution

Five per cent of all intracranial aneurysms are giant aneurysms [57]. They become clinically manifest after the age of 45 in half of the cases and are a little more common in women (60%) than in men.

Their topographic distribution compared with that of intracranial aneurysms regardless of size is shown in Fig. 17. This diagram only gives a rough idea of their average topographic distribution, for the following two reasons:

1. Percentages differ substantially from one series to another depending on the make-up of each particular author's caseload. For instance, Morley and Barr [57] give a predominant place to intracavernous aneurysms (22%) in their series, whereas in Drake's series [25] the incidence of vertebrobasilar aneurysms is much higher (61%), as this author has devoted special attention to them.

2. A precise anatomical identification of neck implantation is often difficult to achieve using neuroradiology and sometimes even on surgical exploration, the more so as the neck can arise from two adjacent arterial segments. This is particularly true for supraclinoid, juxtaclinoid, and vertebrobasilar aneurysms.

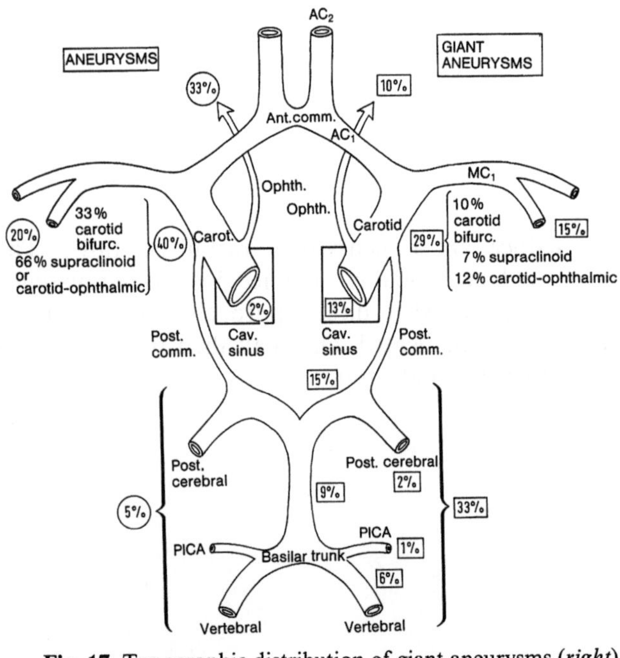

Fig. 17. Topographic distribution of giant aneurysms (*right*) compared with general distribution (*left*). *PICA*, posterior-inferior cerebellar artery

Topographic Types

It is important to differentiate intracavernous from subarachnoid aneurysms, for clinical and therapeutic reasons [51, 63, 64, 65, 83, 88, 91, 93, 94].

Intracavernous Aneurysms

Unlike small cavernous sinus aneurysms which commonly rupture, giving a spontaneous carotidocavernous fistula, giant intracavernous aneurysms rarely bleed. For example, in Morley and Barr's 11-case series [57], only one ruptured. *Hemorrhage* in the subarachnoid space can occur when the aneurysm perforates the cavernous sinus roof [44].

Such aneurysms most often behave like expanding lesions (Fig. 18) responsible for *pseudotumoral syndromes* [20, 23, 46, 70, 73]. Most of them are revealed by progressive neurological signs, while others, rarely, are revealed by acute symptoms, as in Fig. 1a. They usually manifest by chronic retro-orbital pain, fluctuating diplopia, and surrounding bone erosions in the sella turcica

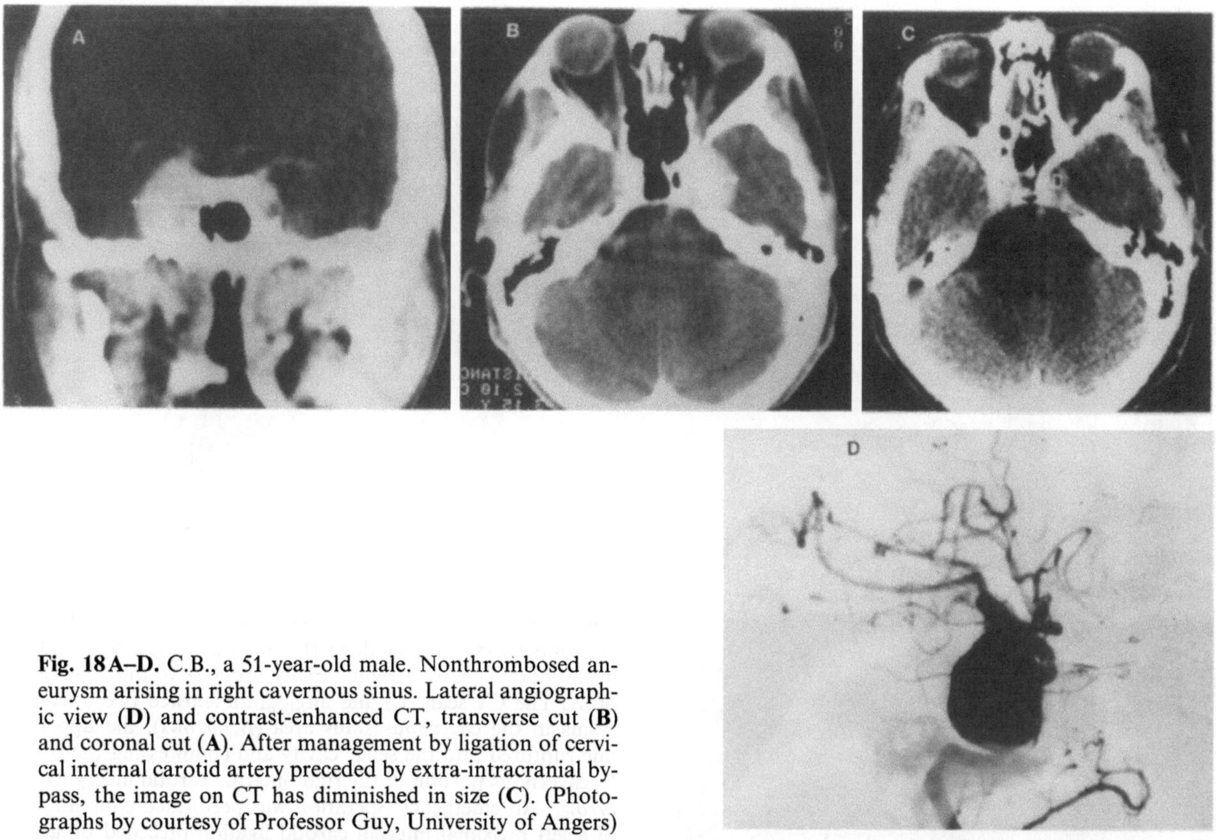

Fig. 18A–D. C.B., a 51-year-old male. Nonthrombosed aneurysm arising in right cavernous sinus. Lateral angiographic view (**D**) and contrast-enhanced CT, transverse cut (**B**) and coronal cut (**A**). After management by ligation of cervical internal carotid artery preceded by extra-intracranial bypass, the image on CT has diminished in size (**C**). (Photographs by courtesy of Professor Guy, University of Angers)

and/or the superior orbital fissure. In the more advanced forms, aneurysms can massively erode the skull base either at the petrous [2, 49, 56, 61] or the sphenoid region and then spread to the nasopharynx, sometimes causing massive epistaxis, as reported by Morley and Barr in one case.

A few rare bilateral intracavernous giant aneurysms have been reported [28, 38, 48, 75].

Subarachnoid Aneurysms

These aneurysms can exhibit three classic clinical manifestations:

1. *Hemorrhagic rupture*, occuring in 20–70% of cases, depending on the series, with an average of 40% (Fig. 20). Of practical importance is the fact that some hemorrhagic ruptures did occur in cases of apparently totally thrombosed aneurysms [82].

2. *Ischemic manifestations* [1, 10, 15, 27, 32, 35, 40, 55, 69, 79, 80], estimated at 4% of the cases and including embolism to distal arteries arising from intrasaccular thrombi as well as extensive parent artery thrombosis (see Fig. 65).

3. *Pseudotumoral syndromes* amounting to 50–75% according to the series. These can be divided into three main groups.

The first group consists of the aneurysms located in the carotid-ophthalmic junction, the posterior communicating and the anterior communicating arteries. These types can cause optic nerve and chiasma compression [1, 13, 29, 34, 36, 62, 74, 86] and, more rarely, hypothalamic-pituitary syndromes [5, 45, 58, 68, 77, 84, 85, 89] (Fig. 21A).

The second group is represented by carotid bifurcation and middle cerebral artery aneurysms, which present with basal hemispheric compression syndromes, inaugurated in 66% by seizures [9, 41, 53, 90] (Fig. 21B).

Posterior cerebral fossa aneurysms belong to the third group. Such types give rise to various clinical pictures [14, 18, 50] depending on the localization of the aneurysm. Most of them simulate tumors, mainly of the third ventricle [8, 72] or the brainstem [14, 18, 24, 59]. These lesions give early cranial nerve palsies and frequent obstructive hydrocephalus [7, 14, 16, 17, 22, 30, 39, 41, 42, 54, 66, 71, 76, 78, 92] (Fig. 21C).

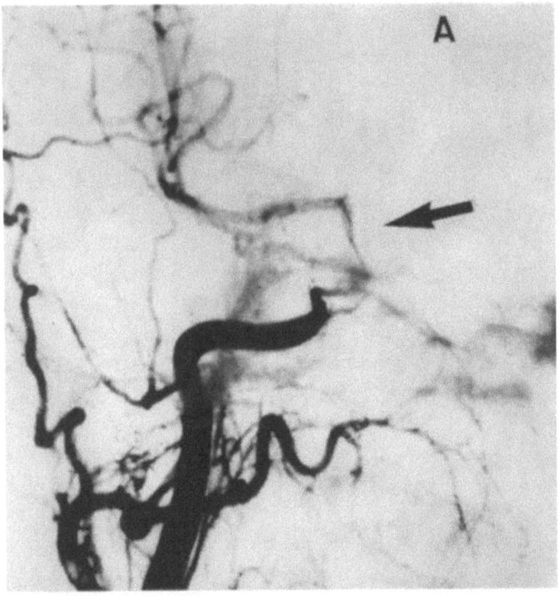

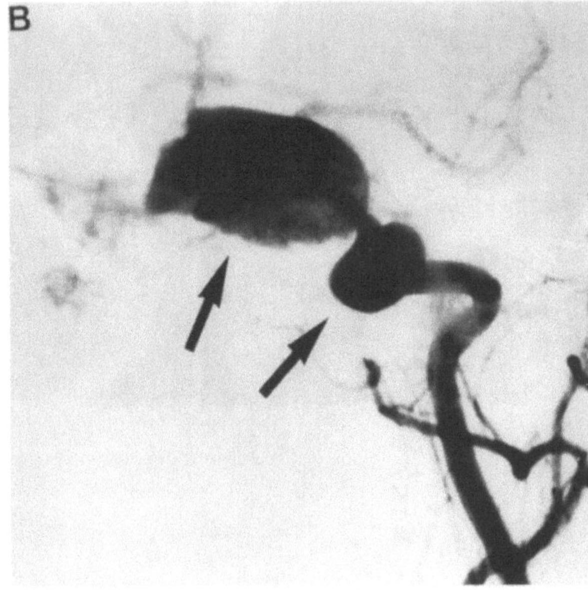

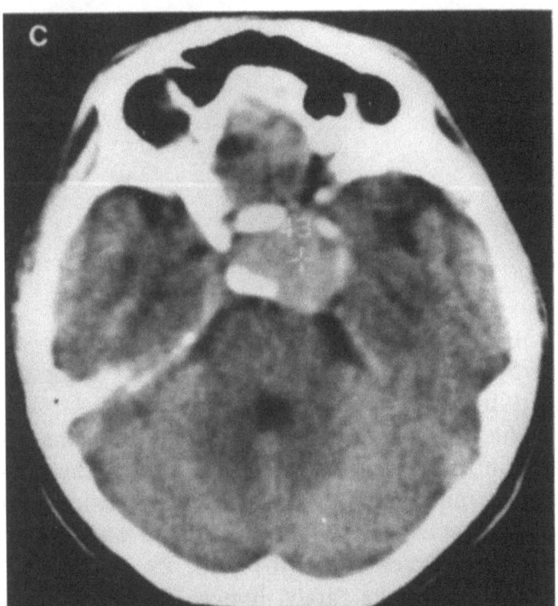

Fig. 19 A–C. C.W., a 24-year-old female, was referred in November 1985 for a sudden left ophthalmoplegia, followed in the next days by a right rapidly progressive third nerve palsy. The CT scan (**C**) and angiogram showed two aneurysms in the cavernous sinus area (**B**, *arrows*), the upper one ruptured into the sellar cavity and compressing the intracavernous portion of the right internal carotid artery (**A**, *arrow*). An emergency operation was performed consisting of a left proximal internal carotid ligation preceded by an extra-intracranial bypass using an interposed saphenous graft, as the superficial temporal artery which fed an angioma of the scalp was not available. Unfortunately, in the early postoperative phase the bypass thrombosed, probably because of technical difficulties encountered in performing the proximal end-to-side anastomosis at the common carotid artery level, due to the fragility of the arterial walls which were dysplastic. Simultaneously with the bypass thrombosis there occurred a left hemiparesia; this was presumed to be connected with the extrinsic stenosis of the right carotid artery. An emergency ST-MCA anastomosis was performed on the right side. Three months after operation, the patient was free of symptoms and the follow-up angiogram showed on the right side a normal caliber carotid feeding both hemispheres as well as a clear extra-intracranial anastomosis, while the left bypass remained thrombosed

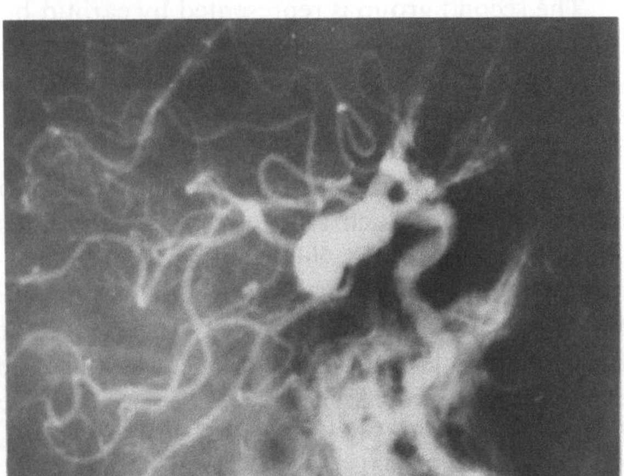

◁**Fig. 20.** R.L., a 71-year-old female. Right carotid-posterior communicating artery aneurysm, nonthrombosed, hemorrhagic type, managed by neck clipping

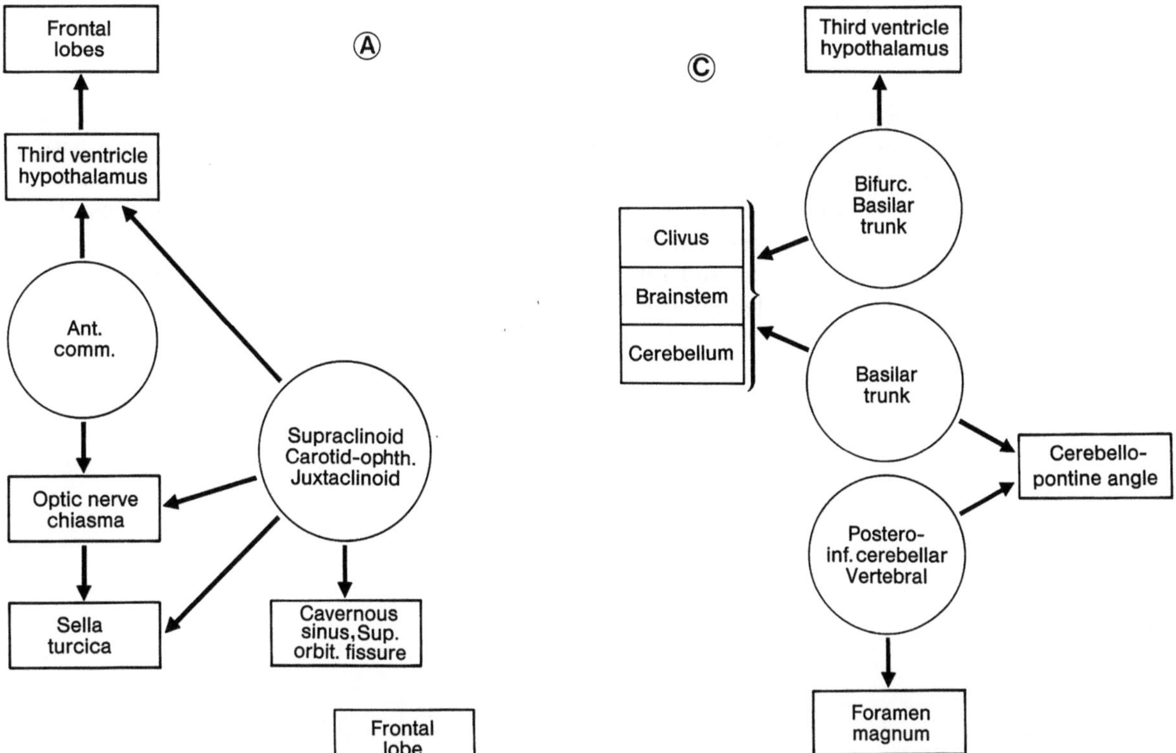

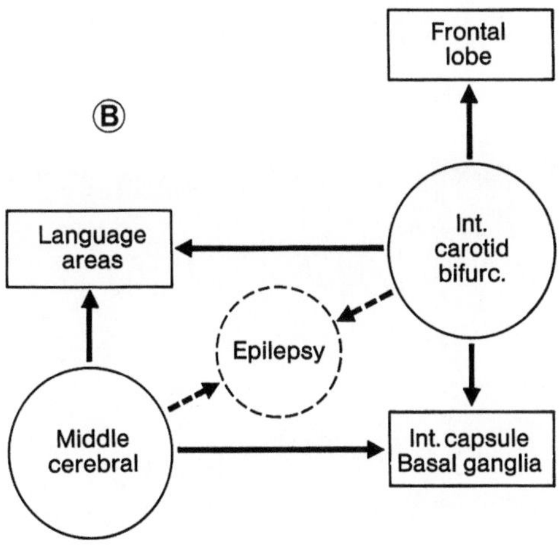

Fig. 21 A–C. Clinical manifestations according to topographic type

Giant Intracranial Aneurysms in Childhood

Intracranial aneurysms of all sizes are rare in childhood (less than 1% of all aneurysms; [4, 43]) and are exceptional before 1 year of age [87].

Seventeen cases of giant aneurysms with indication of size have been reported in *children more than 1 year old* [3, 6, 11, 12, 21, 26, 31, 33, 38, 47, 60, 67, 81]. For those with data concerning their localization, three arose from the *intracavernous portion of the carotid artery*. The first was astride both the intrapetrous and intracavernous carotid segments [67]. The second developed in the intrasellar region [3]. The third was a case of bilateral aneurysm in a 3-year-old child [38]. The right aneurysm was successfully operated on by a direct approach during extracorporeal circulation. As the follow-up angiogram showed an enlargement of the controlateral aneurysm, it was also treated by direct approach, with satisfactory clinical results.

Four other giant aneurysms were located in the *carotid system*: one in the internal carotid artery [26] and three in the middle cerebral artery [11, 21, 60].

Five aneurysms arose from the *vertebrobasilar system* [6, 12, 31, 47]. The case of Bhushan et al., located at the basilar trunk, was successfully treated by bilateral vertebral artery ligation [6]. Concerning the two cases reported by Ganti et al. [31], one, arising from the basilar trunk, was wrapped, with a good immediate result; the other – partly thrombosed, and located at the vertebro-basilar junction – was treated in two stages, a right vertebral ligation and neck clipping, but the outcome was poor. Finally, in the case reported by Carillo et al. [12], the aneurysm which arose from the right posterior cerebral artery that fed an arteriovenous fistula was successfully treated by occlusion of the parent artery.

Two cases of giant aneurysm have been reported in *children less than 1 year old.* Both were located in the posterior circulation. One was a giant aneurysm (6 cm × 5 cm) of the posterior-inferior cerebellar artery, discovered at autopsy [37], while the other was a giant aneurysm of the posterior cerebral artery successfully operated on by clipping–excision [87].

Neuroradiological Features

As the plain radiographic and angiographic descriptions of giant aneurysms are well known [26, 45], this chapter – which is based on analysis of the our own series as well as many detailed reports in the literature – will be mainly devoted to their CT and MRI features.

Plain Skull Radiographs

Giant aneurysms may present with calcifications and/or bone erosions, sometimes only visible on tomography. Egg-shell *calcifications* are characteristic, as are granulation clusters corresponding to calcium deposits in old intrasaccular thrombi (Fig. 22). In the more advanced lesions, *bone erosions* can extend to the sella turcica (Fig. 23), the orbital apex (Fig. 24) or, although more rarely, to the sphenoid sinus, pyramid and middle cerebral fossa.

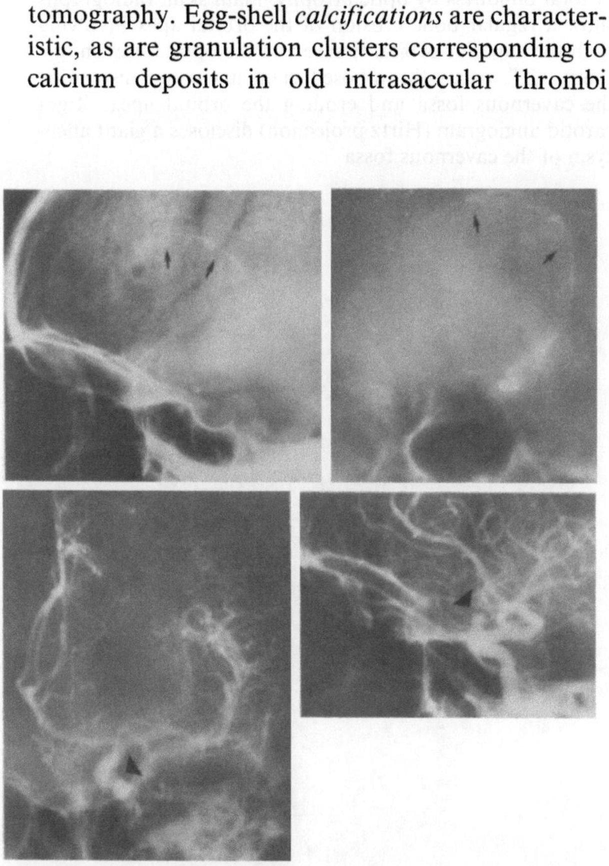

Fig. 22. L.F., a 58-year-old male. Left carotid-ophthalmic aneurysm of the supraoptic variety, pseudotumoral type with shell calcification (*arrows*), totally thrombosed except at attachment site of neck on carotid artery (*arrowhead*)

Angiography

Angiographic exploration of giant aneurysms requires images of excellent quality, as it is of paramount importance for therapeutic strategy. At the present time, it can be performed more safely than before, using microcatheters and digital subtraction to yield a well-defined image with a small quantity of contrast medium.

Angiographic exploration provides three kinds of information:

1. The *site and type of the neck implantation* on the parent artery. This can be sometimes difficult to define exactly, especially when the aneurysm is extensively attached to two contiguous arterial segments or is bullous-shaped (Fig. 25).

2. Evaluation of the *degree of thrombosis*. In the nonthrombosed type, the sac is ordinarily reg-

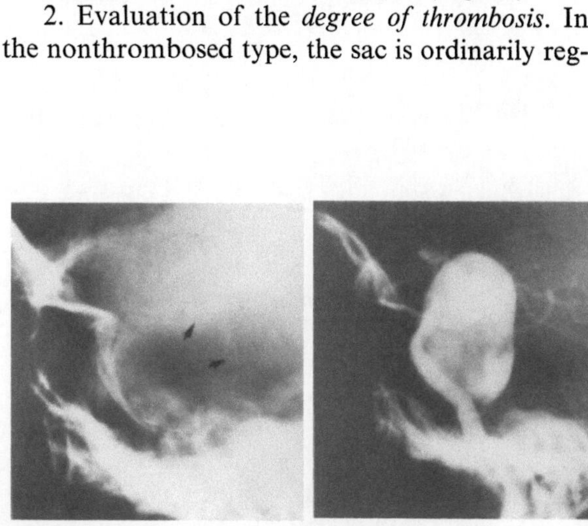

Fig. 23. M.G., a 59-year-old female. Nonthrombosed, pseudotumoral type of intrasellar aneurysm (pituitary insufficiency). Radiographs show destruction of the sella turcica and curved calcifications (*arrows*). Left carotid angiogram, lateral view, shows a giant intrasellar aneurysm

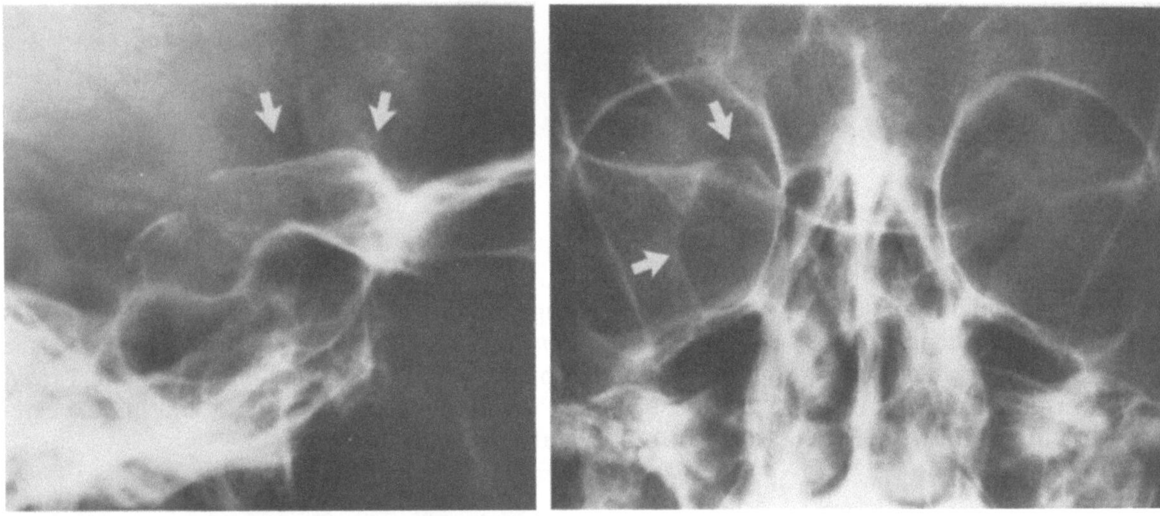

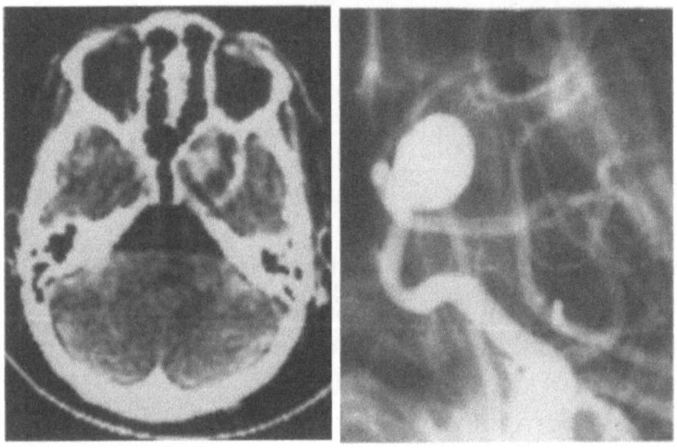

Fig. 24. B.G., a 25-year-old male. Partly-thrombosed, pseudotumoral aneurysm of the right cavernous sinus. Two years' progressive history of right-sided headache and deterioration of vision, with rapid development within 15 days of total blindness by optic atrophy. Plain skull radiographs show a regular bone erosion of the orbital apex involving both the superior orbital fissure and the optic foramen (*arrows*). C.T. partly-thrombosed giant aneurysm distending the cavernous fossa and eroding the orbital apex. Right carotid angiogram (Hirtz projection) discloses a giant aneurysm of the cavernous fossa

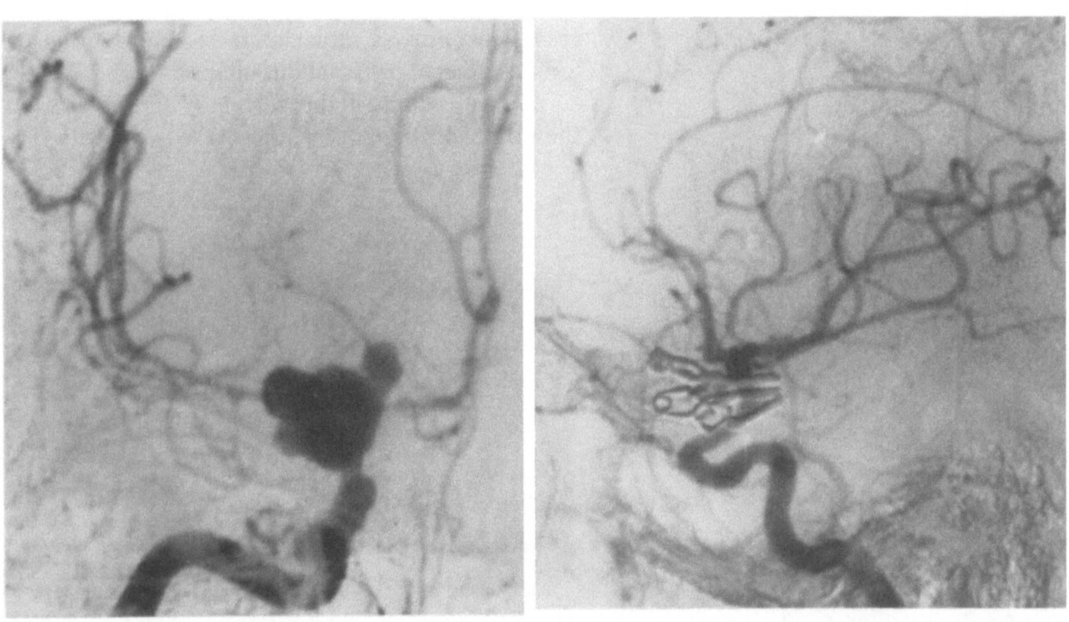

Fig. 25. J.T., a 49-year-old male. Hemorrhagic supraclinoid carotid artery aneurysm with triple localization. It is difficult to conclude from the angiogram whether this is a polylobulated aneurysm or three different aneurysms. Microsurgical dissection of the supraclinoid carotid artery revealed three separate necks and permitted their successful clipping. (Photographs by courtesy of Professor Houtteville, University of Caen)

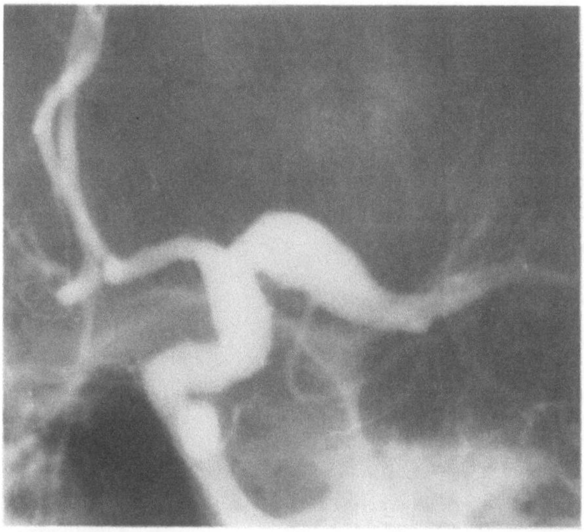

Fig. 26. A.C., a 46-year-old male. Fusiform aneurysm of left intracranial carotid bifurcation in a patient presenting, in addition, two right internal carotid artery aneurysms and one middle cerebral artery aneurysm (not visible in the angiogram)

ular and in perfect volumetric concordance with CT (Fig. 29). In the partlythrombosed type, walls are irregular and the sac smaller in size compared to the CT image (Fig. 30). In certain cases of aneurysms considered to be totally thrombosed, it is not unusual to note a small stumped image at the site of the neck attachment to the parent artery (see Fig. 22).

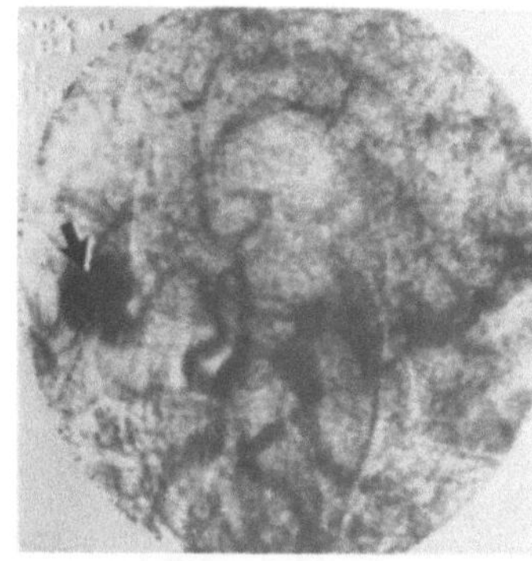

Fig. 27. M.B. Venous digital subtraction angiography shows a partly thrombosed giant aneurysm of the right middle cerebral artery (*arrow*)

3. Morphological as well as hemodynamic evaluation of the *whole cerebral circulation*. This requires an injection of four cervical pedicles together with compression tests, so as to study (a) the patency of both carotid and vertebral arteries, (b) the functional supply of the anterior and posterior communicating arteries (c) the quality of the parenchymal arterial network and (d) the caliber of the external carotid artery branches in view of a potential extra-intracranial bypass.

Besides the three main classical types of giant aneurysms (non-, partially, and totally thrombosed), *serpentine aneurysms* deserve a special place as they constitute a distinct entity. They correspond to partly-thrombosed aneurysms but with

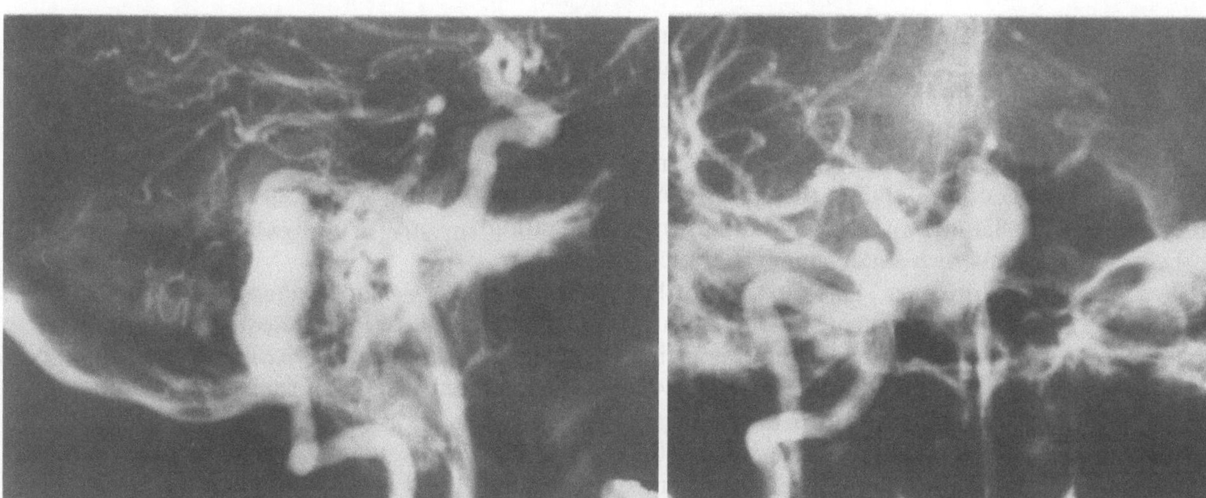

Fig. 28. P.D., a 25-year-old male. Partly-thrombosed, hemorrhagic type of serpentine aneurysm of the right vertebral artery. *Left* Sudden onset of subarachnoid hemorrhage with posterior fossa focal signs. The angiogram shows a voluminous, partly-thrombosed aneurysm of the right vertebral artery. *Right* Management by ligation of cervical portion of right vertebral artery. Loss of respiratory autonomy in the postoperative period, without impairment of consciousness or localizing signs. Complete recovery after 3 months

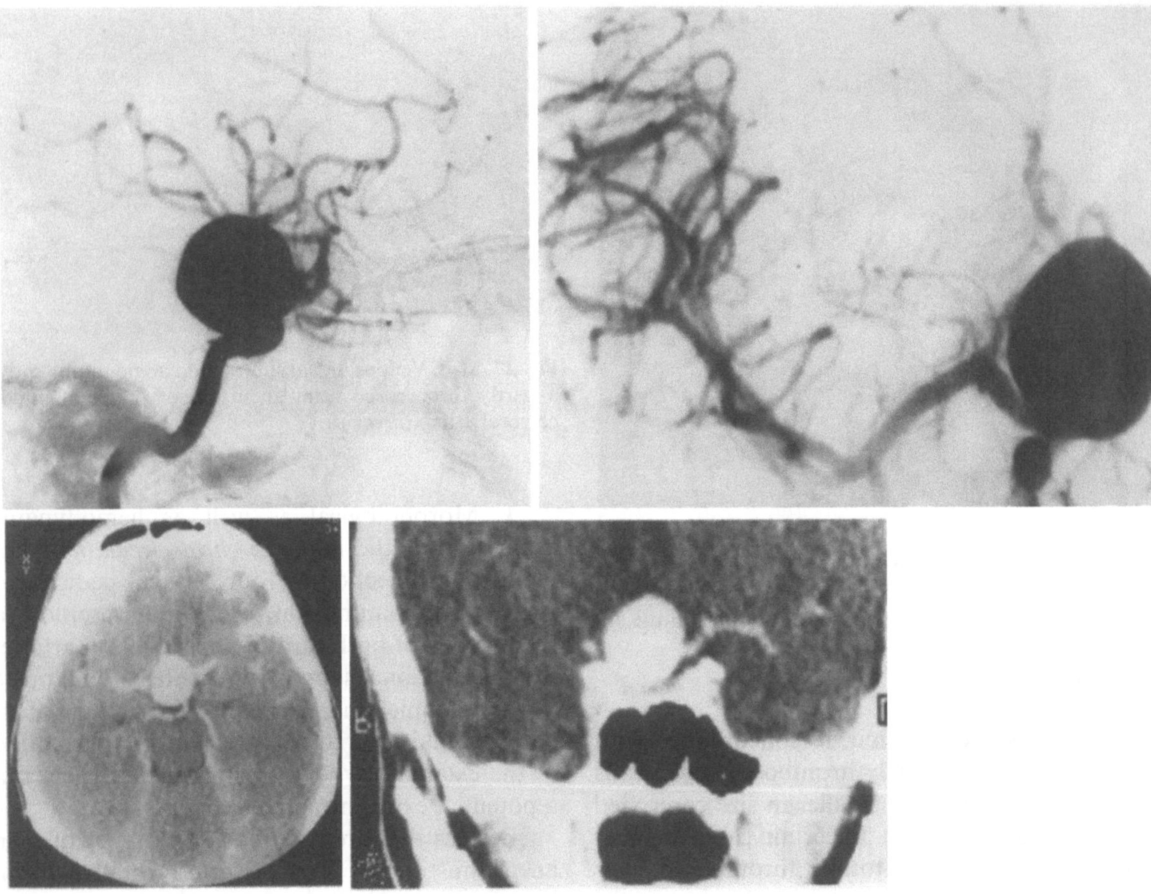

Fig. 29. D.V., a 33-year-old female. Carotid-ophthalmic aneurysm. *Top* Anteroposterior and lateral internal carotid angiograms confirming the giant aneurysm. *Bottom* Axial and coronal contrast-enhanced CT scans showing no thrombus within the aneurysm. The size and mass effect are well demonstrated

a tortuous intrasaccular vascular channel. From a histopathological point of view, serpentine aneurysms present with fairly constant features: (a) relatively thick fibrous walls (1–4 mm) with loss of elastic muscular fibers and neo-vessel formation, and (b) an organized intraluminal thrombus containing a vascular channel without any normal endothelium and from which small channels branch off in a disorganized manner. This type is mostly encountered in the Sylvian system; in fact, 11 out of 16 serpentine cases published in the literature were located in the middle cerebral artery [7, 24, 34, 43, 48, 52, 54, 57], whereas two others were situated in the posterior cerebral artery [15, 30] and the last three in the internal carotid artery [13, 26, 53]. This topographic distribution can be explained by the fact that these aneurysms, which most often arise from small arteries, have a relatively thin neck and low intrasaccular blood flow, thus favoring progressive thrombosis of their sac. Such lesions have characteristic neuroradiological features, so that the combination of angiography and CT permits an almost pathognomonic diagnosis (Fig. 28).

Such types should be differentiated from *fusiform aneurysms* which correspond rather to arterial dilatation, mostly of dysplasic origin [1, 23] (Fig. 26).

Tomographic angiography, in certain exceptional circumstances and if adequate equipment is available, may help to define the morphology of the neck and locate its exact implantation site [44].

Venous digital subtraction angiography, on the other hand [11] (Fig. 27), although not so reliable as arterial, may be useful for checking total thrombosis of the sac after indirect surgical or conservative treatment of the malformation. It is of particular interest for ensuring that space-occupying lesion, previously regarded as a tumor, is not actual-

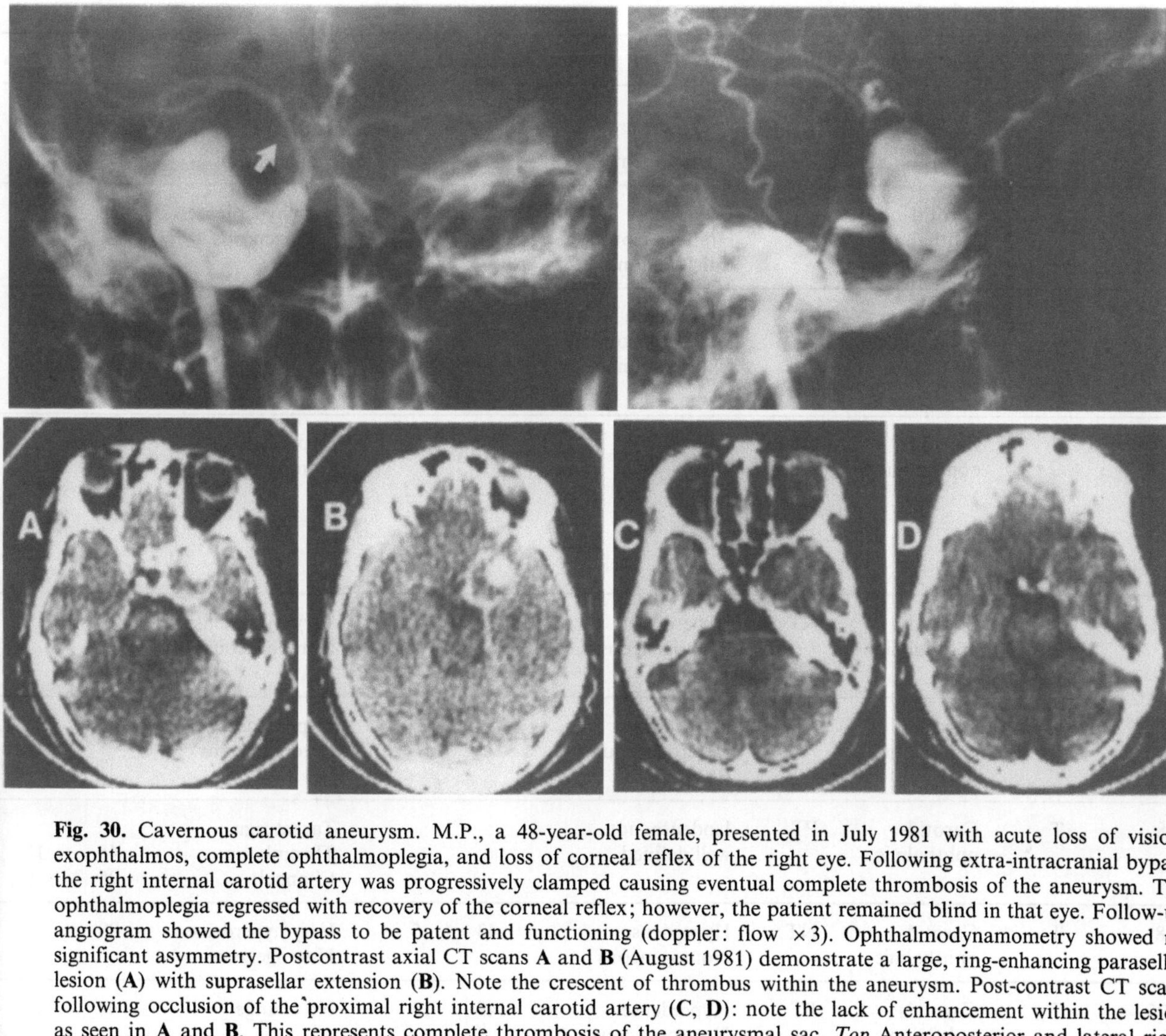

Fig. 30. Cavernous carotid aneurysm. M.P., a 48-year-old female, presented in July 1981 with acute loss of vision, exophthalmos, complete ophthalmoplegia, and loss of corneal reflex of the right eye. Following extra-intracranial bypass the right internal carotid artery was progressively clamped causing eventual complete thrombosis of the aneurysm. The ophthalmoplegia regressed with recovery of the corneal reflex; however, the patient remained blind in that eye. Follow-up angiogram showed the bypass to be patent and functioning (doppler: flow ×3). Ophthalmodynamometry showed no significant asymmetry. Postcontrast axial CT scans **A** and **B** (August 1981) demonstrate a large, ring-enhancing parasellar lesion (**A**) with suprasellar extension (**B**). Note the crescent of thrombus within the aneurysm. Post-contrast CT scans following occlusion of the proximal right internal carotid artery (**C**, **D**): note the lack of enhancement within the lesion as seen in **A** and **B**. This represents complete thrombosis of the aneurysmal sac. *Top* Anteroposterior and lateral right common carotid angiograms demonstrating the huge cavernous aneurysm displacing the middle cerebral artery (*arrow*)

ly a giant aneurysm. This is of paramount importance for masses in the sellar region.

Computed Tomography

The advent of computed tomography (CT) has greatly contributed to the diagnosis, therapeutic planning, and follow-up of cases of giant intracranial aneurysm.

In 1975, Pressman et al. [42] were the first to report the usefulness of CT in exploring 4 cases of giant aneurysms. Since then, several large series have appeared in the literature: Petit-Perrin et al. [36, 37, 38] with 14 cases, Pinto et al. [39] with 21 cases, and Whittle et al. [60] with 22 cases.

In this chapter we will review the significant findings that have been published in the literature, along with our personal experience of 20 cases since 1977.

Method

All CT examinations were performed on a first-generation EMI 1010 CT scanner. Both pre- and postcontrast images were obtained. Contrast was enhanced by the intravenous bolus injection of 60 cc of a water-soluble contrast medium. Multiple

Table 1. Computed tomography data in giant aneurysms

No., Sex, Age	T/H	Topography	Preoperative CT						
			Anatomy	Before contrast enhancement	D	(S)	After contrast enhancement	D	(S)
1.F 59	T	Carotid-ophthalmic	NT	Hyperdense Homogeneous Calcifications	43	8	Very hyperdense homogeneous	91	10
2. F 64	T	Carotid-ophthalmic	PT	Hyperdense Heterogeneous Calcifications	63	45	Target sign	69	43
3.F 49	T	Carotid-ophthalmic	NT				Hyperdense Homogeneous		
4.F 50	T	Carotid-ophthalmic	NT	Hyperdense Homogeneous			Very hyperdense Homogeneous		
5.M 72	H	Carotid-ophthalmic	PT	Hyperdense Heterogeneous Bone lysis	51	12	Hyperdense Heterogeneous	55	23
6.F 48	T	Carotid-ophthalmic	PT	Isodense, not well defined			Target sign Thrombosis Channel	 45 95	 12 9
7.F 68	T	Carotid-ophthalmic	NT	Hyperdense Homogeneous	43	5	Very hyperdense Homogeneous	90	8
8.M 25	T	Carotid-ophthalmic	PT	Hyperdense Heterogeneous Bone lysis	49	14	No change	44	10
9.F 49	T	Carotid-ophthalmic	NT	Hyperdense Homogeneous	52	10	Very hyperdense Homogeneous	91	9
10.F 54	H	Carotid-ophthalmic	NT	Hyperdense Homogeneous	41	5	Very hyperdense Homogeneous	91	9
11.M 40	H	Carotid-ophthalmic	NT	Hyperdense Homogeneous	55	7	Very hyperdense Homogeneous	84	8
12.F 67	H	Middle cerebral	NT	Calcified shell Very hyperdense	153	108			
13.F 44	H	Middle	NT	Hematoma masking aneurysm					
14.M 50	T	Middle cerebral	PT	Heterogeneous Hyperdense Parietal hypodensity			More hyperdense		

Therapy	Postoperative CT								Results
	Timing	Anatomy	Before contrast enhancement	D	(S)	After contrast enhancement	D	(S)	
Internal carotid ligation	4 months	TT	Isodense with hyperdense ring	45	10				+
EC–IC bypass Internal carotid ligation	45 days	TT	Fresh hypodense thrombus	60	39	No change	59	45	
	2.5 years	TT	Heterogeneous calcifications			No change	65	57	+
Internal carotid ligation	5 months	PT	Heterogeneous	31	4	Hyperdense channel	103	5	
			Hypodense			Hyperdense ring	31	5	
			Isodense channel	38	4	Hyperdense thrombosis (target sign)			
	2 years	TT	Hypodense	28	6	Slightly hyperdense	47	8	+
EC–IC bypass Internal carotid ligation	15 days		Hyperdense Homogeneous	38	8				•
EC–IC bypass Internal carotid ligation	2 months	?	Unchanged aspect						•
EC–IC bypass Internal carotid ligation	1 month	TT				Thrombosed channel	43	8	+
						Old hypodense thrombus	29	6	
Internal carotid ligation	1 month	TT	Hyperdense Heterogeneous	57	13	No change	55	11	–
EC–IC bypass Internal carotid ligation	1 month	?	Unchanged aspect	46	20	No change	45	19	+
Internal carotid ligation									– (Death at 6 months)
EC–IC bypass Internal carotid ligation	15 days	TT	Hyperdense	64	7				
	1.5 years	PT	Homogeneous						
			Smaller, less dense	55	8	Target sign	74	16	+
EC–IC bypass Internal carotid ligation	12 days	TT				Heterogeneous Less dense	49	10	+
Wrapping									•
Excision									+
Excision EC–IC bypass									+

Table 1 (continued)

No., Sex, Age	T/H	Topography	Preoperative CT						
			Ana-tomy	Before contrast enhancement	D	(S)	After contrast enhancement	D	(S)
15.F 74	H	Middle cerebral	NT	Hyperdense Homogeneous			Very hyperdense		
16.M 70	H	Middle cerebral	PT	Hyperdense Homogeneous	54	7	Hyperdense Heterogeneous	59	11
17.F 66	H	Basilar trunk	NT	Hypodense Homogeneous	30	8	Hyperdense Homogeneous	46	9
18.F 58	H	Carotid-ophthalmic	NT	Bone lysis Dense homogeneous			Hyperdense Homogeneous		
19.F 54	H	Carotid-ophthalmic	PT	∅ 6 cm Hyperdense Heterogeneous Hydrocephalus Perifocal hypodensity	48	10	Hyperdense Target sign	60	12
20.F 70	H	Carotid-ophthalmic Serpentine	PT	Hyperdense Very hetero-geneous	39	8	Very hyperdense peripheral ring	47	13

T, pseudotumoral type; *H* hemorrhagic type; *NT*, Nonthrombosed; *PT*, partly thrombosed; *TT*, totally thrombosed; *D*, average density; *S*, standard deviation; *Ther*, therapeutic method. Results: + = good; ● = stabilisation; − = bad

+ 1000	
+ 400	Bone
+ 100	
	Hematoma
	Gray matter
	White matter
	Edema
	Cerebrospinal fluid
0	Water
− 100	Fatty tissue
− 1000	
	Air

Fig. 31. Densities in Hounsfield Units (HU)

density measurements were made of the different regions of the aneurysms using the ROI (range of interest) computer program, located by the smallest area cursor available. The measurements are expressed in Hounsfield units (HU; Fig. 31), followed by the standard deviation. The density value represents an averaged number mathematically calculated from the raw data provided to the computer by the detectors of the CT scanner. The standard deviation (SD) is a reflection of the non-homogeneity in the images of the aneurysms.

Our series included 15 females and 5 males between the ages of 25 and 72. The average age was 57 years. Ten cases presented with subarachnoid hemorrhage, while the other ten presented with symptoms of a space-occupying mass. The aneurysms had the following distribution: 14 in the internal carotid artery, 5 in the middle cerebral artery, and 1 in the basilar artery. The clinical, angiographic, and CT data relating to the patients are listed in Table 1.

Therapy	Postoperative CT								Results
	Timing	Anatomy	Before contrast enhancement	D	(S)	After contrast enhancement	D	(S)	
Clipping									+
Clipping									–
									– (Death after 1.5 years)
									– (Death on 9th day)
									– Progressive deterioration
									•

Clinical Observations

Preoperative Aspects

Correlation of the angiograms with the CT images permits the patients to be divided into two groups: 12 with nonthrombosed aneurysms and 8 with partially thrombosed aneurysms. We have not encountered any case of a patient presenting with a completely thrombosed giant aneurysm.

Nonthrombosed Aneurysms (Cases 1, 3, 4, 7, 9, 10, 11, 12, 13, 15, 17, 18; Figs. 18, 29, 32)

The unenhanced CT appearance of giant aneurysms is one of a round, sometimes multilobulated, well-defined mass, slightly hyperdense (average 49.6 HU) when compared to the surrounding parenchyma and usually very homogeneous (SD 7.45 HU). After injection of contrast medium, the aneurysm becomes very hyperdense (average 79.1 HU) but remains homogeneous (SD 9.92 HU).

In case 12, the wall of the aneurysm was almost entirely calcified (153 HU) while its contents showed areas of low density, causing a wide SD of 108 HU. Following contrast injection, the entire sac of the aneurysm becomes enhanced.

Partially Thrombosed Aneurysms (Cases 2, 5, 6, 8, 14, 16, 19, 20; Figs. 24, 30, 33)

Due to the varying amounts of thrombus, these aneurysms appear larger on CT than in the angiograms. They have an heterogeneous appearance on noncontrast studies (SD 16.2 HU), with a mean density of 51 HU. Most present with some degree of calcification of the wall of the aneurysm, which is well demonstrated on CT (Fig. 33). Contrast enhancement defines the extent of thrombosis by showing the low-density thrombus outlined by the enhanced residual lumen of the aneurysm (Fig. 34). This may produce Kricheff's "target sign", cited by Schubiger et al. [46]. The image corresponds to the enhanced ring around the wall of the aneurysm, the nonenhanced mural throm-

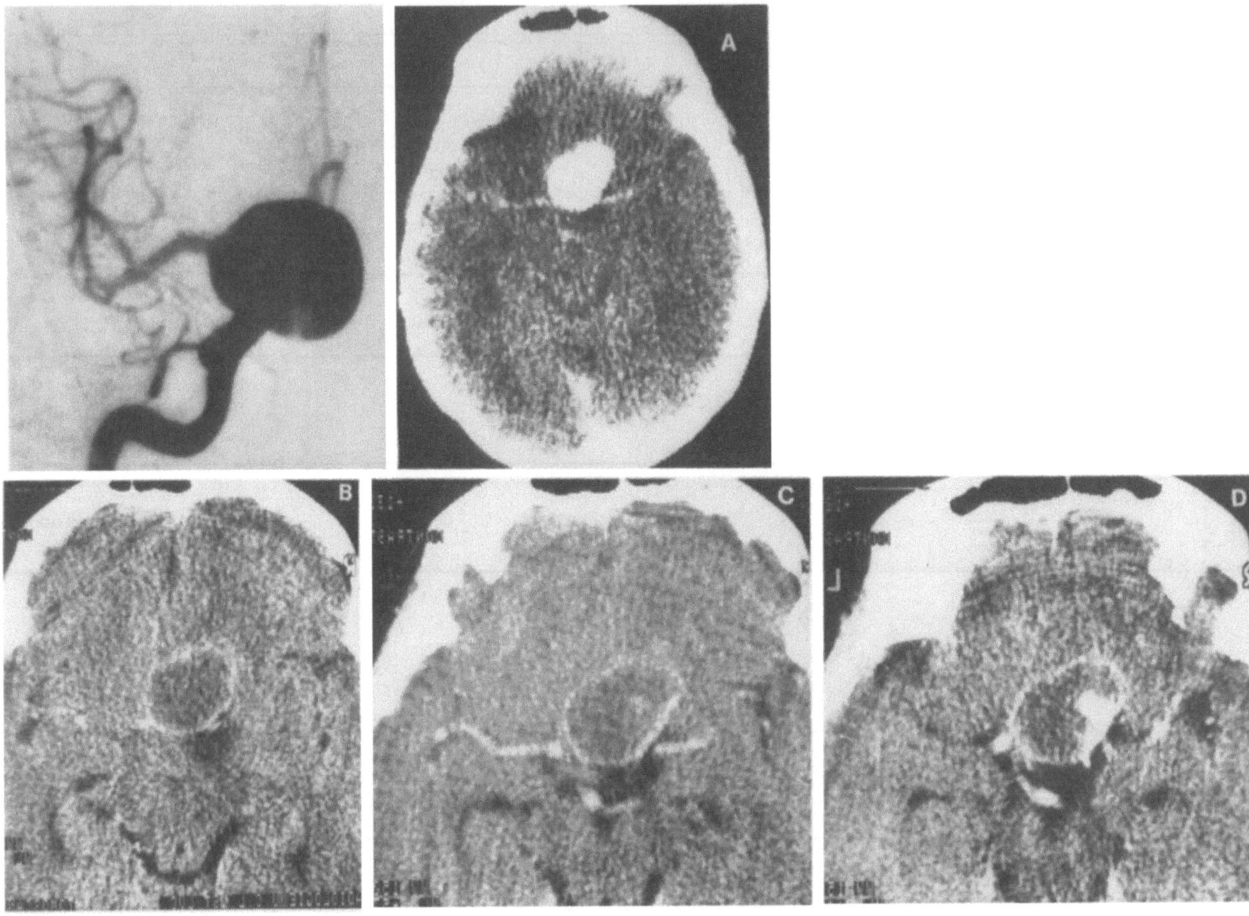

Fig. 32. Carotid-ophthalmic aneurysm. D.B., a 62-year-old female presented in January 1983 with decreasing vision in the right eye since 1981 and now with acute loss of vision in left eye (1/20). Right ICA ligation was well tolerated. Two months later the patient's vision has slightly improved (3/10). *Top left* Right internal carotid angiogram confirming the giant aneurysm. **A** postcontrast axial CT: no thrombus is seen within the aneurysm. **B–D.** Postcontrast axial CT scans following carotid occlusion: near complete thrombosis with small enhancing residual channel at the base (**D**) of the aneurysm. (Images courtesy of Prof. G. Stroobandt, Catholic University of Louvain)

bus, and the enhanced central region of residual blood flow. The density of the thrombus varies from patient to patient owing to the age of the thrombus. Initially it is hyperdense, then within a few months it becomes low-density as the clot organizes; it may eventually show areas of calcification.

Postoperative Aspects

Seven patients treated by proximal occlusion of the internal carotid artery were followed up with CT to monitor the progress of thrombosis, and change in size of the aneurysm. Three out of four nonthrombosed aneurysms eventually thrombosed totally, the other showing only partial thrombosis (see Fig. 32). In the partially thrombosed group two out of three patients' aneurysms totally thrombosed (see Fig. 30). The other case showed additional thrombus but never completely occluded. The degree and evolution of the thrombus are very well demonstrated by CT. Comparison with earlier CT studies allows the delineation of subtle changes within the aneurysm. CT is currently the method of choice for evaluating the true size of the aneurysm. Only two of our cases (see Figs. 18, 69) showed reduction in size following thrombosis.

Other Uses of Computed Tomography

CT also provides analysis of surrounding structures:

1. Bony erosions of the sella or skull base are easily identified (see Fig. 24).

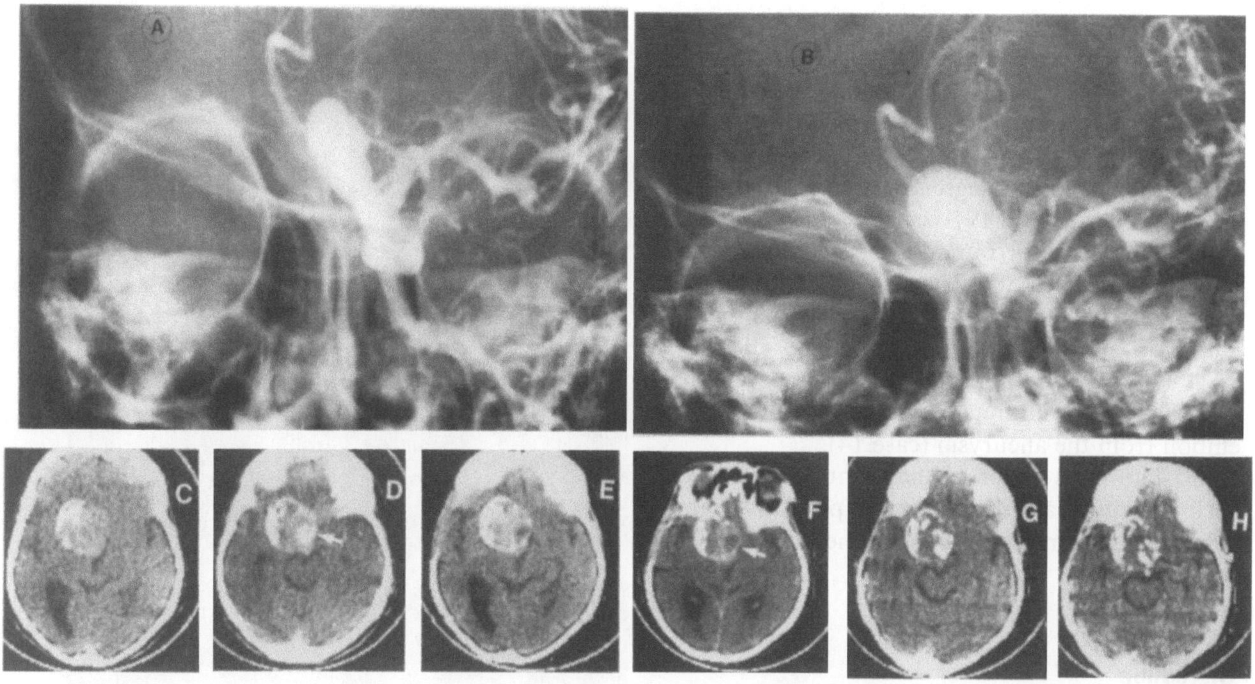

Fig. 33A–H. Carotid-ophthalmic aneurysm. M.E., a 64-year-old female, presented in 1977 with left craniofacial pain, loss of consciousness associated with falls, amnesia and behavioral changes, and pituitary dysfunction. Angiography (**A**) confirmed the giant aneurysm. She was rehospitalized in August 1979 for aggravation of the same symptoms. Repeat angiogram (**B**) shows slight enlargement in the size of the aneurysm. Precontrast axial CT scan (**C**) shows the calcifications in the aneurysm. Postcontrast CT (**D**) shows the large amount of thrombus present with the small, patent channel along the medial border of the aneurysm (*arrow*). In September 1979 an extra-intracranial bypass and carotid ligation were done. Follow up CT scans (**E, F**) show acute thrombosis of the previously patent channel (*arrow*). Patient's neurological exam was unchanged; however, the headaches had decreased. New hospitalization in March 1982 for progressive mental deterioration. Pre- and postcontrast CT scans (**G, H**) show calcification of the thrombus with no evidence of enhancement, indicating the aneurysm has remained completely thrombosed. The patient died in April 1983. Post mortem (see Fig. 1) confirmed the thrombosed, heavily calcified giant aneurysm to be compressing the diencephalon

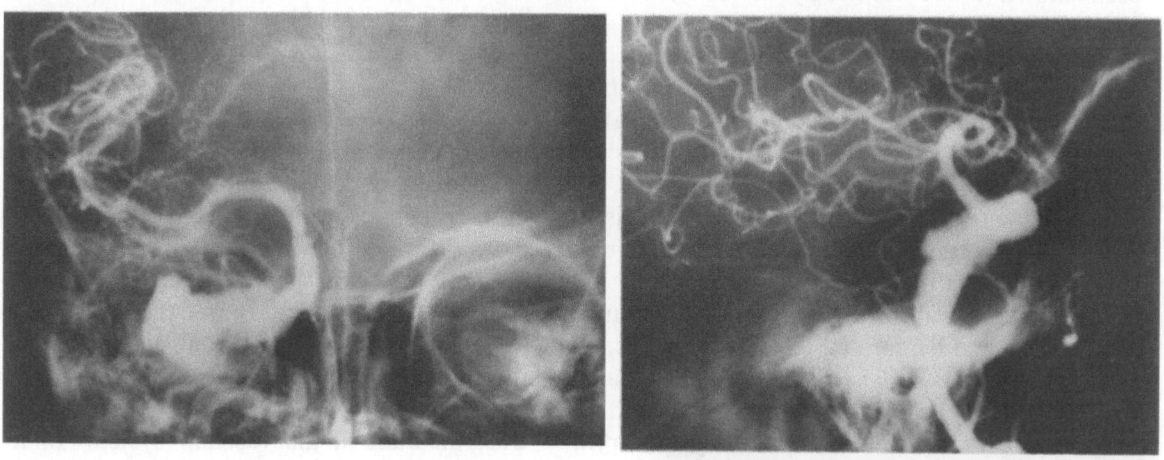

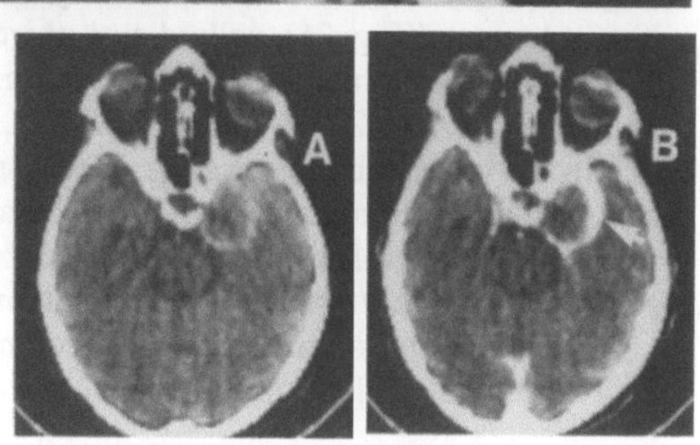

Fig. 34. Cavernous carotid aneurysm. G.G., a 70-year-old male, presented in July 1981 with subarachnoid hemorrhage (SAH). He developed a sixth cerebral nerve palsy in June 1982. In July 1982, total ophthalmoplegia with recurrent SAH. Patient considered inoperable due to poor general condition and advanced age. AP and lateral right carotid angiograms: large cavernous aneurysm. **A, B** Pre- and postcontrast axial CT scans demonstrating a partially thrombosed giant aneurysm. Note the crescent-shaped residual lumen (*arrow*)

2. Calcification of the aneurysmal wall or thrombus may be identified. These calcifications may sometimes be seen on plain radiographs (cases 1, 2), but CT is much more sensitive in detecting them. The presence of calcification does not correlate with the size or degree of thrombosis of the aneurysm (cases 1, 2, 19).

3. Absence of surrounding parenchymal edema may be established, which is helpful in differentiating giant aneurysms from tumors such as meningiomas.

4. The cerebral hemispheres can be evaluated for existence of infarcts secondary to thrombotic emboli from the aneurysm (case 14).

5. The mass effect of the giant aneurysm on such structures as cranial nerves, pituitary gland, orbit, and cerebral and cerebellar hemispheres can be evaluated.

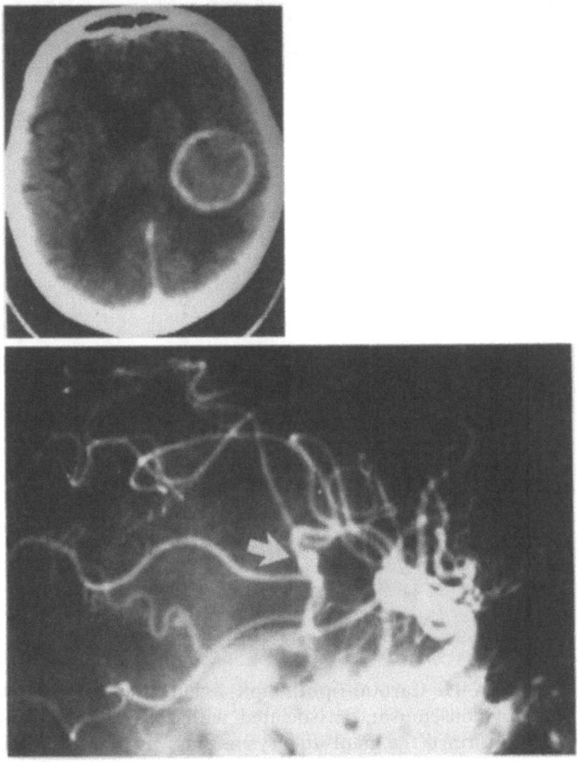

Fig. 35. R.B., a 67-year-old female. Middle cerebral aneurysm. This patient had complete excision with clipping of the neck parallel to the trunk of the parent artery, preserving patency. Uneventful postoperative course. Postcontrast axial CT scan demonstrates the large (5 cm) middle cerebral artery aneurysm to be completely thrombosed. Lateral internal carotid artery angiogram showing filling of the neck of the aneurysm (*arrow*). (Images courtesy of Professor Pansini, University of Florence)

Discussion

A review of the literature (covering 125 cases in total) confirms our experience with the CT appearance of giant aneurysms [12, 17, 18, 22, 31, 35, 36, 42, 46, 47, 60]. Each article emphasizes the typical characteristics of nonthrombosed and partially thrombosed aneurysms. The "target sign" was reported in approximately 50% of the cases. The ring enhancement of the aneurysmal wall has been shown to be secondary to newly formed blood vessels which occur with progressive clot resorption and formation of scar tissue [22, 31, 39, 60]. Thus, the presence of a peripheral contrast ring indicates a thrombus undergoing organization [54, 60]. All authors agree that angiography is still necessary to confirm the diagnosis, but that CT shows the true size and degree of thrombosis [9, 49]. A totally thrombosed aneurysm may only show mass effect on the angiogram (Fig. 35). CT is also helpful in differentiating poorly vascularized tumors and hematomas from aneurysms, for which they may otherwise sometimes be mistaken [10]. The differential diagnosis of giant carotid aneurysms must take account of meningioma, pituitary adenoma, (Fig. 36), colloid cyst, third ventricle glioma, chordoma, and craniopharyngioma [4, 5, 16, 17, 18, 19, 21, 27, 29, 32, 33, 41, 45, 58, 62]. In the vertebrobasilar system, aneurysms, neurinomas, and meningiomas may have a similar appearance [17, 56]. Most of these cases can be distinguished by the pattern of contrast enhancement. CT metrizamide cysternography, as recommended by Naheedy et al. [28], is not diagnostic and still requires angiographic confirmation. However, as in the case of Lavyne et al. [22], it may help to differentiate a carotid aneurysm mimicking a pituitary adenoma for which the patient was operated upon by the trans-sphenoidal approach.

Pinto et al. [40], and after them several others [2, 3, 20, 59, 64], report their experience using a rapid sequence of CT images during contrast injection. This demonstrates the progress of the contrast medium in the vascular system. In fact, it is possible to get a graphic analysis of the density of the contrast medium in various structures at different intervals. Thus Pinto found that the curve obtained for a giant nonthrombosed aneurysm is identical to that of the normal large arteries supplying or constituting the circle of Willis, and that there is a recirculation peak which is absent in all other suprasellar lesions, including meningiomas. They believe that "dynamic" scanning is as

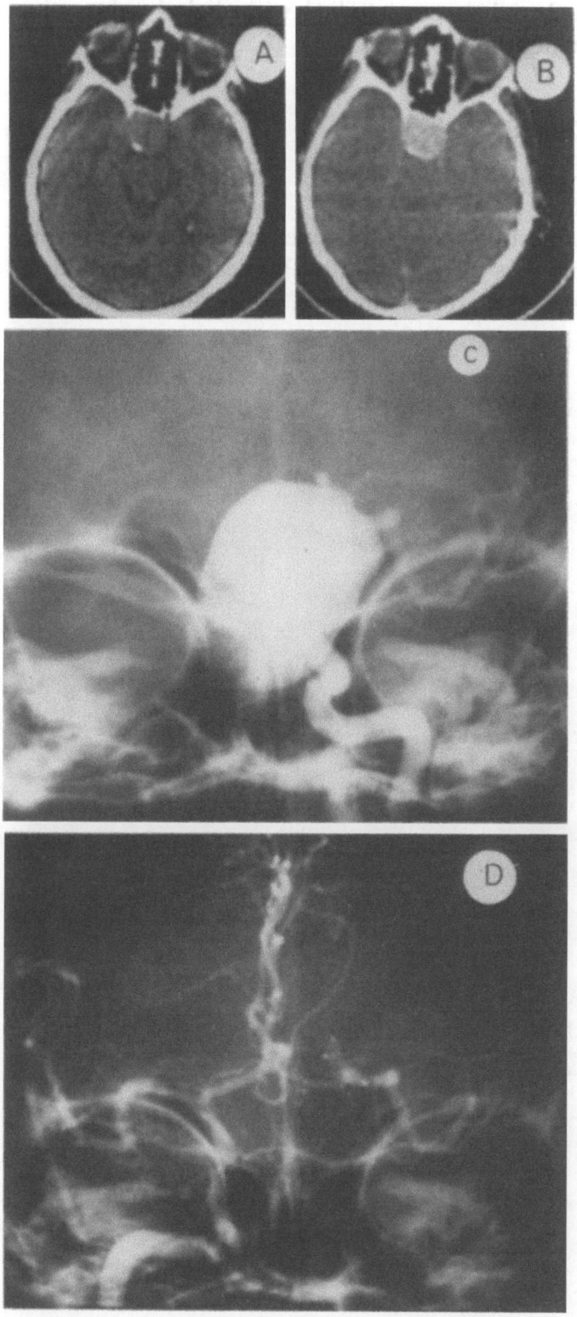

Fig. 36 A–D. Intrasellar carotid aneurysm. M.G., a 59-year-old female, was hospitalized for difficulty in walking, and frequent falls. Physical examination revealed an akinetic-hypertonic syndrome with diminished vision and bilateral optic disk atrophy without visual field disturbance. Laboratory tests revealed anterior pituitary insufficiency. Plain radiographs showed destruction of the sella turcica and curvilinear calcifications. Pre- and postcontrast axial CT scans (**A**, **B**) confirm the diagnosis of an enhancing intrasellar mass. AP left carotid angiogram (**C**) confirms the giant intrasellar aneurysm. **D** AP right carotid angiogram shows no filling of aneurysm with cross compression. This case illustrates the problem differentiating these lesions by CT alone

reliable as angiography in diagnosing giant aneurysms. However, most authors believe, as we do, that angiography or at least a venous digital subtraction angiogram is still indicated (see Fig. 36).

Finally, CT appears to be the best method for following up giant aneurysms. Both their size and the degree of thrombosis can be easily evaluated [8, 50, 51, 55, 61]. Pinto et al. [40] believe that the use of dynamic CT enables one to totally dispense with follow-up angiographic examinations. However in our experience, it is not possible to rule out the possibility of a small patent channel existing inside a freshly thrombosed aneurysm solely on the basis of the CT scan. This is especially important as partial thrombosis does not eliminate the risk of recurrent subarachnoid hemorrhage [10, 14, 60, 65].

Conclusion

CT is an excellent method of diagnosing and evaluating giant intracranial aneurysms. Unlike angiography, pre- and post-contrast CT accurately determines the presence or absence of calcification and thrombus within the aneurysm, as well as the aneurysm's true size. CT is also useful for evaluating the mass effect on adjacent structures, and identifying bony erosions and embolic infarctions. Serial CT examinations demonstrate subtle changes in size and in the evolution of the thrombus. Angiography is still considered to be necessary for absolute diagnostic confirmation, but CT is now the method of choice for monitoring the long-term course of these lesions.

Magnetic Resonance Imaging

Magnetic resonance imaging (MRI) is a simple, noninvasive technique for demonstrating the presence of flow within large intracranial aneurysms, as well as for differentiating recent from organized thrombi.

Four clinical examples are presented with CT and angiographic correlation. These cases demonstrate that rapid and/or turbulent flow gives no signal on short (T1-weighted) spin echo sequences, but may show a central phase artefact on longer (T2-weighted) echoes.

Recent thrombosis, as may be seen within the aneurysm following endovascular occlusion, gives a bright echo on both sequences. The etiology of the various signal intensities are discussed along with their clinical potential.

All patients were studied with a 0.5 Tesla Thomson CGR Magniscan 5000 using various spin echo sequences to obtain T1- and T2-weighted images in 5-mm slices. Pre- and post-contrast enhanced CT was done before and after contrast enhancement in all cases. The first case was studied with conventional angiography. Cases 2, 3 and 4 were studied with digital subtraction angiography (DSA).

Clinical Observations

Case 1

L.B., a 35-year-old female, presented with vertigo and loss of equilibrium. Physical examination revealed no abnormalities. Subsequent CT study

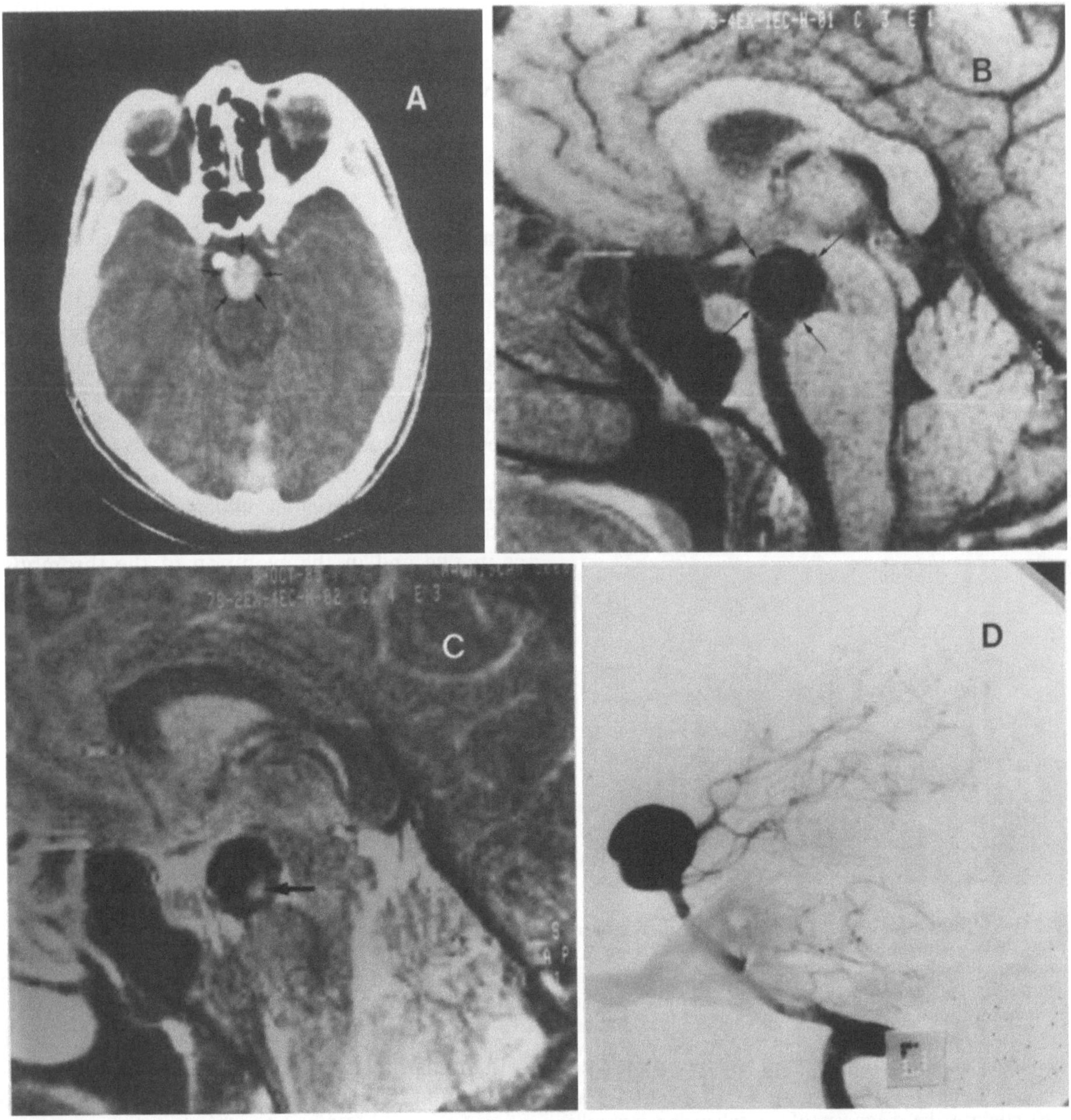

Fig. 37 A–D. Basilar artery aneurysm. **A** CT: Axial scan at the level of the midbrain demonstrating a large, enhancing mass (*arrows*) in the interpeduncular cistern. No calcium or thrombus is shown. **B** MRI: T1 (TE 28/TR 300) sagittal image showing a large, circular area of absent signal (*arrows*) corresponding to the mass on CT. **C** MRI: T2 (TE 40/TR 2000) sagittal image showing the central artifactual bright signal (*arrow*) **D** Lateral vertebral angiogram confirming the large aneurysm of the basilar artery

(Fig. 37A) revealed a large, well-defined, homogeneously enhancing mass in the interpeduncular cistern. A basilar artery aneurysm was suspected. MRI (Fig. 37B, C) showed the lesion to give no signal on the short echo (T1-weighted) images, but on the long echo (T2-weighted) images there was a central irregular region of increased signal. DSA (Fig. 37D) confirmed the large aneurysm at the tip of the basilar artery and demonstrated rapid turbulent flow without thrombosis.

Case 2

D.D., a 55-year-old female, presented with headaches and galactorrhea. Neurologic examination revealed no abnormalities. A CT study (Fig. 38A) to evaluate for a suspected pituitary adenoma revealed a large enhancing mass extending upwards in the left cavernous sinus with a densily calcified rim. The pituitary fossa was normal. MRI (Fig. 38B, C) demonstrated the aneurysmal dilatation of the left ICA as a no-signal area. There was a slightly increased signal in the lateral and upper margin of the aneurysm on both T1- and T2-weighted images, suggesting recent thrombus. DSA (Fig. 38D, E) confirmed the aneurysm of the cavernous portion of the left ICA. Also found were small saccular aneurysms of the right anterior choroidal and posterior communicating arteries, mild aneurysmal dilatation of the right cavernous ICA, and generalized arteriosclerotic vascular disease.

Case 3

C.D., a 12-year-old female, presented with headaches and vomiting. The physical and neurological examinations revealed no abnormalities. The symptoms resolved within 48 h and she was discharged. Nine days later, she was readmitted with the same symptoms as well as photophobia. She now had a right sixth cranial nerve palsy. A CT scan (Fig. 39A) showed a huge multilobulated enhancing mass in the right cavernous sinus extending superiorly.

There was a curvilinear low density in the lateral margin of the mass, suggesting mural thrombus. DSA (Fig. 39B) confirmed the giant cavernous carotid aneurysm and demonstrated rapid flow within the lesion. The patient was embolized with two latex detachable balloons, one placed across the neck of the aneurysm, and the other placed more proximally in the carotid siphon as "insurance." MRI (Fig. 39C, D) performed 1 month later showed an almost completely homogeneous high signal throughout the thrombosed aneurysm on T1-weighted image. The T2 images showed marked signal loss from the mural thrombus while the recent thrombus remained bright. Two months later an intravenous digital angiogram documented no flow within the aneurysm.

Case 4

F.B., a 71-year-old female, presented with diplopia. Physical examination showed a left third cranial nerve palsy, along with left-sided ptosis and anisocoria.

A CT scan (Fig. 40A) demonstrated aneurysmal enlargement of the left cavernous sinus. There was also evidence of old mural thrombus on the enhanced images. MRI (Fig. 40B) demonstrated high-velocity signal loss with artefactual enhancement on the T2 images, as in case 1. The old mural thrombus was also observed to behave as in case 3. DSA (Fig. 40C) confirmed the large saccular aneurysm of the left internal carotid artery. The patient was treated as in case 3, with the placement of two latex detachable balloons completely occluding the aneurysm, and distal left internal carotid artery.

Discussion

The first case demonstrates the effect of turbulent flow in a large, saccular aneurysm. The initial T1 images show no signal due to high-velocity signal loss. This happens because the excited protons are washed downstream before they can emit a signal in the section being imaged. The T2 images show an irregular area of increased signal in the center of the lesion (see Fig. 37C). This artefactual enhancement is thought to be secondary to two independant processes. The first, described by Mills et al. [25], is that there is a maintenance of a subpopulation of excited protons due to the turbulent, circular flow within the aneurysm. The second explanation, proposed by Bradley et al. [6], suggested that the signal is due to a rephasing of the even echoes in a multiecho sequence.

All the cases show the expected high-velocity signal loss in the central portions of carotid aneurysms. In cases 2 and 4 a crescent-shaped mural thrombus was identified on CT which corre-

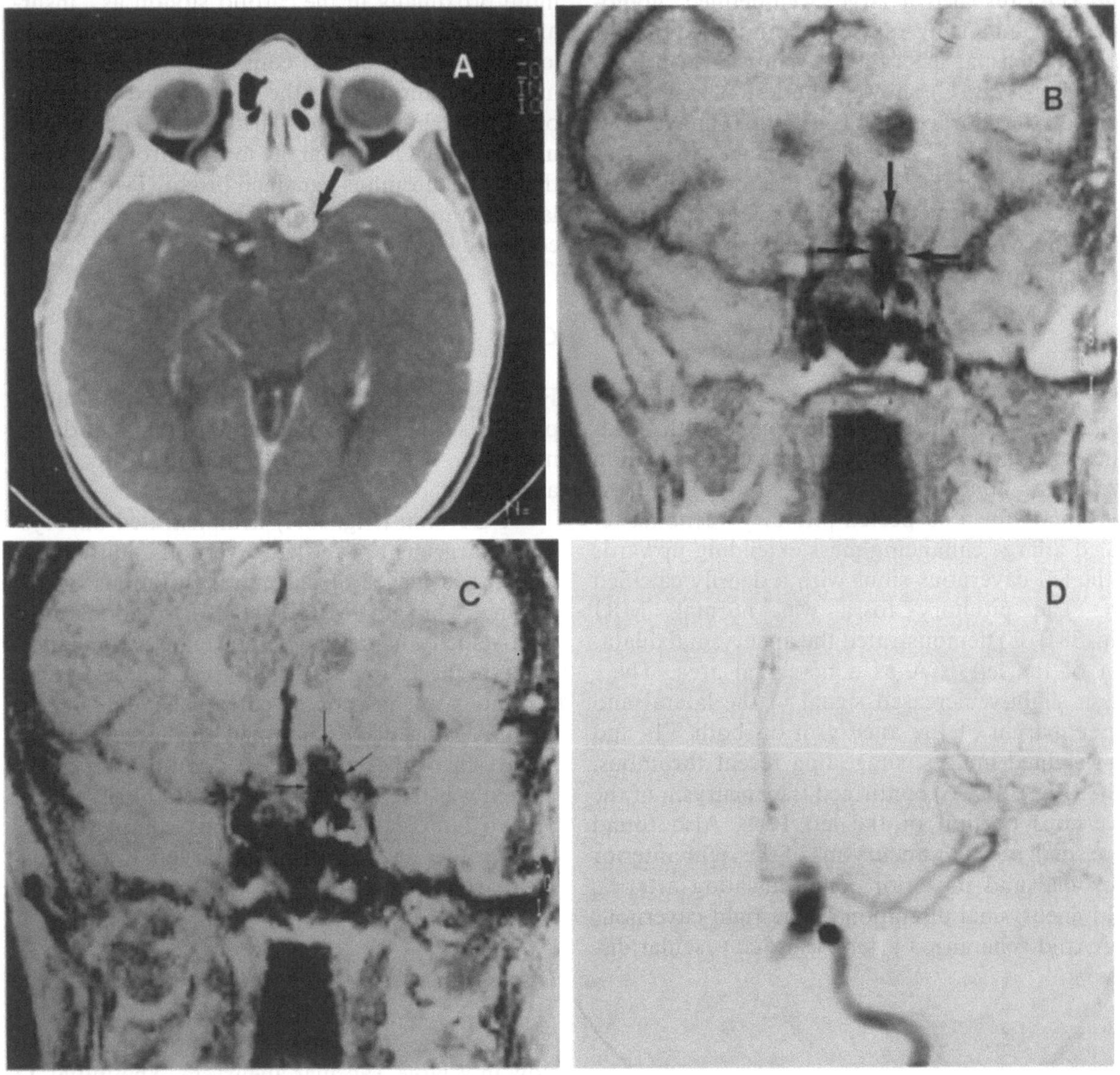

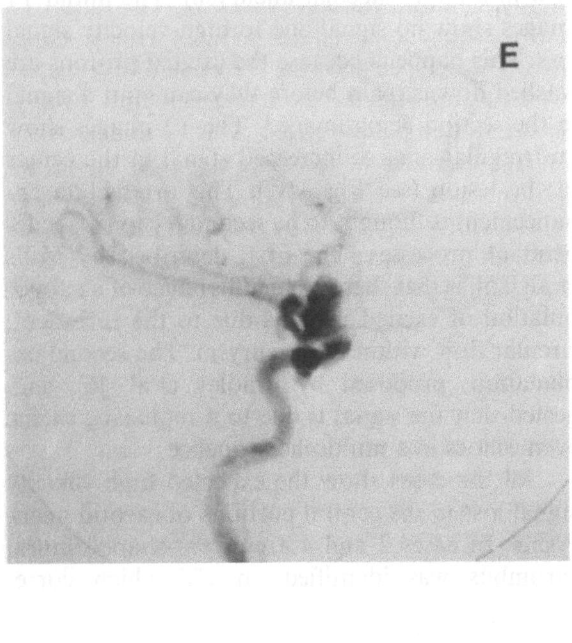

Fig. 38 A–E. Supraclinoid carotid aneurysm. **A** CT: axial scan just above the sella demonstrating a heavily calcified, enhancing mass on the left of midline (*arrow*). **B, C** MRI: coronal T1 (TE 28/TR 400) and T2 (TE 60/TR 1500) images through the sella, showing a multilobulated area of absent signal above the left cavernous sinus (*arrows*). Notice the rim of increased signal in the superior margin, showing no change in intensity on the two sequences. This is most likely due to recent mural thrombus in the aneurysm. **D, E** DSA: AP and lateral views of a selective left internal carotid artery injection confirming the supraclinoid aneurysm

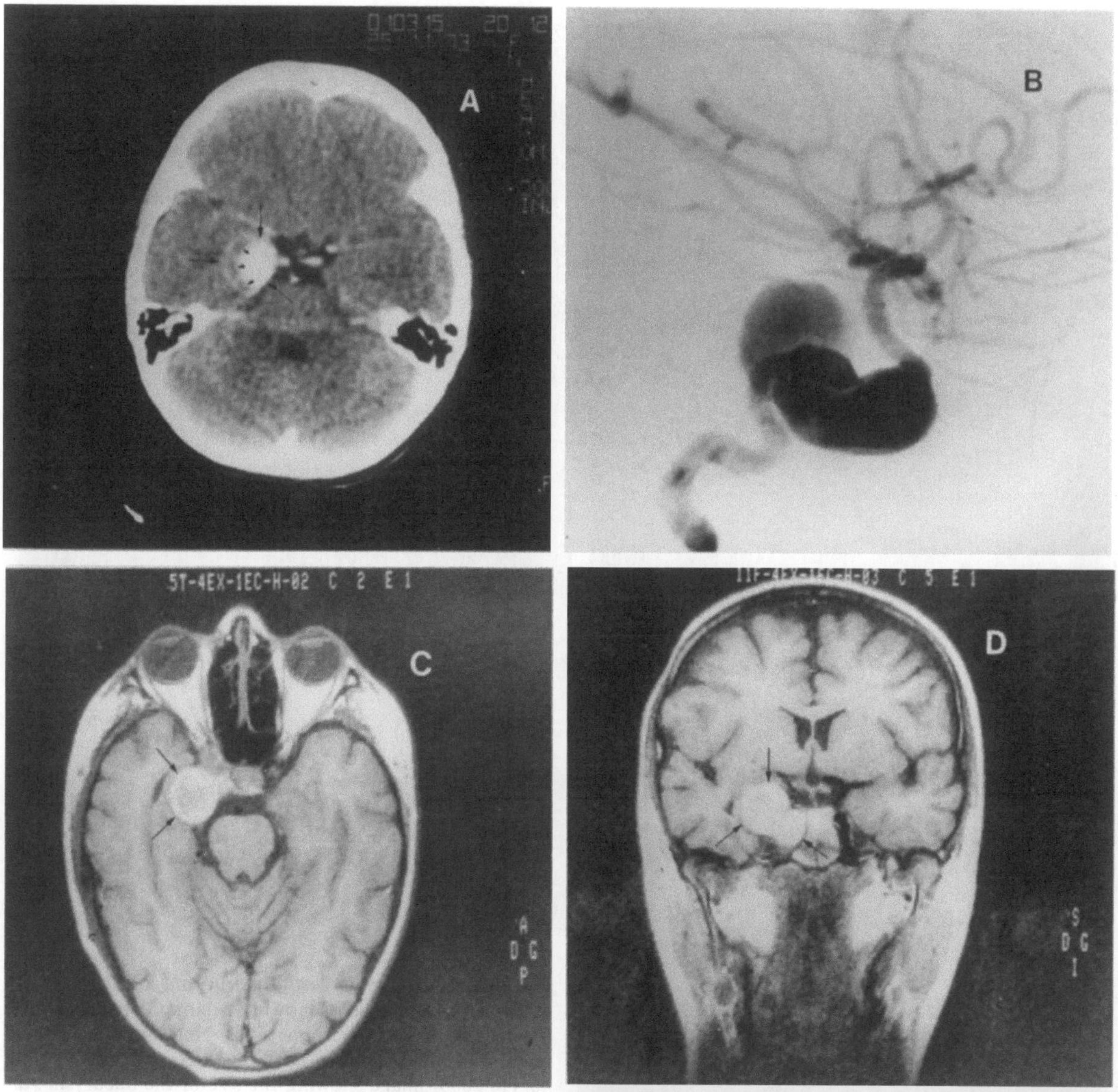

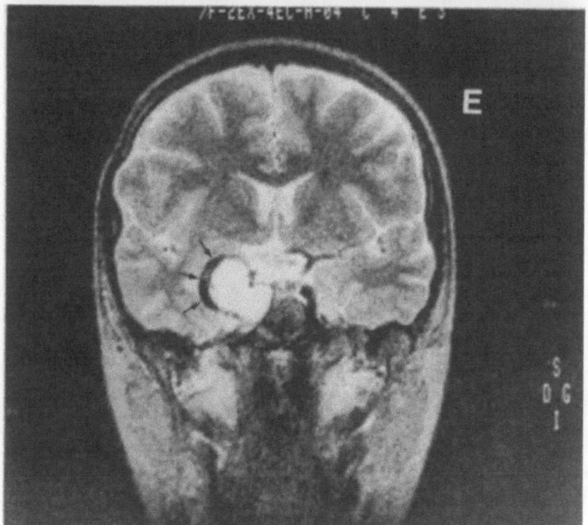

Fig. 39 A–C. Cavernous carotid aneurysm. **A** Preembolization CT: axial scan at the level of the sella showing a large enhancing mass on the right (*arrows*) consistent with a carotid aneurysm. Note the crescent of mural thrombus in the lateral portion of the aneurysm (*arrowheads*). **B** Preembolization DSA: Lateral view of selective right internal carotid artery injection confirming cavernous aneurysm. **C, D** Postembolization MRI: axial and coronal T1 (TE 28/TR 300) images showing the lobulated aneurysm (*arrows*) to be of bright signal. The inhomogeneity in the center of the aneurysm on the axial image is due to flow artefact. **E** Postembolization MRI: coronal T2 (TE 60/TR 2000) image showing the recent thrombus to remain increased in signal while the crescent-shaped mural thrombus shows no signal (*arrows*). This is probably due to absorption of the water from the old thrombus, leaving fewer protons available for excitation

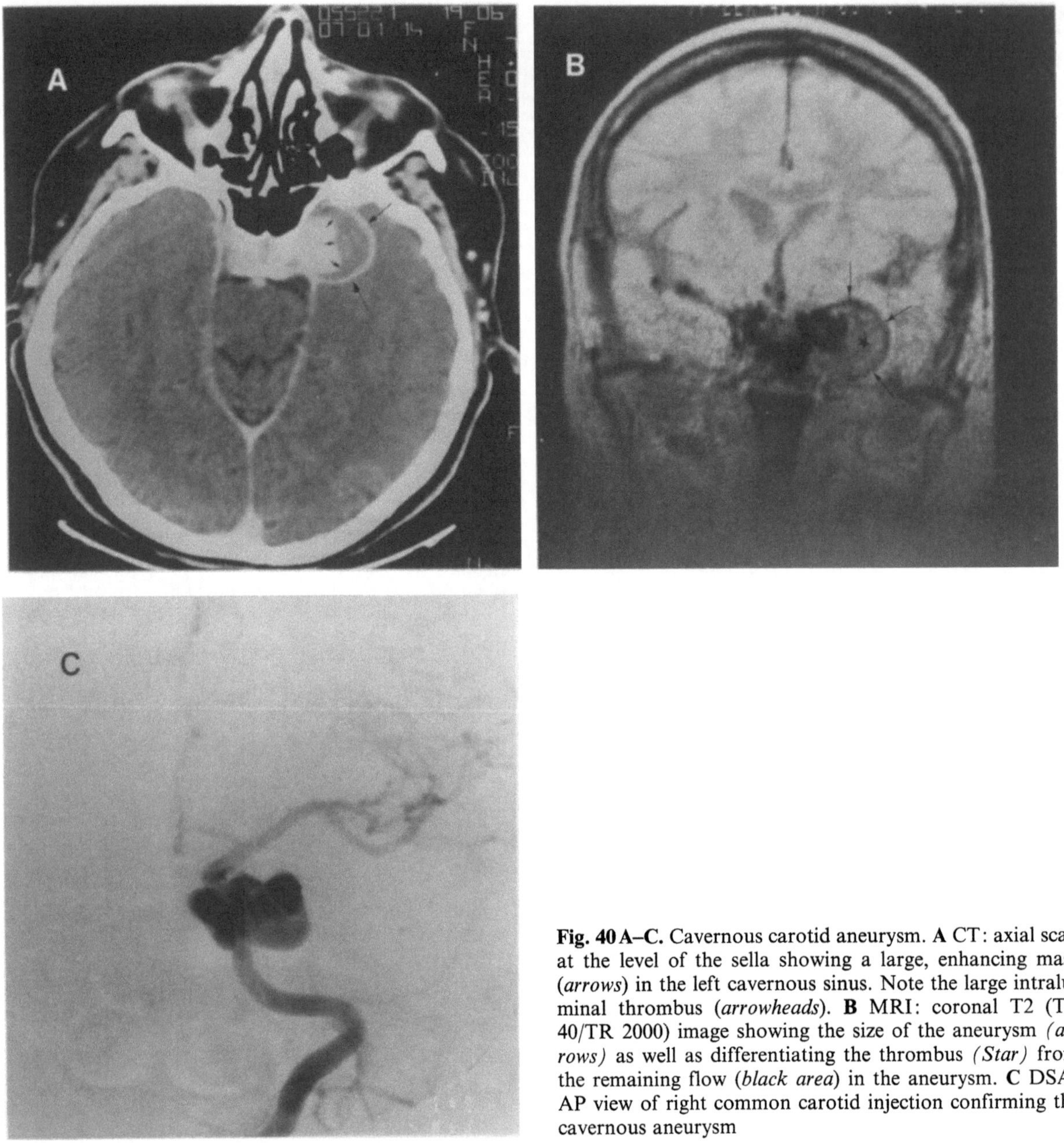

Fig. 40 A–C. Cavernous carotid aneurysm. **A** CT: axial scan at the level of the sella showing a large, enhancing mass (*arrows*) in the left cavernous sinus. Note the large intraluminal thrombus (*arrowheads*). **B** MRI: coronal T2 (TE 40/TR 2000) image showing the size of the aneurysm (*arrows*) as well as differentiating the thrombus (*Star*) from the remaining flow (*black area*) in the aneurysm. **C** DSA: AP view of right common carotid injection confirming the cavernous aneurysm

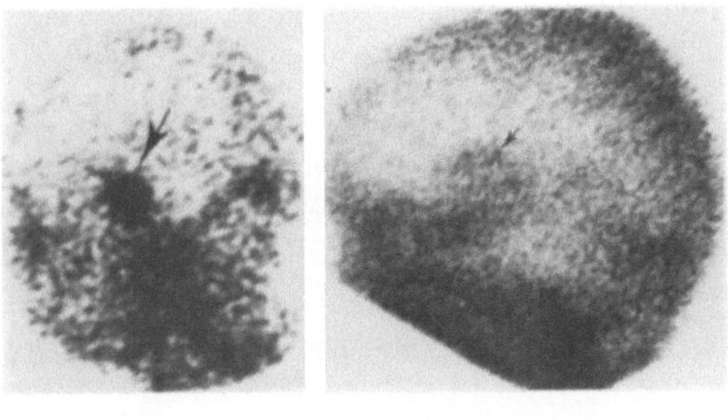

Fig. 41. Radionuclide brain scan. *Left* Lateral view of a giant nonthrombosed carotid-ophthalmic aneurysm (*arrow*). *Right* Delayed scan of a partially thrombosed carotid-ophthalmic aneurysm (*arrow*)

sponded to an identically shaped region of medium signal on the T1 image. This same area showed marked loss on the T2 image. The recent thrombosis within the aneurysm of the third case gave a completely different signal to that of the old mural thrombus. The recent clot remained bright on both T1 and T2 images, although the signal became slightly less intense and inhomogeneous on the later echo. The apparent conclusion is that, as the water is reabsorbed from the organizing clot, its signal becomes less and less intense, as there are fewer hydrogen protons remaining for excitation.

The clinical potential of MRI in large intracranial aneurysms lies not only in the excellent demonstration of neuroanatomic relationships, but also in the evaluation of intraluminal flow. Worthington et al. [63] demonstrated very well the ability of MRI to recognize giant carotid aneurysms. We agree that MRI provides an excellent method not only of identifying the lesions, but also of following their regression in size, mass effect, and evolution of the intraluminal thrombus.

Radionuclide Brain Scanning

Cerebral radionuclide tomography, when used in the diagnostic assessment of atypical neurological disease, has most often proved to be positive in dynamic study of nonthrombosed aneurysms (Fig. 41, left) and in static study whatever the degree of thrombosis (Fig. 41, right), exhibiting a limited increase uptake zone located next to the skull base. However, such nonspecific characteristics make this form of examination of little interest in practice.

Direct Surgical Treatment by Neck Occlusion

Selective occlusion of the neck by direct approach is the ideal treatment of giant aneurysms, as it preserves normal blood flow in the parent artery. It also allows decompression of the mass by opening of the sac.

General Technical Considerations

General

Practicability of Neck Occlusion in Giant Aneurysms

Except in certain special cases, the practicability of this operation can only be estimated on the basis of direct exploration of the malformation. Angiography does not make it possible to predict with any certainty whether or not the neck is suitable for occlusion.

The clips in current use, having wide openings, long blades, and many different shapes, have extended the indications for neck occlusion (see pp. 47–51). Nevertheless, this technique most often presents difficulties because of the anatomical characteristics of the neck and intrasaccular pressure.

Size of the Neck

Neck size can be reduced by first positioning a ligature to produce a circumferential reduction of the neck caliber, collapsing it with a large-jaw forceps, or shrinking its wall by either bi- or monopolar electrocoagulation. When bipolar coagulation, highly advocated by Yasargil et al. [60, 134, 136, 137], cannot be employed because of the large size of the aneurysm and the thickness of its walls, recourse may be had to unipolar coagulation applied tangentially at different points of the sac, as recommended by Pertuiset et al. [85]. These techniques, commonly used in large berry aneurysms, are difficult or even impracticable in giant aneurysms, especially if they are thrombosed, or when their walls are thick, atheromatous, and/or calcified, or else very thin and fragile.

In some of these wide-necked aneurysms where the clip or ligature fails to produce a complete occlusion of the neck, some authors prefer to leave them in situ waiting for a reduction in volume and partial thrombosis of the sac, as reported in four cases by Bonnal [11], rather than performing a forced ligation which might result in sectioning of the neck at the site of its implantation in the parent artery (see Fig. 45).

When the diameter of the neck remains large, it is essential that the clip be placed at a certain distance from the parent artery so as not to reduce its caliber, which can be underestimated in cases of major hypotension or temporary clamping (Fig. 42).

Walls of the Neck

When the walls of the neck are particularly thick, the blades of the clip may not be occlusive at their distal extremity, as they do not lie parallel and their strength is reduced. For such cases Drake

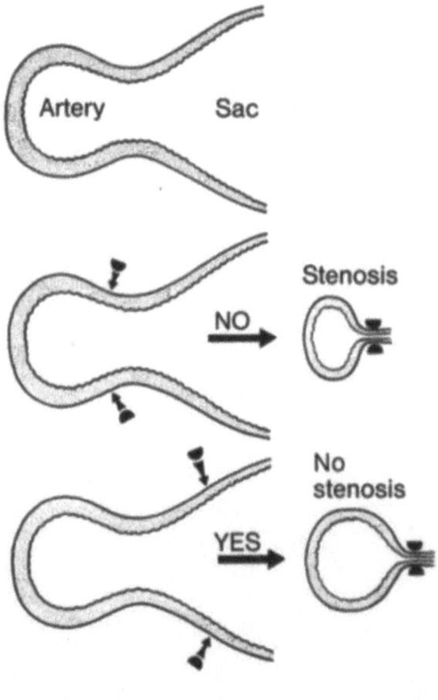

Fig. 42. Incorrect and correct technique of clip application

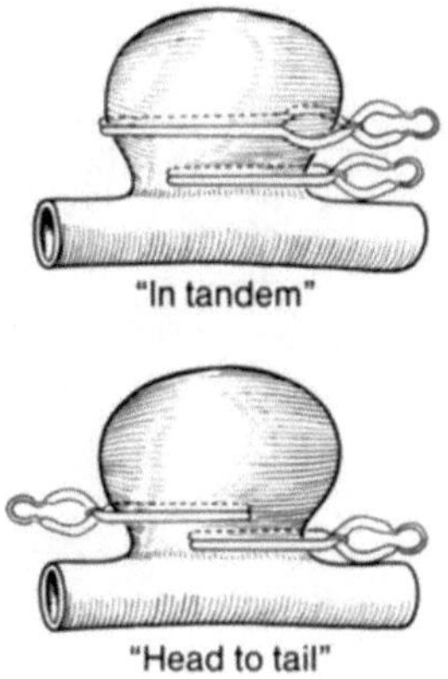

Fig. 43. Techniques to improve the gripping pressure of clips on wide-necked aneurysms

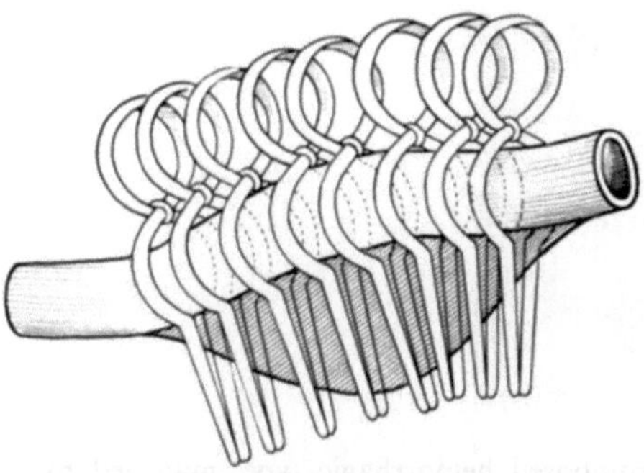

Fig. 44. Several clips placed close together along a fusiform aneurysm to reduce the lumen of the parent artery

proposes the technical artifice of clips placed "in tandem" or "head to tail" (Fig. 43) or even "piggy back", which can double the occlusive pressure. In cases of fusiform aneurysm, several clips can be placed close together so as to reduce the lumen of the parent artery (Fig. 44).

Another tool – helpful for thick-walled giant aneurysms – is the Sundt's booster clip, used as an additional clip to secure closure of the primary one. These booster-clips, which were designed to encircle the primary clip and close upon its jaws, were used by this author in 19 giant aneurysms operated on from March 1982 to June 1983 (ref. 24 in chapter "Clips and Giant Aneurysms").

In cases of atheromatous plaque or mural thrombus located at the neck, application of the clip can be dangerous, for various reasons. The clip can slip, cut the neck, or slide towards the parent artery and stenose it. Collapsing the neck with large-jaw forceps prior to clip application can be helpful but must be done gently, as this can tear the neck at its implantation in the parent artery or produce insults to the tunica intima, which can be factors of secondary thrombosis or embolism. In certain cases, recourse may be had to endarterectomy or to excision of the atheromatous plaque and/or mural thrombus, after opening of the sac, in order to reduce the rigidity of the neck before applying the clip. The same techniques must be carried out before performing endoaneurysmorrhaphies or reconstruction of the parent artery, although this can be difficult owing to the poor quality of the arterial walls. During these surgical manipulations, hemorrhages can be prevented or controlled by moderate or low arterial hypotension or temporary clamping.

Intrasaccular Pressure

Dissection of the aneurysm and collapse of its neck can be greatly facilitated by reducing the intrasaccular pressure. This can be obtained by the classic method of systemic arterial hypotension. Pertuiset et al. [86], studying brain blood volume under controlled hypotension, have shown that cerebral autoregulation maintains good cerebral protection until a mean systemic arterial pressure of 40 mmHg is reached. Moreover, their clinical experience with more than 500 cases of vascular malformations has confirmed that it is possible to induce hypotension of the order of 30 mmHg mean pressure without harmful consequences, provided that it does not last more than 30 min.

Proximal Temporary Clamping

Because of their particular problems, the management of giant aneurysms calls for a somewhat frequent use of temporary proximal clamping or even trapping of the parent artery. This can be done at the level of the internal carotid artery either by cervical clamping or, possibly (if the operating room is equipped for intraoperative angiography), by temporary endovascular occlusion using a balloon catheter. Intracranially, proximal occlusion can be performed with the newly designed temporary clips. Owing to the risk of distal ischemia associated with clamping, caution is essential with the systematic use of arterial hypotension. Any temporary proximal clamping (or trapping), even of short duration, should prompt the anesthesist to reestablish normal arterial pressure or even to moderately raise it so as to improve anastomotic collateral circulation. Great care must be taken as to the duration of temporary clamping. According to Drake [28], it can become dangerous in *nor-*

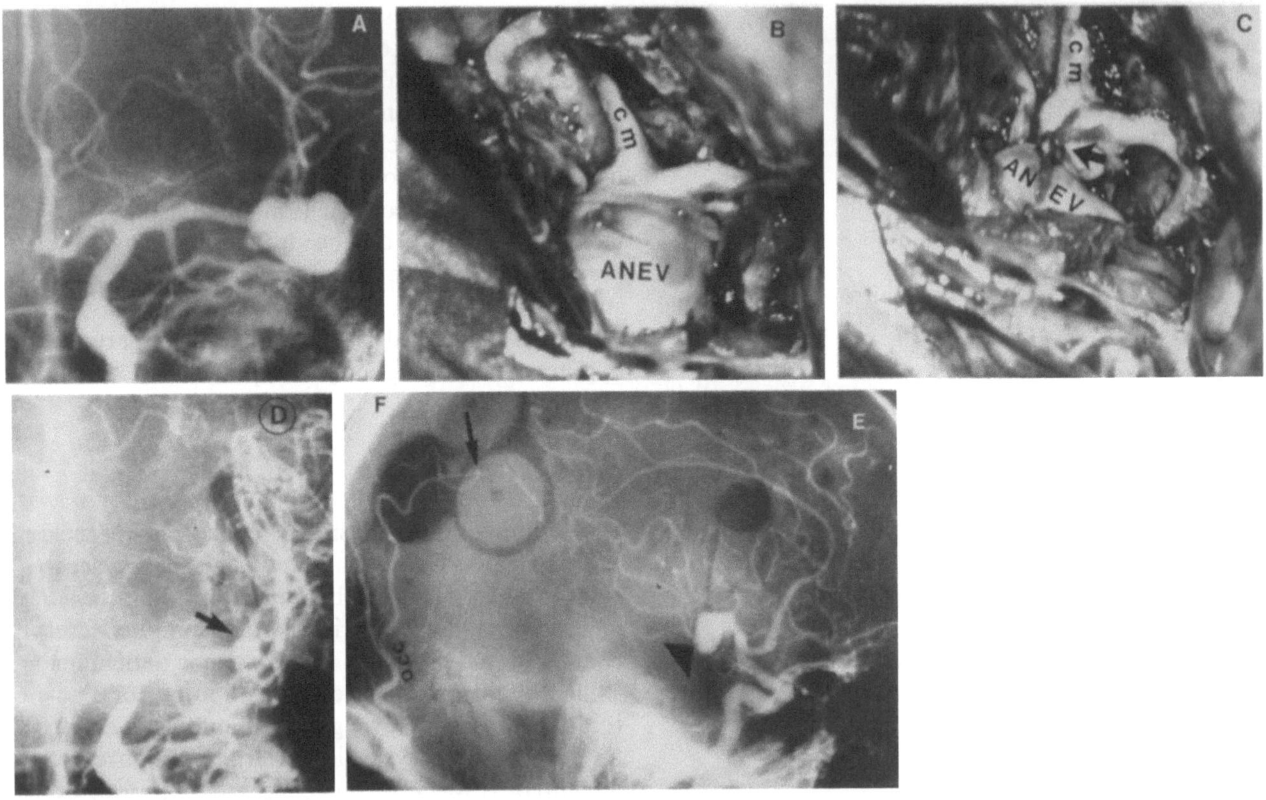

Fig. 45 A–E. V.B., 70-year-old male. Left sylvian aneurysm (*ANEV*) nonthrombosed hemorrhagic type, managed by ligation of the neck; unsuccessful. Subarachnoid hemorrhage with transitory dysphasia by rupture of a left sylvian aneurysm 25 mm wide at its largest diameter (**A**). On operation, it is felt that owing to its size and morphology, the neck is more suited to ligation than to clipping (**B**). A temporary clamp is then placed on the sylvian trunk (*cm*) for 4 min, so as to produce collapse of the sac and create a thinner neck by bipolar coagulation. A ligature of the neck (*arrow*) is then effected with linen thread, without incident (**C**). The sac is punctured in order to ensure imperviousness of the ligature. Uneventful postoperative course. Follow-up angiogram after 10 days (**D**) shows the good quality of the ligature (*arrow*).

Two months later, the patient is readmitted for a new subarachnoid hemorrhage. Left carotid angiogram (**E**) shows refilling of the sylvian aneurysm (*arrowhead*). It is decided to reoperate after making an extra-intracranial bypass between the occipital artery and a posterior parietal branch of the left sylvian artery (*arrow*), the patency of which is checked by angiography (*F*); functionality is checked by Doppler sonography (flow × 2).

Direct approach of the sylvian valley reveals a fibrinous inflammatory magma with fibrous adherences to the surrounding vascular structures, dissection of which leads to a hemorrhage which can only be controlled by trapping of the sylvian bifurcation. Postoperative death secondary to a sylvian infarct, which bypass could not prevent

mothermia beyond 3 min, whilst in Hosobuchi's experience [47] temporary clamping was left for 5–8 min without any postoperative complications, especially in giant aneurysms of the middle cerebral artery, with the help of barbiturate protection.

In *hypothermia* at 29° C, temporary clamping can be left for about 10 min. Beyond that, only deep hypothermia (15° C) with extracorporeal circulation offers some protection against severe ischemic complications (see pp. 79–84). But this can lead to complications which are specific to the method, notably that of heparin therapy, which is responsible for hemorrhagic infarcts. Therefore, Drake recommends the use of hypothermia with circulatory arrest only in the most exceptional circumstances, and instead advocates recourse to deep narcosis by barbiturates in conjunction with moderate hypothermia; according to his experience, this permits prolongation of temporary occlusion for about 20 min.

Temporary proximal occlusion or trapping of the parent artery permits safe opening of the sac and evacuation of the thrombus contained, thus facilitating occlusion of the neck by a suitable clip. In doing this, Symon was able to perform a selective direct occlusion of the aneurysm in 80% of his 36 cases, with 8% mortality and only 6% poor results. In addition, decompression of the sac led

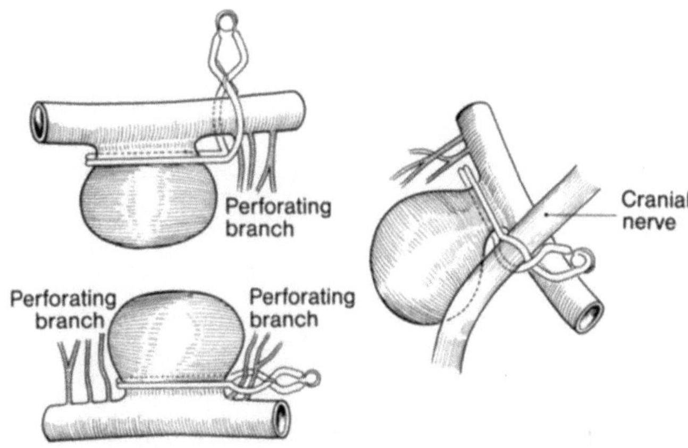

Fig. 46. Fenestrated clips

in his series to an improvement of visual loss in 6 out of 7 patients and of disturbed eye movements in 4 out of 7 [121].

Continuous Aspiration of the Sac

In order to facilitate clip application, intrasaccular pressure and volume of the sac can be diminished by continuous aspiration. This can be made by a punctiform incision at the dome of the sac and the application of an aspirating cannula on the breach, according to Laine's technique, or by the introduction into the sac of a needle with a catheter connected to continuous aspiration, according to Flamm [30]. In order better to collapse the sac, others have proposed associating aspiration with a temporary trapping, the better to dissect out and preserve the adjacent vessels [104].

Recent Clips Adapted to Giant Aneurysms

Use of the more recent clips adapted to giant aneurysms, such as those perfected by Drake, Yasargil, and Sugita (long clips, wide-opening jaws, various shapes; see pp. 47–51), undoubtedly improves the possibilities of clipping. Fenestrated clips make it possible to preserve the parent artery, as well as adjacent perforating arteries and surrounding cranial nerves (Figs. 46, 47).

Excision of the Malformation

The development of microsurgical techniques allows in certain cases excision of the whole aneurysmal malformation and reconstruction of the arterial wall, either by resuturing the edges of the implantation site or by patching the defect in order to preserve the lumen caliber. Such reconstructions have been reported by several authors, in particular by Donzelli and De Divitiis in animal experiments [23], and Artero et al. in fresh human cadavers at the level of the anterior communicating artery complex and the middle cerebral artery [6]. In humans, excision of giant aneurysms followed by arterial reconstruction have been performed by Yasargil in the anterior communicating artery [137], and Dolenc at the level of the intracavernous portion of the internal carotid artery [21] and the posterior inferior cerebellar artery [20]. Recently, we successfully excised a giant aneurysm of the second portion of posterior cerebral artery and reconstructed it with a graft taken from the superior temporal artery.

Decompression of the Sac

Direct approach of giant aneurysm makes it possible to achieve decompression of the sac. This is of prime importance, as these voluminous lesions almost always exert a mass effect on nearby structures and lead to a local or even general decrease in cerebral blood flow as shown by Hosobuchi [47] and observed in several cases treated by the authors.

Using Bloor et al.'s technique [10], Hosobuchi measured the intravascular pressure of the distal arteries by direct puncture, during trapping of the parent artery of giant aneurysms, before and after decompressing the aneurysmal sac. These measurements have shown that distal pressure, which drops from 110/60 mmHg to 50/30 mmHg after trapping, rises to 90/50 mmHg after decompression of the sac.

The type of decompression of the sac depends on its anatomical shape:

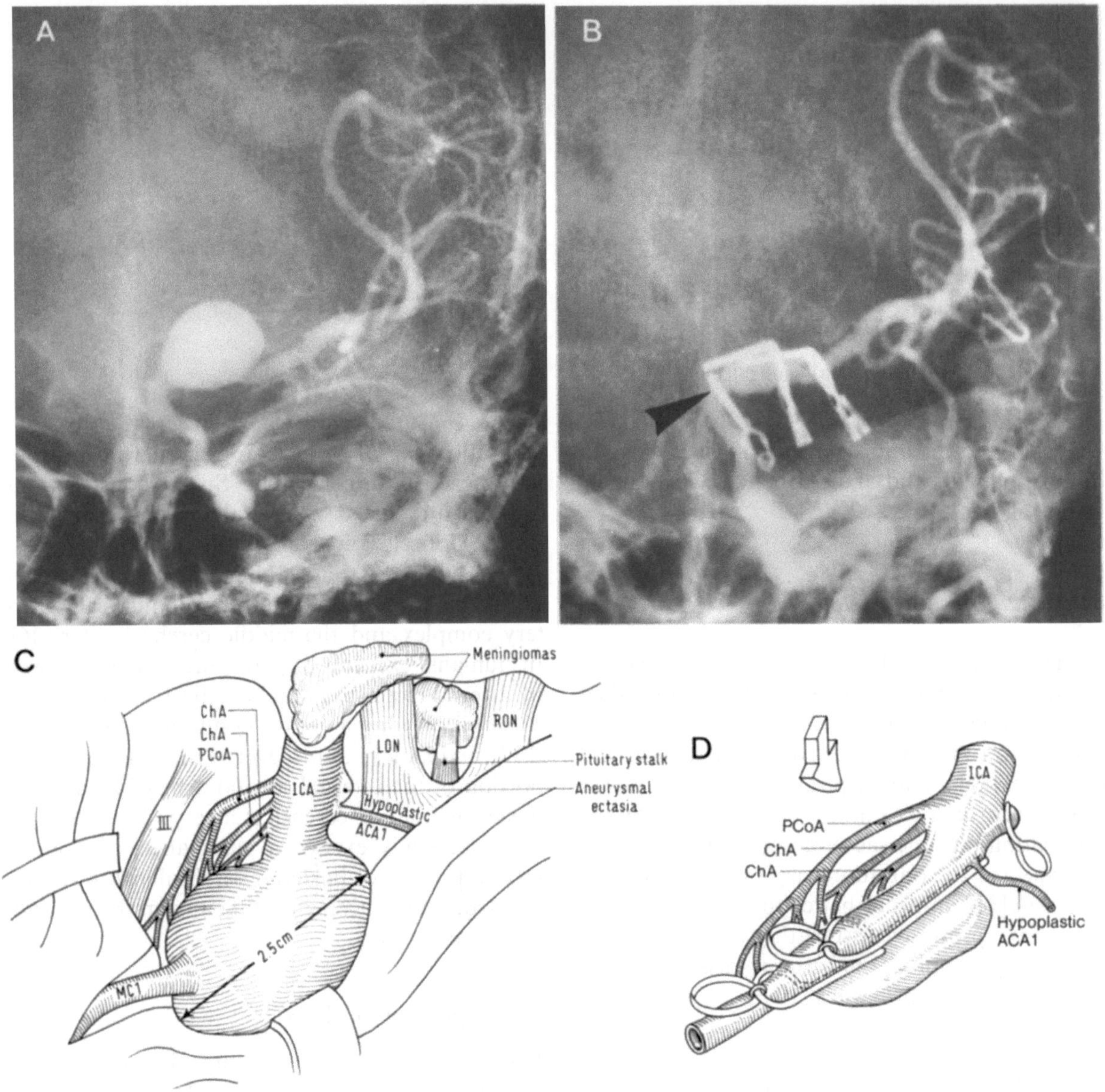

Fig. 47 A–D. Use of Sugita's angled fenestrated clip for obliterating large fusiform necks of giant aneurysms and protecting the caliber of the lumen of the parent artery. In this 65-year-old female referred in January 1986, two such clips (**B**, **D**) were applied to the giant aneurysm at the junction of the left internal carotid and middle cerebral arteries (**A**, **C**). Another, straight clip was used to obliterate a small sessile aneurysm of the dorsal aspect of the supraclinoid carotid artery (*arrowhead*). Note that two asymptomatic small distinct meningiomas (one inserted on the left anterior clinoid process, the other on the diaphragm sellae) were discovered at surgery through this left pterional approach

In *nonthrombosed* aneurysms it is sufficient, after occlusion of the neck, to aspirate the blood by puncture of the sac. This also makes it possible to check that the occlusion is complete.

In *partially thrombosed* aneurysms the mass must be decompressed by thrombectomy. This must be carried out with great care in order to avoid tearing the walls of the neck to which the thrombus adheres. The thrombus can be removed piece by piece or, more recently, with ultrasonic aspiration [2].

In *totally thrombosed* aneurysms the mass must be excised, leaving in place part of the neck in order to avoid hemorrhage. The tightness of the neck can be reinforced with a clip, a ligature, or even plastic coating.

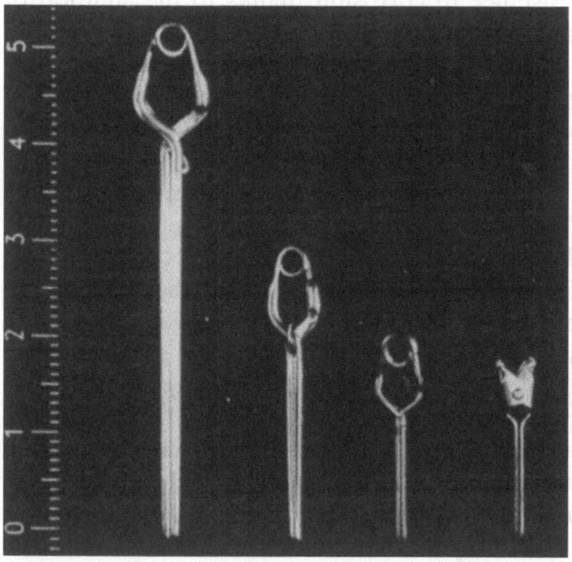

Fig. 48. Lengths of the largest currently available models of Sugita, Yasargil, McFadden, and Heifetz clips (from *left* and *right*). (Since acceptance of this manuscript, new Yasargil clips up to 41.5 mm long have become commercially available.)

Alternatives to Neck Occlusion

When exploration shows that occlusion of the neck is impracticable, or even hazardous the direct approach makes it possible to perform a trapping, or simply a proximal occlusion by means of a ligature, a clip, or, better, the tourniquet method, associated or not with an extra-intracranial bypass. Other possibilities are an intravascular thrombosis or a wrapping (see pp. 74–78).

Clips and Giant Aneurysms

The anatomic peculiarities of giant aneurysms (e.g., large necks, thick walls, fragility of the implantation of the base into the affected artery, development of collaterals at the walls or the neck) make them difficult to treat by clipping. For these reasons, we have made some studies regarding the technology of the clips used in current practice for giant aneurysms: the shape and opening angle of their blades, the solidity of the metal used, and the strength and tightness with which they close.

Shape

All the clips mentioned here (details of which are given in [25]) are available in different blade-lengths. The longest straight clips can be seen in

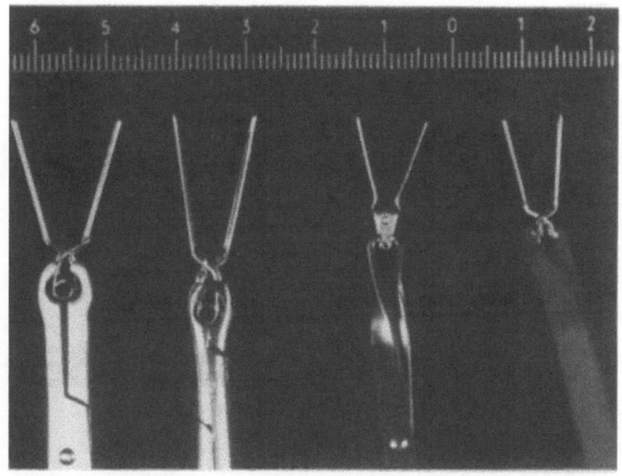

Fig. 49. Maximum opening angle of four large clips, almost similar in size: Sugita, Yasargil, Heifetz, and McFadden (from *left* to *right*)

Fig. 48. Long blades are useful, not only for aneurysms with necks of considerable diameter, but also to reach those that are located deep in an area of restricted operative maneuvrability, as is the case with aneurysms at the branching of the basilar artery [23].

The great variations in the seat and the axis of the neck, with respect to the direction of the operative approach, have led to the design of clips of various curvatures or of bayonet shape.

The close relationships of these aneurysms with essential vascular and nervous structures, particularly carotido-ophthalmic or vertebrobasilar aneurysms, have led certain authors even in the presence of a previous clip, to propose clips with straight fenestrated blades [4] and, later, curved ones [20, 22]. For example, fenestration diameters thus vary from 3.5 to 6 mm in Sugita's clips [21].

Opening Angle

The maximum opening angle of the blades, a crucial point with wide-necked aneurysms, is a function of the length and shape of the blades (for example, Sugita's fenestrated clips, with blades all the same length, have a maximum opening distance varying from 14 mm for the straight clips to 7 mm for the right-angled ones; [22] Fig. 49).

The clips most often used are those with crossed blades. They were developed by Mayfield from Schwartz's temporary clip and are based on the ductility of stainless steel 301 [13]. However, the fatigue induced by repeated opening of the blades has led Heifetz to design a spring clip, not

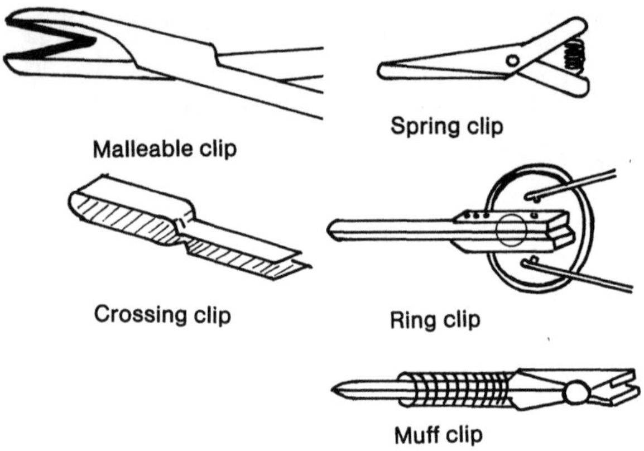

Fig. 50. Different clip mechanisms (from Fox [9])

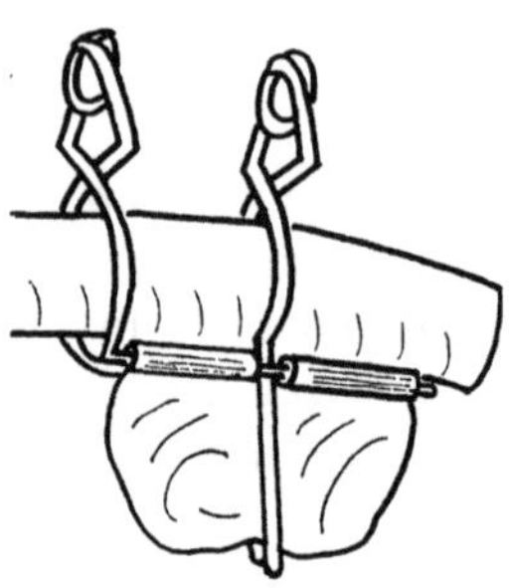

Fig. 51. Fenestrated clips: example of a clinical application (from Sugita [20, 22])

subject to fatigue [10]. Since then, other crossed-blade clips made of different metals have found their way into use (Drake, Yasargil, Sugita; Fig. 50).

When the opening angle is not wide enough, the size of the aneurysmal sac may nevertheless by reduced by the prior application of a clip with triangular blades, or else by a straight clip placed on the axis of the neck (the later crossing over, with the clip positioned onto the neck, being anticipated by covering the blades with silastic fragments (Fig. 51).

Solidity

The solidity of a clip depends on the resistance of the alloy used with respect to mechanical constraints and electrolytic corrosion by the environment, the latter being related to its chemical composition (notably its acidity and polarity); these different factors increase with time. The most commonly used alloys are as follows:

Stainless steels (iron alloyed with chromium), known as austenitic (of the series 300), show good resistance to corrosion thanks to the addition of molybdenum (steels 316, 317). But such steels are subject to carbon precipitation and thus to intergranular corrosion. In this group, steels with a low carbon content are preferred (steels of the series L, for example 316 L, 317 L).

High precipitation stainless steels, designated by "Ph" and referred to as semiaustenitic, are highly ductile and slightly less resistant to corrosion than the steels of the series 300; but they can be improved by the addition of molybdenum (as with steel Ph 15–17 Mo). The rare cases of clip rupture [3, 8, 11, 12, 15, 17] have occured in only one type of these steels, stainless steel 17–7. Ph. Metallurgic analysis [12] has led to the conclusion that its structure was too granular and had too high a content of iron, which made it very susceptible to electrolytic corrosion.

Nickel or cobalt superalloys, containing molybdenum (MP35N, Algiloy, Vitallium) have much greater solidity and resistance to corrosion, due above all to the absence of nonmetallic substances. However, the technical difficulties involved in the production of the alloys are such that the finished item is of somewhat variable quality. Thus, the blades of a straight bayonet clip of 18 mm made of Elgiloy do not close completely after an opening and closing test repeated 30 times. The same test repeated 100 times on a curved bayonet clip of 19 mm (of the same alloy) shows an alteration of the opening strength from 140 to 80 mmHg. These changes have not been observed in the other stainless steel clips tested, except for steel 301–304 [2]. In another experiment, no fatigue deformation was detected in the same clips after 1000 openings [10].

Resistance to corrosion is not as good when different parts of the clip are made of different alloys (galvanic pile formation) or if the clip does not consist of only one piece (interfaces between parts of the clip made of the same alloy lead to electrolytic stagnation and oxygen impoverishment, which favor corrosion) [2, 14]. Moreover, the solidity of the clip depends not only on its caliber but also on its design. As a matter of fact, to obtain a uniform distribution of the closing force along the length of the blade, closure must begin at the distal end of the blades and then be smoothly carried towards their proximal parts. This way, the joint strength of the clip and with the blade resistance converges towards one only point: the hinge between the clip body and the blades, which is a preferred site for rupture. This "hinge" effect is greater for spring clips, in which the arm lever is longer, than that of crossed-blade clips, where the arms and blades are opposed on either side of the opening plane at the level of the hinge.

Closing Force

The quality of clipping of giant aneurysms depends upon the closing strength of the clip, which is difficult to evaluate.

The force that can produce a 1-mm opening at the extremity of the blades can be measured by introducing the gauge of a dynamometer between the two tips and submitting them to a known force strong enough to separate them to the chosen distance [1].

The force producing the opening (from 0.3 mm to the maximal opening) can also be measured at each point along the entire length of the blade with a very fine thread attached on one side to a traction engine and on the other to a set of weighing scales (Fig. 52). The opening force is thus read in grams. It decreases from the base towards the extremity of the blades and varies in the same way as the opening angle (Fig. 53) [19].

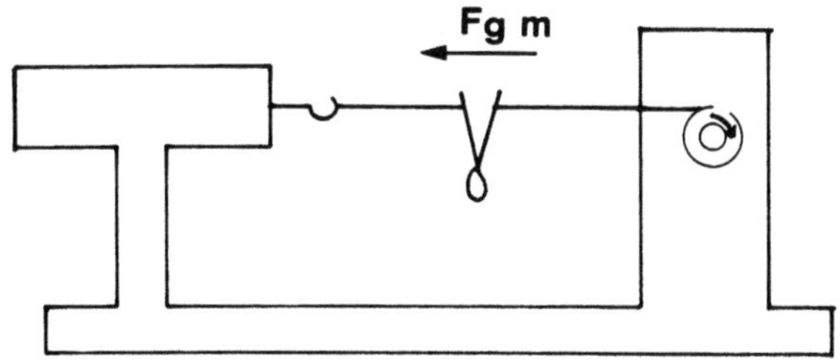

Fig. 52. Measurement of the opening force of clips (from Sugita [19])

So, in order to retain sufficient force at the distal extremity of the blades, the tension of long clips is sometimes considerable at their proximal extremity (about 800–1100 grams for Sugita clips of 30, 35, and 45 mm with a distal force of 180–200 grams).

This can be a source of lesions of the neck leading to its rupture [23].

Imperviousness

The imperviousness of a clip could until now be evaluated only with simple model in which the clip was placed perpendicularly to the parent artery [7, 16].

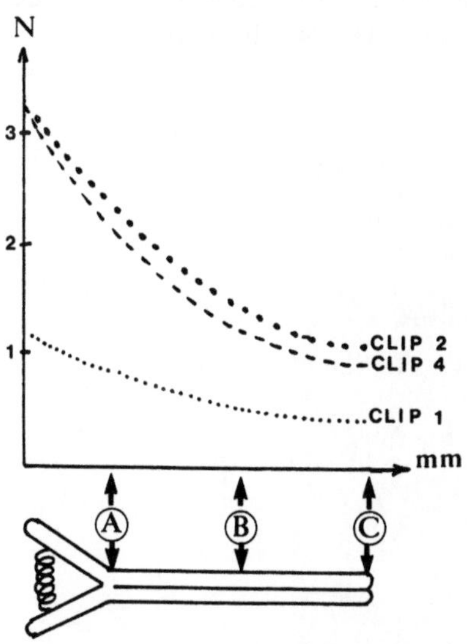

	A	B	C
	Force at the hinge (N)	Force at the mid-point of the blades (N)	Force at the end of the blades (N)
1) Straight Yasargil clip Cat. no. FD 791 code no. 577037 Length = 29 mm	1.18	0.60	0.41
2) Straight Sugita clip Cat. no. 18 Lot no. GG 10-29 Length = 25 mm	3.28	1.59	1.05
3) Curved Sugita clip Cat. no. 2 Lot no. G7–40 Length = 26 mm		0.95	
4) Straight Heifetz clip Cat. no. 659107 no. 1 C 1098 Length = 15.3 mm	3.30	1.45	0.93

Fig. 53. Closing force of four large clips. The forces applied to the two extremities and the middle of the blades of four large clips have been measured for an opening angle very close to zero. Measurement by: CETIM, 52 av. Felix Louat, 60304 Senlis, France. The comparative measurements enable one to establish that:

1. For a comparable sizes (25 and 29 mm respectively), the force measured at the two extremities and in the middle of the blades is almost three times greater for the straight Sugita clip than for the straight Yasargil clip tested.

2. The force measured in the middle of the blades is almost twice as weak for the curved Sugita clip tested as for the straight Sugita clip, despite an almost identical length (26 and 25 mm).

3. The force measured at the hinge, in the middle, and at the distal extremity of both straight Sugita and Heifetz clips is about equal, despite a difference in size (29 mm vs. 15.3 mm)

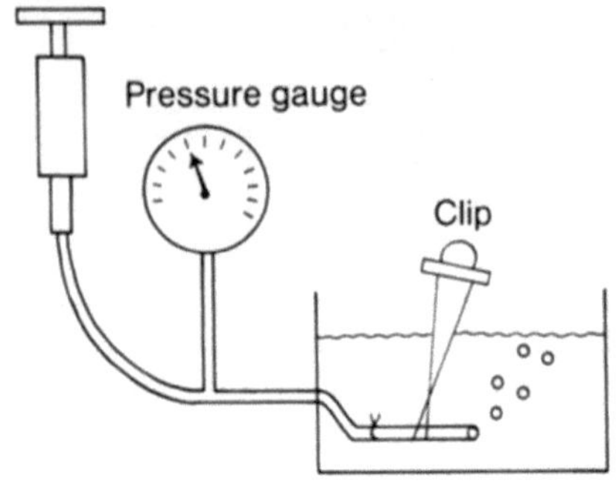

Fig. 54. Measurement of the opening pressure of clips (from Rosenbaum [16])

The pressure required to open the clip ("opening pressure") is measured by injecting air into a tube, the pressure of which is known, and which is connected to a fragment of a clipped vessel immersed in water. If air bubbles appear, the clip has opened, and the pressure read corresponds to the opening pressure of the tested clip (Fig. 54). The opening pressure can also be evaluated by Laplace's law (see pp. 12–17).

Thus, the opening pressure is low for large vessels subjected to low arterial pressure and high for small vessels with high pressure values. Exceptions observed are linked to irregularities in thickness and elasticity of the arterial wall. The opening pressure can vary considerably (±50 mmHg) if the clip is removed and then replaced at practically the same place [16].

The minimum occlusion force of an artery – a rat aorta, for example – in relation to its diameter, to the arterial pressure, and to the width of the clip blades, has been accurately measured with a variable force gauge-clamp. These studies were correlated to an electron scanning microscopy study of endothelial lesions after 1-h clamping [7]. The endothelial lesions, initially limited to an increase of the fold for the minimum occlusion force, become amplified in the form of thrombi, craters, and even, when the force of the clamp is increased, real endothelial fractures revealing the tunica media.

The intensity of the closing force definitely plays a significant role in the sliding of the clip (a case of this was reported by Drake and Allcock [4]). *The sliding force of a clip* can be studied by applying the latter to a vessel fragment linked by a very fine thread to set of scales [19]. The sliding force – that is, the force it is necessary to exert on the clip to made it slide – is very variable, depending on the arterial pressure, the caliber, and the nature of the walls of the vessel tested. It increases proportionally to the opening force of the clip. A number of solutions have been proposed to diminish the risk of sliding, such as notching the blades; crossing the blades at their distal extremity [13]; perforation of the distal extremity of the blades to allow a thread to be passed through; indentation of the aneurysmal edge of the blade to increase adherence [18], welding the distal ex-

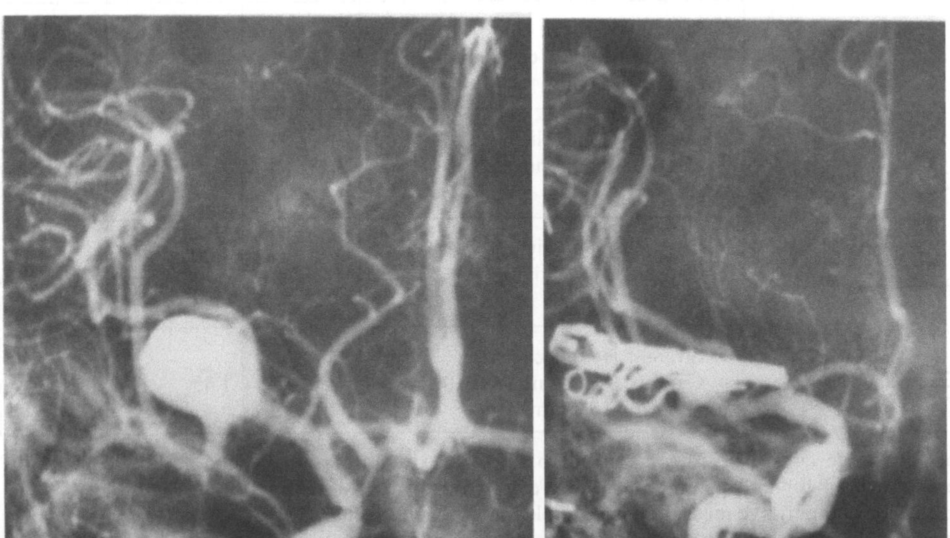

Fig. 55. Clipping of a giant right sylvian aneurysm, partly thrombosed, requiring the positioning of several kinds of clips. Two medium-sized clips are first placed to reduce the size of the aneurysmal sac. Another large clip permits exclusion of the major part of the aneurysm. To finish, a new neck is created by the positioning of a fenestrated clip

tremities once the clip is positioned; incorporation in the fenestration of a vessel which will restrain the clip [5]; or the booster clip [24].

Open Questions

The study of clip technology leaves a number of questions unanswered. Some are specific to giant aneurysms, notably how to define the optimal length and shape of the blades according to the diameter of the aneurysm neck and its orientation with respect to the parent artery, and the optimal closing force of the clip in relation to each aneurysm. Others are common to all aneurysms, especially regarding the fact that they are made of metal (causing) artifacts in follow-up CT scanning, or rotating or even slipping under the effects of MRI [6]).

Magnetic sensibility is nil in austenitic steels (Sugita, McFadden, Yasargil, and Scoville clips) and highest in martensitic steels, which form part of the composition of Heifetz clips (90%) and, to a lesser extent (35%), of Mayfield clips.

The surgeon should be familiar with these physical properties so as to be able to choose the most appropriate clip for each case under treatment (Fig. 55).

Direct Surgical Approaches According to Topographic Type

In this section, the results of the main literature series are developed under separate headings according to the different topographic varieties of aneurysm. Only aneurysms managed by a direct approach (neck occlusion by means of a clip or ligature or by intra-aneurysmorrhaphy) are discussed here.

Analyzing the literature covering giant intracranial aneurysms managed by the direct approach raises serious problems. Some publications do not distinguish giant from normal-sized aneurysms, although their illustrations clearly show aneurysms with diameters greater than 25 mm [32, 53, 61, 83, 90, 92, 108, 118, 135, 138, 139, 144].

The results obtained by direct approach with neck occlusion are set out in Tables 2, 3, 4 and 5. It must be mentioned that they do not always faithfully reflect the exact clinical events. For example, postoperative deaths related to the surgical intervention and deaths due to rebleeding are often grouped together due to lack of precise information. Furthermore, it has not always been easy to distinguish between postoperative sequelae secondary to the operation from those related to the severity of the preoperative condition. Therefore, we have only included under the heading "morbidity" patients whose condition was aggravated by the operation.

Aneurysms of the Carotid Artery

This group comprises three main varieties.

1. *Carotid-ophthalmic aneurysms,* which arise from the medial aspect of the infra- and/or juxtaclinoid part of the carotid artery, between the origin of the ophthalmic artery to the emergence of the posterior communicating artery [59, 124].

2. *Aneurysms of the posterior communicating artery* (also called carotid-posterior communicating artery aneurysms), which arise at the level of the supraclinoid carotid artery, most often on its posterior aspect, distal to the emergence of the posterior communicating artery and/or at its origin

3. *Carotid bifurcation aneurysms*

Associated with this group are *aneurysms of the cavernous sinus,* which will be considered in a special section at the end of this chapter.

Carotid-Ophthalmic Aneurysms

These aneurysms arise from the inner wall of the internal carotid artery and are thought to originate from vestigial aneurysms developed from the prechiasmatic anastomotic network described by Dawson [18]. Three subgroups may be identified:

1. *The infraoptic-chiasmatic type* is by far the most frequent (two out of three of the cases). It corresponds to the superior-median variety described by Drake. The aneurysm originates in the angle between the carotid and ophthalmic arteries, under the anterior clinoid process. The neck passes under the homolateral optic nerve and the dome of the sac frequently compresses the lower face of the chiasma and the contralateral optic nerve (Fig. 56). In the most voluminous types, the aneurysm may shift the pituitary stalk and hypothalamus backwards. It must emphasized that the exact origin of the neck is often difficult to identify on angiograms and sometimes even intraoperatively.

2. In *the supraoptic-chiasmatic type,* the neck passes above the optic nerve.

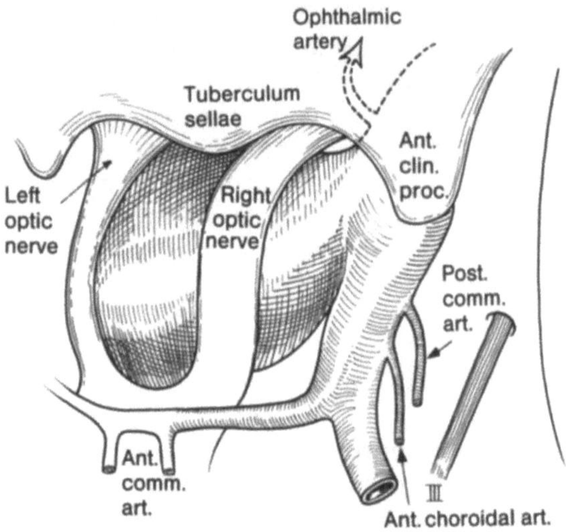

Fig. 56. The infraoptic-chiasmatic type of carotid-ophthalmic aneurysm, in which the neck passes above the optic nerve

3. In *the posterior-inferior type*, the sac adheres very closely to the cavernous sinus roof [88]. This type may be difficult to distinguish from the aneurysms which are located astride the cavernous sinus and the subarachnoid space [71, 140]. Nevertheless, these latter must be separately categorized as a specific entity for tactical surgical reasons, as pointed out by Nutik [73] who reported five cases of such aneurysms.

Carotid-ophthalmic aneurysms are the most voluminous aneurysms of the carotid system. They usually compress the optic and chiasmatic pathways; they are more frequently revealed by ophthalmologic signs (75% of the cases; [4, 82]) than by hemorrhagic complications. Although exceptional, endocrine manifestations can predominate, as in the case reported by Verbalis [129], in which the patient's panhypopituitarism regressed after clipping and excision of the malformation.

In this topographic type, bilateral mirror-like aneurysms are not infrequent [15]: 8 out of 24 cases in Drake's series [26] 5 out of 25 cases (all sizes gouped together) in Yasargil's material [140]. Bilateral carotid-ophthalmic aneurysms have also been encountered in cases of numerous multiple localizations [31].

Surgical Approach

Classically managed by carotid ligation [12], giant carotid-ophthalmic aneurysms – or at least some of them – can now be selectively clipped by a direct approach using modern microsurgical techniques.

Because of the difficulty or even impossibility of finding its proximal segment by an intracranial approach as pointed out by Sundt and Piepgras [117], it is generally safer to start the operation by exposing the internal carotid artery at the neck, in order (a) to monitor the carotid circulation if the aneurysm ruptures during dissection, and (b) to evaluate tolerance to clamping by measurements of pressure and flow, in case a trapping procedure should be necessary.

The approach recommended by most authors is the *frontotemporal pterional approach* [133, 141]. The *skin flap* must be made in such a way that it preserves the superficial temporal artery and its two branches, in case an extra-intracranial bypass becomes necessary.

Once the pterional approach has been performed, with as large a resection as possible of the small wing of the sphenoid bone up to the orbital periosteum and the outer edge of the superior orbital fissure, direct intradural exploration of the aneurysm will determine whether a *resection of the anterior clinoid process* should be done carried out (Fig. 57). Drake rarely found it necessary, but did not hesitate to carry it out when needed. By contrast, several authors, especially Sundt and Piepgras [117], believe that clinoid removal must be effected systematically, in order to free the internal aspect of the infraclinoid carotid artery and especially to expose the ophthalmic artery properly (Fig. 58). Dolenc [21] and Yasargil [140] recommend opening the optic canal and removing the anterior clinoid process for better manipulation of the optic nerve, so as to enlarge the operative field.

After exposing the carotid-ophthalmic region, the relations between the aneurysm and the surrounding vascular and nervous structures must be appraised in order to ascertain (a) the precise location of the implantation of the aneurysm, (b) the connections of its neck with the ophthalmic artery, and (c) the relationships of both the neck and the sac with the optic-chiasmatic complex as well as with the anterior choroidal and the posterior communicating arteries, which have generally been shifted laterally.

The possibilities for clipping (Fig. 59) are related not only to the softness of the neck and to the depressibility of the sac, but also to its adherence to the duramater of the tuberculum and diaphragm sellae. The relations of the aneurysm with the homolateral optic nerve as well as the ophthalmic artery (especially in the infraoptic-chiasmatic varieties) are particularly important to con-

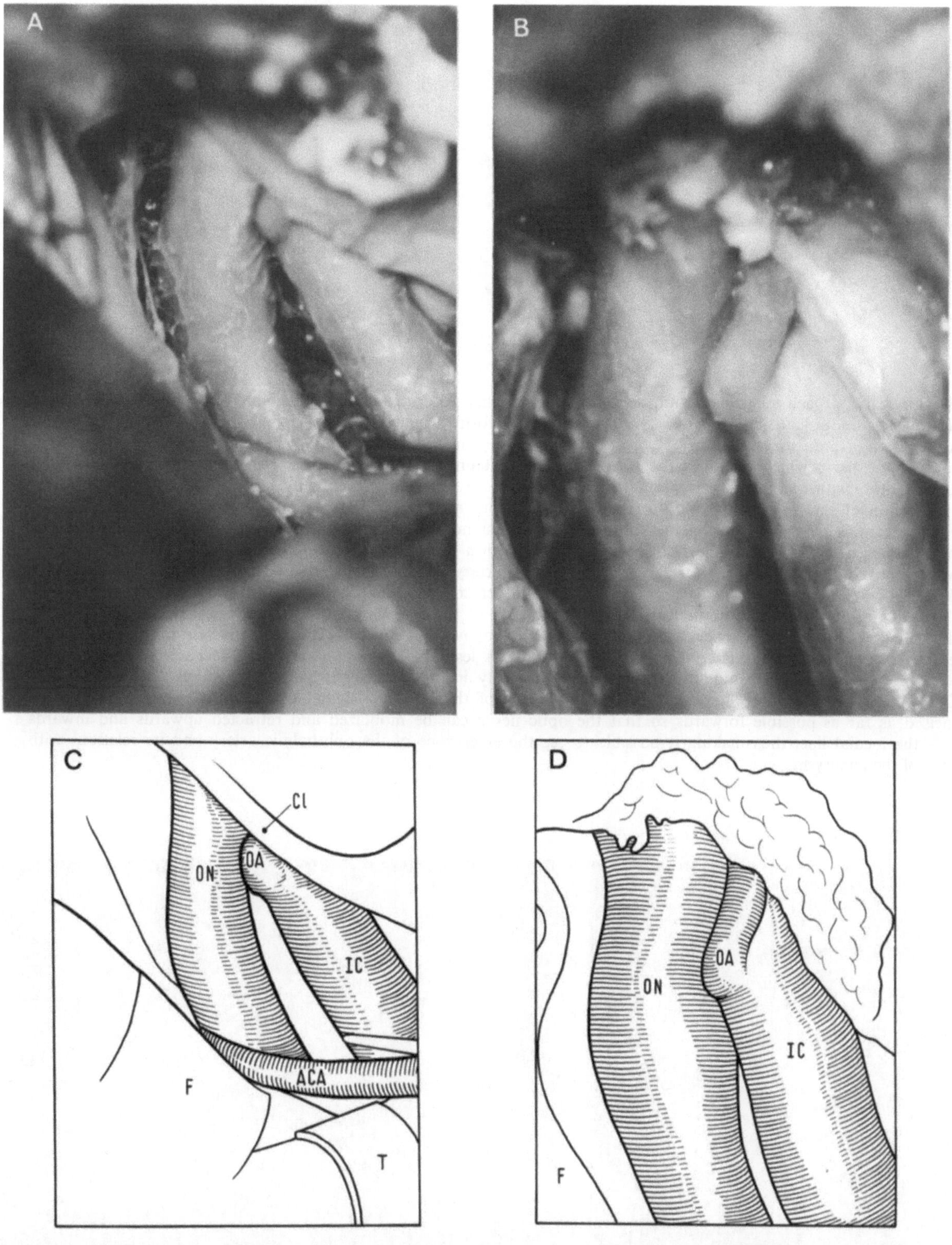

Fig. 57 A–D. Anatomical preparation of the internal aspect of the infraclinoid carotid and exposure of the ophthalmic artery (*OA*), before (**A**, **C**) and after (**B**, **D**) removal of the anterior clinoid process (*Cl*) through a right pterional approach. *IC*, supraclinoid internal carotid artery; *ACA*, anterior cerebral artery; *F*, frontal lobe; *T*, temporal lobe. (Courtesy of Dr. P. Mercier, Angers)

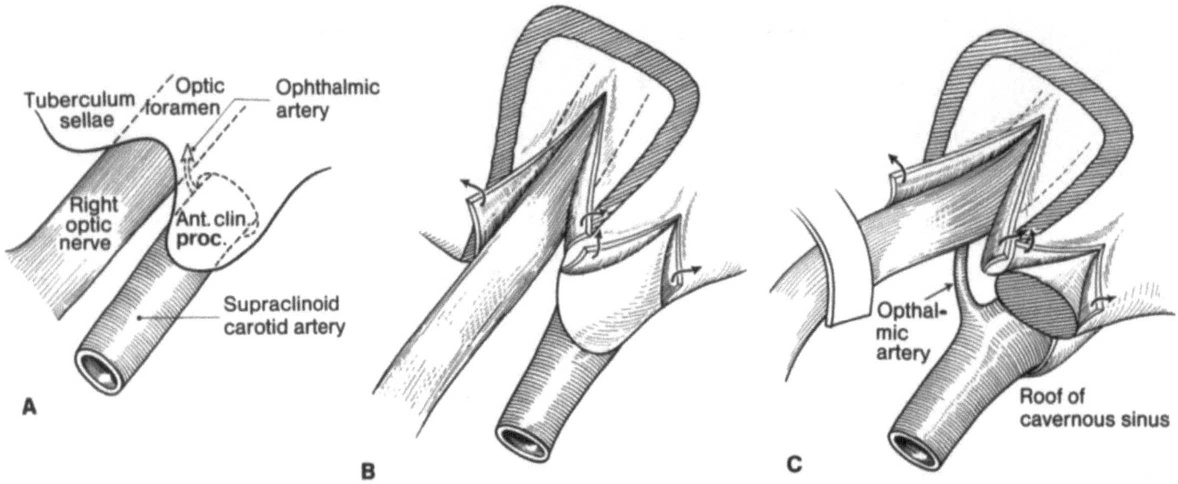

Fig. 58. Surgical approach for giant carotid-ophthalmic aneurysms. After making the classic pterional approach according to Yasargil's technique [136, 139, 140, 141], the operation is performed as described by Dolenc [21].

A *Exposure of the optic nerve: orbitotomy* 1 cm behind the edge of the orbit and resection of the roof of the orbit up to the optic nerve which preserves the periorbitary periosteum: *trephination of the roof of the optic foramen* with a diamond drill, with continuous irrigation with cold serum, in order to prevent any lesion of the nerve caused by heat. Resection of the wall of the optic foramen is carried out superiorly, medially, and laterally. When the wall of the optic groove is removed medially the sphenoid sinus must not be open. In the event of its opening, the mucosa at least must be preserved intact and the opening blocked with a thin layer of wax. When the lateral wall of the optic groove is removed, the ophthalmic artery, the internal carotid artery, and the aneurysmal wall must be carefully avoided.

B *Resection of the anterior clinoid process:* The dura mater covering the anterior clinoid is incised along its whole length (8–10 mm) and then carefully released; the central part of the anterior clinoid process is excavated and its walls are thinned down. In a like manner, the clinoid process is cut without difficulty and detached from the dura mater. Sometimes the removal of the clinoid process can provoke a lesion of the dura mater in the anterior-superior pole of the cavernous sinus. The resulting venous hemorrhage is easily arrested by plugging with Surgicel.

C *Exposure of the ophthalmic artery:* the dural sheaths of the optic nerve and of the infraclinoid carotid artery are incised as far as possible forwards so that the optic nerve can be mobilized and retracted upwards and inwards towards the medial line, thus making it possible to see the emergence of the ophthalmic artery and its relations with the neck of the aneurysm

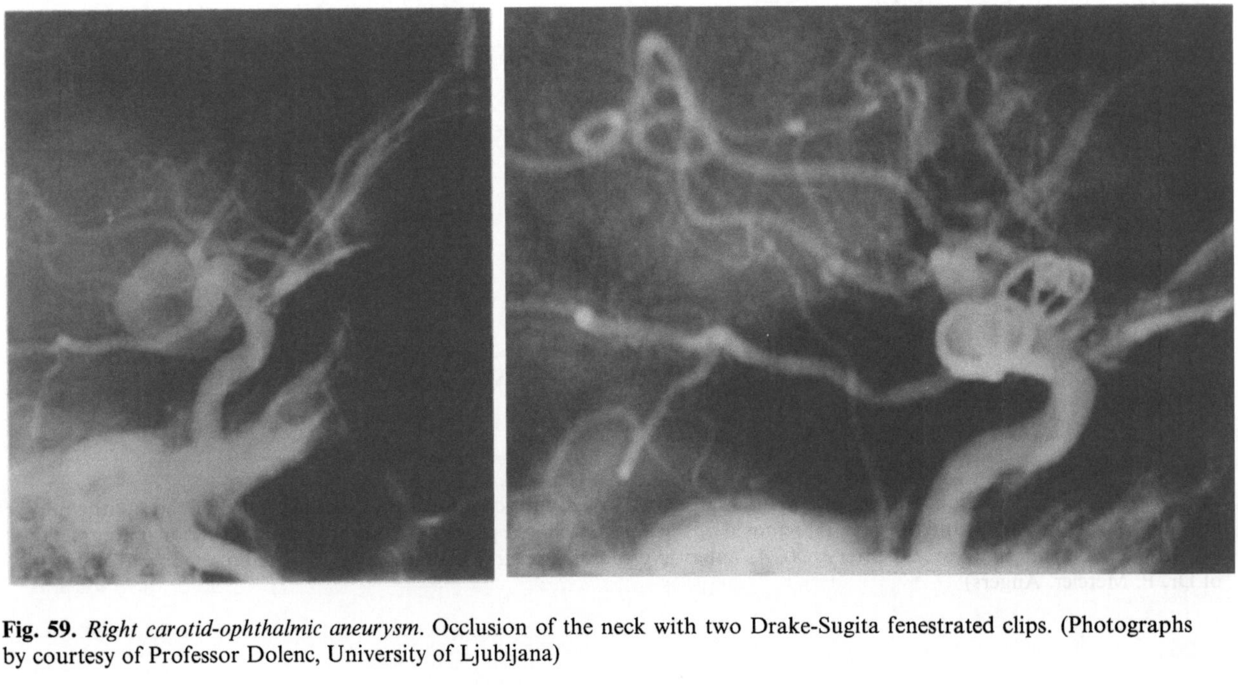

Fig. 59. *Right carotid-ophthalmic aneurysm.* Occlusion of the neck with two Drake-Sugita fenestrated clips. (Photographs by courtesy of Professor Dolenc, University of Ljubljana)

sider. In cases of complete blindness, the nerve may be sectioned if it is an obstacle to clipping; otherwise a Drake-Sugita clip may be used, its fenestration permitting the passage of the optic nerve [115]. The supraoptic-chiasmatic varieties generally cause fewer clipping problems with respect to the relations of the neck with the optic system. Paraclinoid posterior-inferior aneurysms are often impossible to clip, since their neck cannot properly be freed from the posterior-inferior aspect of the carotid artery and from the roof of the cavernous sinus. However, Samii was able to clip two such giant aneurysms with a narrow neck after opening the lateral wall of the cavernous sinus.

Bilateral carotid aneurysms can be operated upon in one procedure, using the bifrontal approach of Pool and Pottas (one case of reported by Garcia-Bengochea [36]), or the unilateral pterional approach on the side of the bleeding or on the right side in the nonhemorrhagic types (five cases reported by Yasargil [140]. Another option is to use the pterional approach in two successive operations, as reported in one case by Fox [31].

Carotid-Posterior Communicating Artery Aneurysms

In these types, the neck is attached to the posterior-inferior aspect of the carotid artery, distal to the emergence of the posterior communicating artery, on which it can also be implanted. The sac compresses the inferior aspect of the temporal lobe and, in the most voluminous types, the brainstem.

Clipping these aneurysms may prove to be hazardous because of the difficulty of identifying the neck at the posterior aspect of the carotid. In these types, two types of clips may be useful: the fenestrated, angled Drake-Sugita clip and the Sundt clip. When occlusion of the neck is impracticable, recourse may be had to occlusion of the parent artery with extra-intracranial bypass if necessary.

Aneurysms of the Carotid Bifurcation

As they develop within the basal ganglia and their neck is surrounded by the anterior perforators, giant aneurysms of the carotid bifurcation are extremely difficult to clip (Fig. 60).

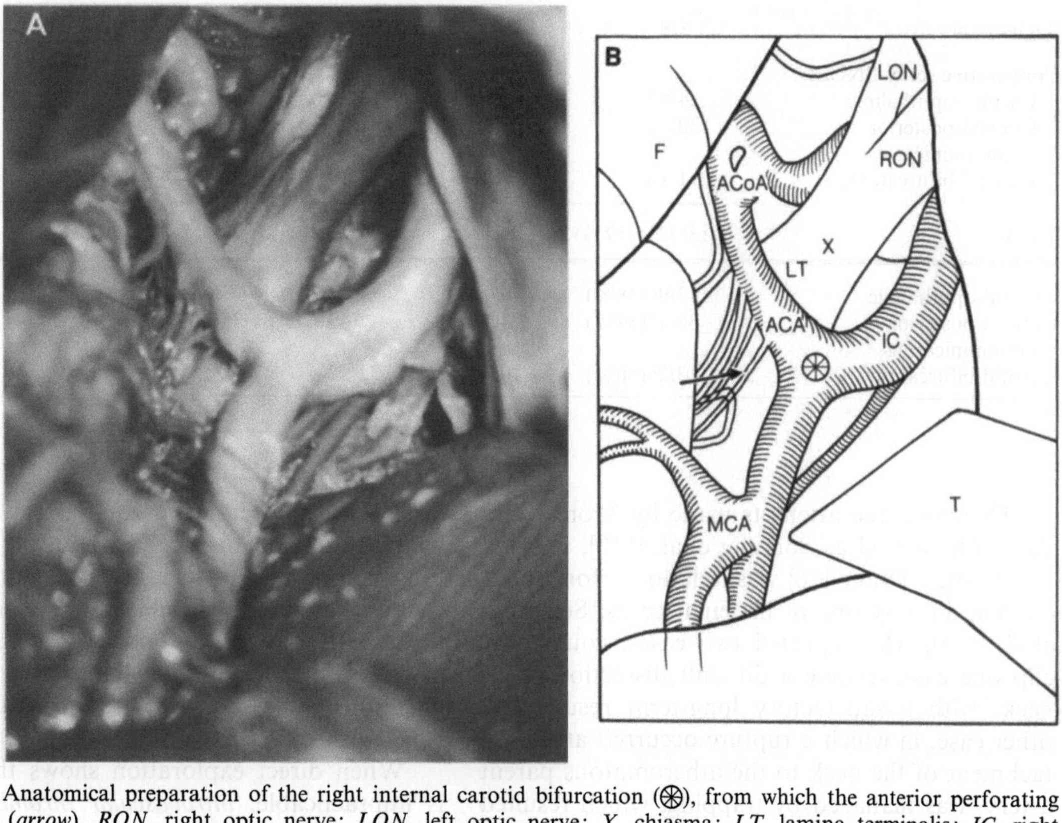

Fig. 60 A, B. Anatomical preparation of the right internal carotid bifurcation (⊛), from which the anterior perforating arteries arise (*arrow*). *RON*, right optic nerve; *LON*, left optic nerve; *X*, chiasma; *LT*, lamina terminalis; *IC*, right supraclinoid artery; *ACA*, right anterior cerebral artery; *MCA*, right middle cerebral artery; *ACoA*, fenestrated anterior communication artery; *T*, retractor on the right temporal lobe; *F*, retractor on the right frontal lobe. (Courtesy of Dr. P. Mercier, Angers)

Table 2. Results in giant carotid intracranial aneurysms managed by neck occlusion. (The cases summarized at the bottom of the table are only those for which a precise localization could be obtained)

	No. operated/ total no.	Mortality	Morbidity	Good results or identical to preop. condition	Remarks
Garcia-Bengochea and Delande	1/1			1	Mirror bilateral type
Sonntag et al.					
Carotid bifurcation	1/2	1			
Drake					
Carotid-ophthalmic	16/24	2	3 Unilateral blindness	11	
Carotid-posterior communicating	6/7	1		5	
Carotid bifurcation	1/8			1	
Fox	1/1		1 Transient amaurosis		4 Multiple bilateral type of aneurysms of which 3 were giant carotid artery aneurysms
Hosobuchi					
Carotid-ophthalmic	3/19	1		2	
Onuma and Suzuki	8/15	3	1	4	
Sundt and Piepgras	28/51	1	3	24	
Sugita et al.	8/8			8	
Cooperative series SNCLF					
Carotid-ophthalmic	24/47	3(12.5%)	6(25%)	15(62.5%)	
Carotid-posterior communicating	30/36	3(10%)	7(23%)	20(70%)	
Carotid bifurcation	11/16	9(80%)	1(10%)	1(10%)	
Total	138/235(59%)	24(17%)	22(16%)	92(67%)	
Carotid-ophthalmic	43/90(48%)	6(14%)	9(21%)	28(65%)	
Carotid-posterior communicating	36/43(84%)	4(11%)	7(19%)	25(70%)	
Carotid bifurcation	13/26(50%)	10(77%)	1(7%)	2(16%)	

Therefore, the attempts made by Morley and Barr [70], as well as Sonntag et al. [110], resulted in fatalities. Drake [26] was able to perform neck clipping in only one of his eight cases. Sengupta et al. [106], who reported two cases, could only clip one case, despite a difficult dissection of its neck, with a satisfactory long-term result. The other case, in which a rupture occurred at the attachment of the neck to the atheromatous parent artery, was managed by trapping, which resulted in a secondary hemiplegia and dysphasia.

These surgical difficulties explain why a majority of authors prefer *proximal occlusion*, either at the level of the cervical carotid artery or intracranially. Although ligation at the neck has proved to give good results, its efficacy remains uncertain because of the possibility of revascularization through the anterior and posterior communicating arteries. Furthermore, it is liable to ischemic complications, unless prior extra-intracranial bypass is performed.

When direct exploration shows that clipping is impracticable, *intravascular thrombosis* of the sac may be attempted, as reported by Hosobuchi in one case. In the presence of thrombosed and compressive aneurysms, thrombectomy may be

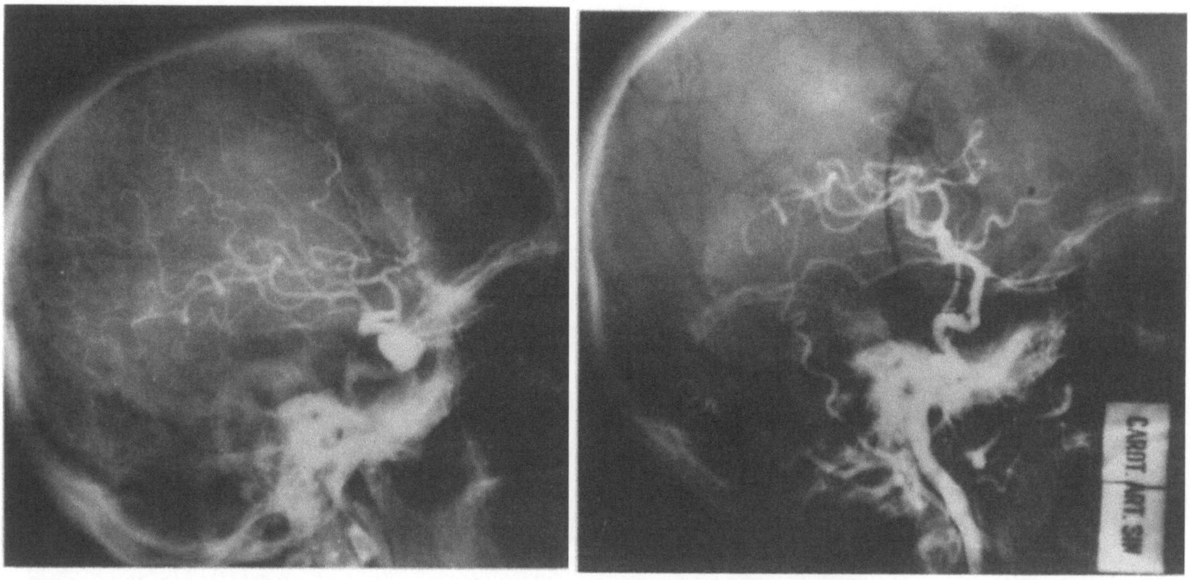

Fig. 61. Partly thrombosed right intracavernous giant aneurysm. Management by the direct approach: resection-suture (*arrow*). (Photographs by courtesy of Professor Dolenc, University of Ljubljana)

carried out with coating of the neck, as performed by Maxwell and Chou [67] in one case of an aneurysm with a diameter of 7.5 cm.

Results

There is a spate of publications devoted to carotid aneurysms, but many of them do not specifically focus on giant aneurysms [3, 9, 39, 44, 67, 69, 72, 75, 107]. The results relating to giant aneurysms strictu-sensu are shown in Table 2. This study, which covers 138 cases operated on by selective neck occlusion, shows that global mortality rose to 17% and morbidity to 16%. The best results were obtained in aneurysms of the posterior communicating artery (70%) and of the carotid-ophthalmic region (65%). By contrast, mortality turned out to be extremely high in the locations at the carotid bifurcation (77%), which is indicative of their great surgical difficulty.

Intracavernous Aneurysms

Giant aneurysms of the cavernous sinus, classically considered to be of atherosclerotic origin, actually most often stem from common saccular aneurysms.

According to Barr et al. [7], they develop at the level of the fork from which one of the three branches of the intracavernous carotid artery emerges. The hypothesis of their malformative origin is supported by observations of bilateral aneurysms [19, 29, 105, 131], especially in young subjects [56], or in association with disorders of the elastic tissue such as Marfan's syndrome [66] or Ehlers-Danlos syndrome [102]. A bacterial infectious etiology was advocated to explain the formation of giant aneurysms in two cases developing after cavernous thrombo-phlebitis [97].

These cavernous aneurysms, whatever their etiology may be, develop in the orbitary apex, towards the suprasellar region or in the sella turcica. They may be responsible for hypothalamic-pituitary insufficiency, simulating a pituitary tumor [130].

Some authors question the justification for surgical intervention on these aneurysms, since many untreated patients can have a long survival period after the onset of clinical signs [7, 55, 68, 70], moreover, oculomotor disorders do not always completely regress after occlusion of the carotid axis. The essential argument in favor of an operation is the presence of unbearable pain which, unlike oculomotor palsies, most often disappears after surgical treatment.

By far the most common treatment is *occlusion of the parent artery*, whether or not preceded by an extra-intracranial bypass. When occlusion does not suppress the compressive symptoms, a direct approach of the aneurysm inside the cavernous sinus can be carried out secondarily, as in the case of Nakahara et al. [71].

Recent advances aiming at preserving the patency of the carotid artery have been achieved for

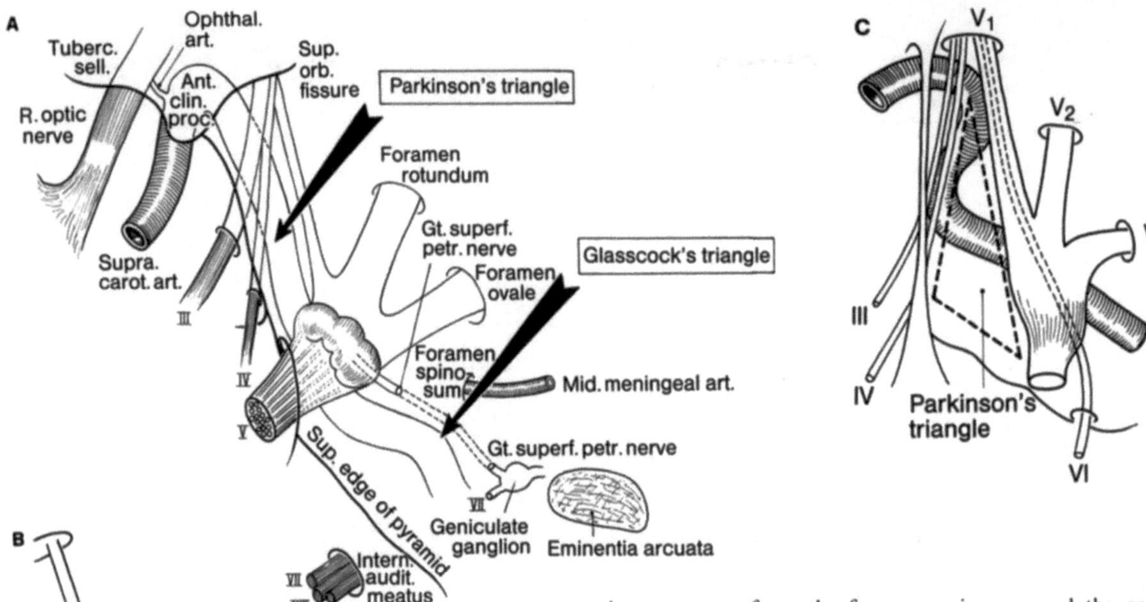

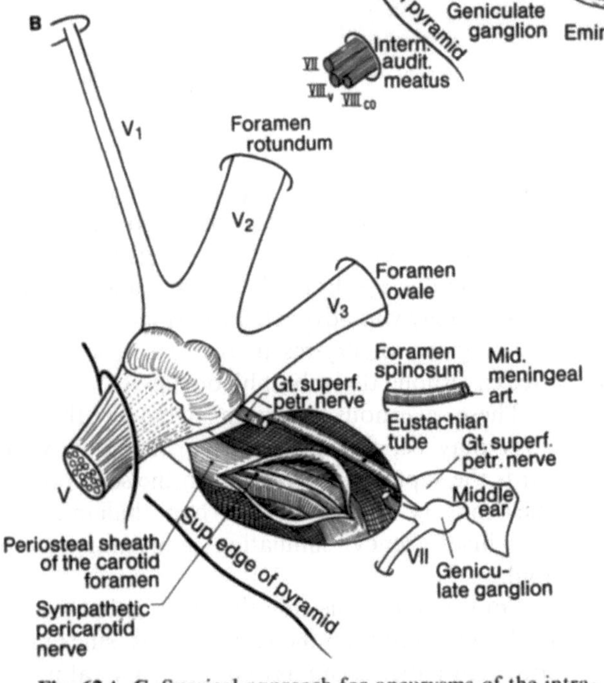

Fig. 62 A–C. Surgical approach for aneurysms of the intracavernous carotid (according to Dolenc). The direct approach of intracavernous aneurysms proposed by Dolenc [21] requires a posteriorly enlarged approach in order to gain access to the temporal fossa and the lateral wall of the cavernous sinus. The management of these aneurysms calls not only for an enlarged approach of the cavernous sinus but also for a check of the proximal and distal segments of the intracavernous carotid artery in the event of temporary or definite trapping being obligatory.

The first part of the operation consists in exposing the infraclinoid carotid artery as has been described for carotid-ophthalmic aneurysms in such a way that all the veins draining into the sphenoparietal sinus are sacrificed.

The second part consists in exposing the intrapetrous carotid artery behind the posterior-inferior pole of the cavernous sinus, at the level of the Glasscock zone [37] (**A**). To do this, the dura mater is released from the middle cerebral fossa and the pyramid up to the outer edge of the cavernous sinus. The middle meningeal artery is ligated at its emergence from the foramen spinosum and the great superficial petrosal nerve is then interrupted to avoid lesions of the geniculate ganglion by traction of the latter; this could lead to a deficit of the facial nerve. The intrapetrous carotid is approached according to the technique proposed by Glasscock [37] (**B**) perpendicularly to the great superficial petrosal nerve, between the foramen spinosum anteriorly and the eminentia arcuata posteriorly. The roof of the horizontal portion of the carotid foramen is resected with the diamond drill up to the periosteum sheathing the artery. This trephination generally leads to an opening of the bony canal of the eustachian tube located laterally from the carotid foramen. Care must be taken to avoid the periosteum of the eustachian tube. The bony canal is closed with a wax plug or muscle in order to prevent the development of a cerebrospinal fistula. After removing the roof of the carotid foramen, resection of the bone surrounding the vessel is continued until a large enough part of the intrapetrous carotid artery is exposed to allow the positioning of a temporary clip, thereby completely interrupting the flow of blood in the carotid artery.

The third part consists in opening the cavernous sinus. The dural incision is made from back to front, at the upper part of the triangle described by Parkinson [76, 77] along the trochlear and oculomotor nerves up to the superior orbital fissure forwards (**A** and **C**). The oculomotor nerve is exposed first, then the trochlear nerve, followed by the ophthalmic nerve, the maxillary, and the mandibular nerves [21]. These nerves can be exposed without opening the cavernous sinus proper, as they are all (except the abducens nerve) located between the two dural sheaths of the lateral wall of the cavernous sinus [42, 81, 96, 127]. All these nerves having been located, the intracavernous carotid artery and the neck of the aneurysm are exposed, and the possibility of clipping is evaluated. If the aneurysm has been accidentally ruptured, a temporary clamp can be made thanks to the prior exposure of the segments proximal and distal to the intracavernous carotid artery.

If the aneurysm is located in the *anterior third of the cavernous sinus*, it is not necessary to expose all the branches of the trigeminal nerve. It is sufficient to uncover nerves III and IV and the first segment of V. With temporary clamping, the blood or the thrombus is drained off from the management of these malformations. Among them, one must mention: endovascular occlusion of the neck by means of *detachable balloons*, direct wire *intrasaccular thrombosis*, and the possibilities of *direct closure of the neck through an intracavernous approach*, introduced by Parkinson (Fig. 62) [76, 77], either during extracorporeal circulation [56] or after temporary clamping of the intracavernous carotid artery, as performed by Dolenc [21, 22] in one case treated by resection of the aneurysm and reconstruction of the internal carotid artery by suture (Fig. 61), and by Fukushima (personal communication) in one case treated by excision of the aneurysm and the parent artery and reconstruction of the intracavernous carotid artery with an interposed saphenous venous graft anastomosed between the intrapetrous carotid artery at the Glasscock triangle and the supraclinoid portion of the carotid.

Aneurysms of the Middle Cerebral Artery

Description

Sylvian aneurysms generally attain a considerable size (up to 12 cm, as in the case of Pianetti et al. [93]), notably on account of the absence of an osteodural structure hindering their development. *Sylvian aneurysms are more frequently thrombosed*

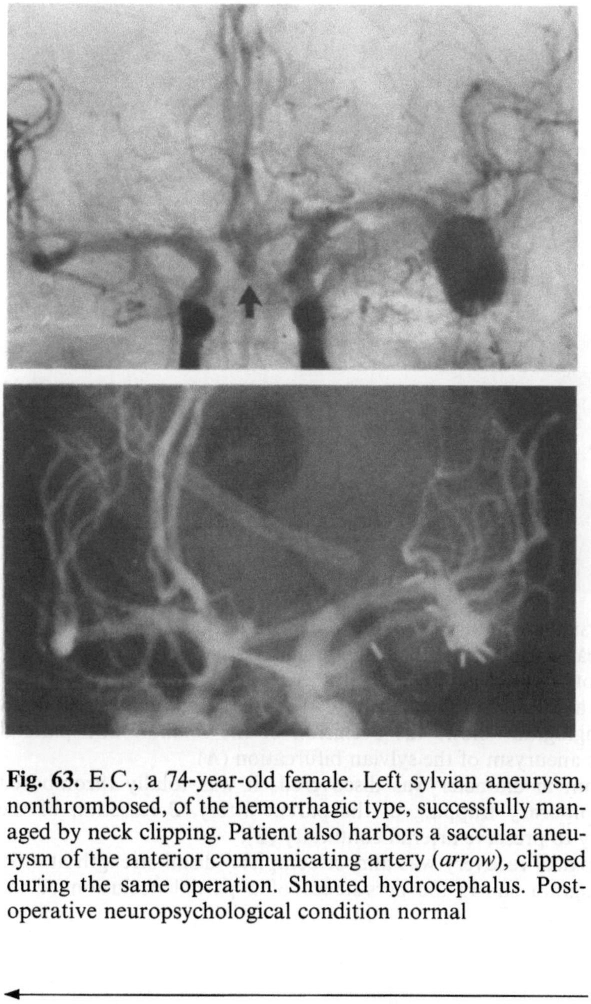

Fig. 63. E.C., a 74-year-old female. Left sylvian aneurysm, nonthrombosed, of the hemorrhagic type, successfully managed by neck clipping. Patient also harbors a saccular aneurysm of the anterior communicating artery (*arrow*), clipped during the same operation. Shunted hydrocephalus. Postoperative neuropsychological condition normal

the aneurysm, then occlusion of the neck is performed with a clip, or resection of the malformation and suture of the vascular wall is carried out.

When the aneurysm is located in the *posterior part* of the cavernous sinus, all branches of the trigeminal nerve and nerves III and IV must be carefully exposed.

Nerve VI, located deeper in contact with the intracavernous carotid artery, is then exposed in order to be preserved. The aneurysm is then managed either be neck clipping or by sac resection with suture of the arterial wall.

Venous hemostasis is often difficult, but is generally controlled in a satisfactory way by filling up the sinus with Surgicel.

When possible, the dural wall of the cavernous sinus is closed with separate stitches

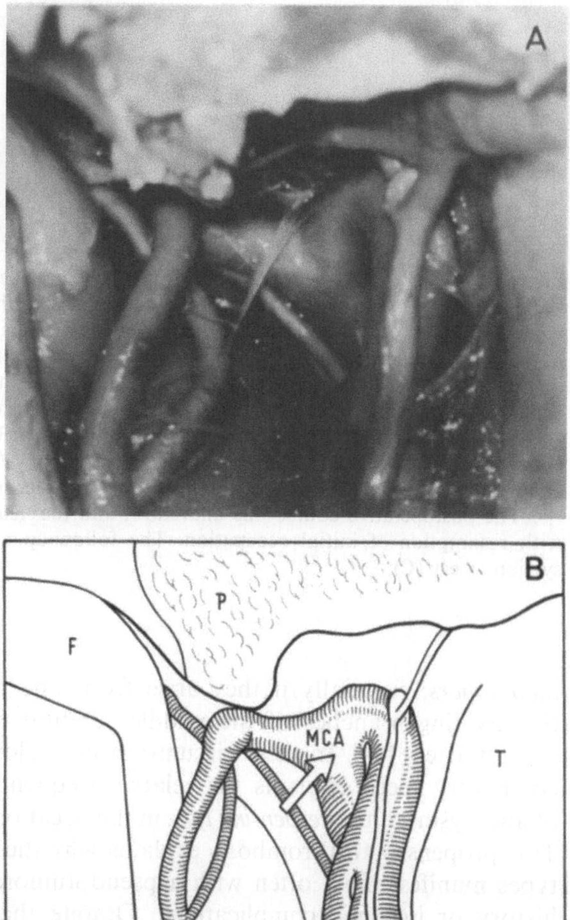

Fig. 64 A, B. Anatomical preparation of the middle cerebral bifurcation (*arrow*), through a right pterional approach. *P*, pterion; *T*, temporal lobe; *F*, frontal lobe. (Courtesy of Dr. P. Mercier, Angers)

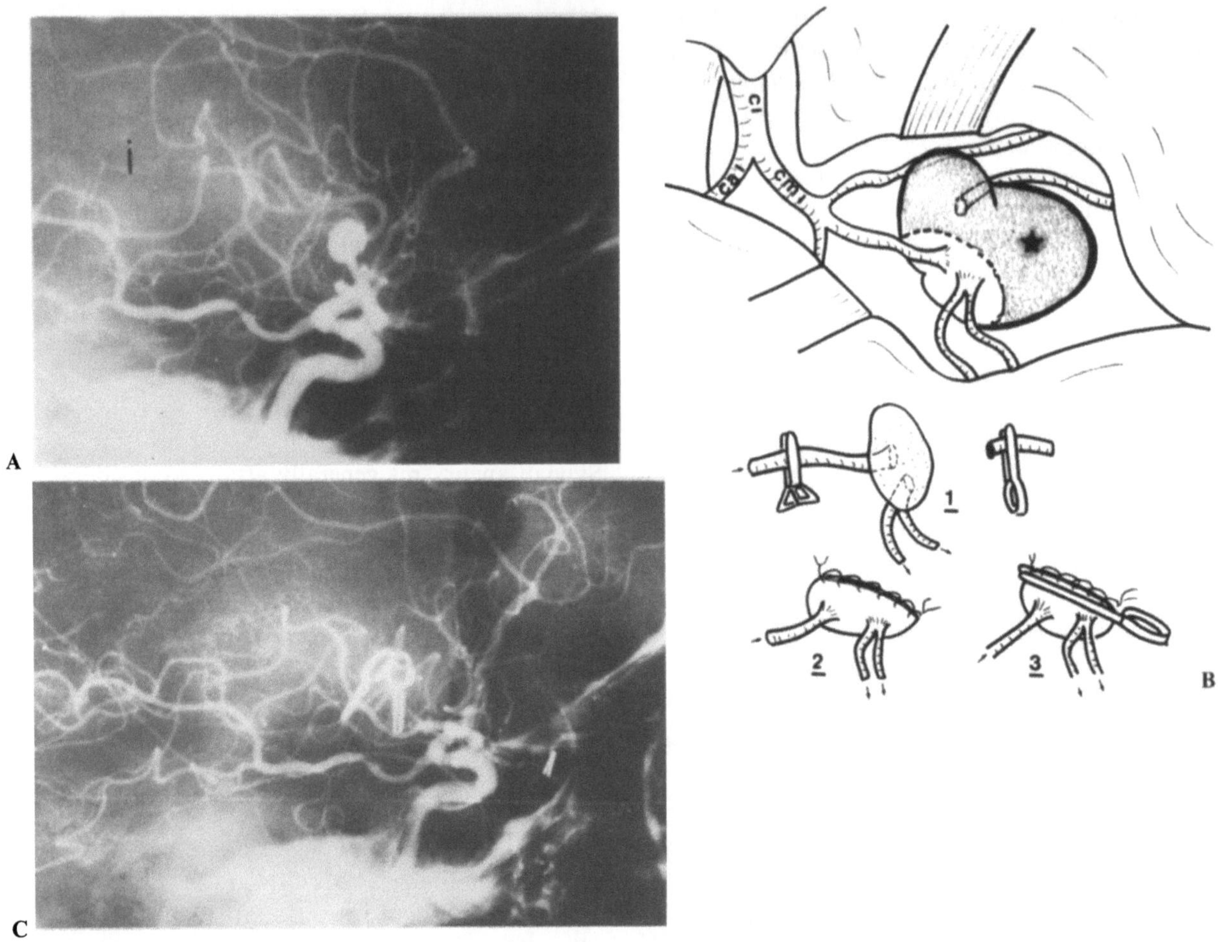

Fig. 65 A–C. J.R., a 51-year-old male. Right sylvian aneurysm, thrombosed, of the pseudotumoral and ischemic type. Patient had a 20-year history of seizures. Acute onset with headaches and left hemispheric deficit syndrome, incompletely regressive. The CT scan showed a heterogeneous image, not well-defined, slightly hyperdense, and weakly reinforced by contrast enhancement in the temporal region, suggesting a glioma: a hypodensity of the *ischemic* type was apparent in the posterior part of the right hemisphere. The right angiogram shows the occlusion of the rolandic and parietal branches of the middle cerebral artery (*i*) and a small saccular aneurysm of the sylvian bifurcation (**A**).

At surgical exploration a voluminous aneurysm ×30 mm in diameter was discovered; it was totally thrombosed (*star*) except at its neck. The operation consisted of: *1* temporary trapping of the parent artery, *2* resection of the aneurysmal mass, and *3 endoaneurysmorrhaphy*, in order to try to preserve arterial continuity (**B**).

The postoperative course was uneventful and the neurological recovery was almost complete (distal strength at 4/5), with resumption of initial occupation. The follow-up angiogram shows the persistence of a partial occlusion of the sylvian artery (**C**)

than others, especially if they arise from one of the dividing branches of the middle cerebral or sylvian artery [34]. In these circumstances, a slow circulatory speed explains the relative frequency of aneurysms of the *serpentine type* in this location. This propensity to thrombosis explains why these types manifest most often with a pseudotumoral history or ischemic complications. Despite their low rate of spontaneous hemorrhagic complications, these serpentine forms must be operated upon because of their tendency to progressively expand, as demonstrated in various publications in which the cases were followed up with repeated angiography and/or CT [5, 80, 125].

Surgical Techniques

As their sac is most often fairly easy to dissect from the adjacent parenchyma and their neck is usually relatively thin, giant aneurysms of the middle cerebral artery are particularly suitable for *management by a direct approach* (Fig. 63) through the pterional approach (Fig. 64). This statement

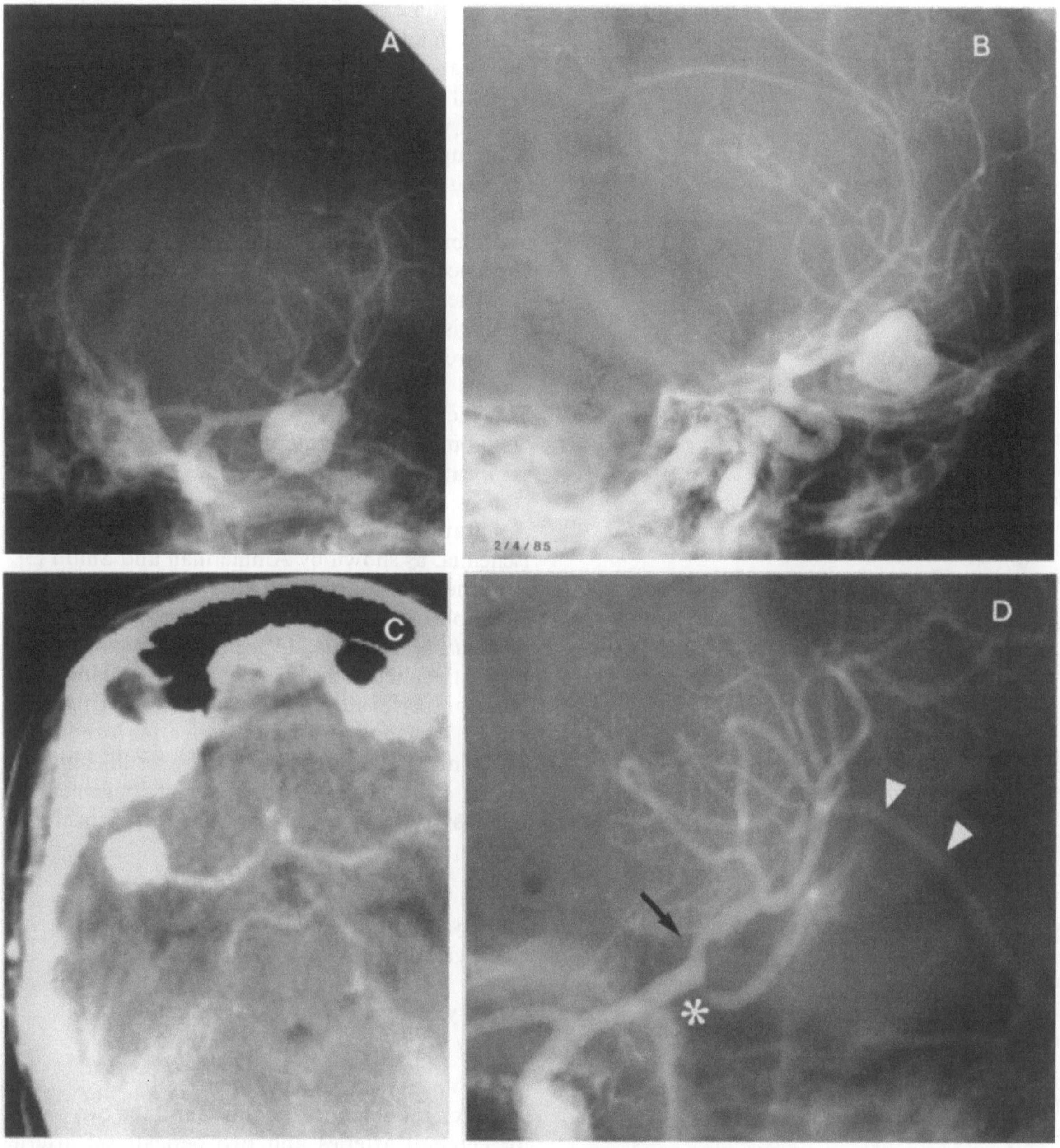

Fig. 66 A–D. Endoaneurysmorrhaphy in an aneurysm of the middle cerebral artery.

After a history of subarachnoid hemorrhage, the CT scan and angiography confirmed the presence of an aneurysm at the bifurcation of the middle cerebral artery (**A–C**). The patient underwent excision of the aneurysm and aneurysmorrhaphy (**D**, *arrow*). At the time of surgery, a stenosis of the inferior branch of the MCA was noted (*star*); for this reason, a superficial temporal-middle cerebral artery anastomosis to this particular branch was performed (*arrowheads*). The postoperative angiogram shows complete reconstitution of flow through the aneurysmorrhaphy and anastomosis (**D**). (Photographs by courtesy of Professor F. Diaz, Henry Ford Hospital, University of Michigan)

must, however, be tempered by the fact that the afferent and efferent parent arteries often enter or leave the sac direct, or at least are closely joined to it.

Clipping or ligation of the aneurysm can easily be carried out if the neck is narrow, or after shrinking it if it is wide, provided that tributaries of the parent artery are not attached to it. *Endoaneurysmorrhaphy* (Fig. 65) or its variant, consisting of resection-reconstruction of the sylvian bifurcation [22], is equally satisfactory. When one of the branches of the middle cerebral artery remains

Table 3. Results in sylvian aneurysms managed by direct approach

	No. of cases	Mortality	Morbidity	Good results or identical to preoperative condition
Neck occlusion				
Sato and Kamitani	1			1
Howe et al.	1	1		
Sonntag et al.	1	1		
Drake	5		2	3
Hosobuchi	1			1
Onuma and Suzuki	3	1	1	1
Sundt and Piepgras	10	1	1	8
Cooperative series SNCLF	37	9	8	20
Subtotal:	59	13(22%)	12(20%)	34(58%)
Endo-aneurysmorrhaphy				
Santini and Gouaze	2			2
Drake	1		1	
Hosobuchi	1			1
Pasqualin et al.	1			1
Dolenc	3			3
Cooperative series SNCLF	8	1	2	5
Subtotal:	16	1(6%)	3(18%)	12(76%)
Serpentine types managed by trapping-excision				
Terao and Muraoka	1	1 intraoperative hemorrhage		
Cambria et al.	1			1
Ammerman and Smith	1			1
Segal and McLaurin	2			2
Steimle et al.	1			1
Tomasello et al.	1			1
Subtotal:	7	1		6
Total:	82	15(18%)	15(18%)	52(64%)

stenotic, an extra-intracranial bypass can be performed in addition at the distal level of this particular branch, as illustrated in Fig. 66. The quality of results is linked both to the condition of the arterial wall tissues and to tolerance of temporary clamping. The more distal the clamping to the perforating branches of the sylvian trunk, and the shorter the clamping period – less than 10 min under barbiturate protection [99] – the higher the tolerance.

When the aneurysm has no identifiable neck and arises from a branch of the sylvian artery, the parent artery cannot be preserved and the lesion is generally managed by *trapping-excision*. This method, used in seven cases in the literature, was completely tolerated in six because of the distal location of these aneurysms. In these circumstances, an extra-intracranial bypass prior to direct exploration can reduce still further the risks of ischemia, as shown by Ammerman and Smith [5].

When the aneurysm does not appear to be clippable or removable, it can be treated by a *tourniquet inserted on the M1 segment*, as near as possible to the aneurysm, in order not to endanger the anterior perforators. This solution was used by Drake in 4 out of 15 cases after performing an extra-intracranial bypass in 3. The results reported in the literature concerning the management of giant sylvian aneurysms by direct approach are shown in Table 3.

Aneurysms of the Anterior Communicating and Pericallosal Arteries

Aneurysms of the Anterior Communicating Artery

These aneurysms are characterized by the fact that the neck is often poorly defined and the two anterior cerebral arteries and two pericallosal arteries most often arise directly from the sac, as do also some of their perforating branches, especially the hypothalamic ones. For these anatomical reasons, clipping these aneurysms may be difficult. The application of the clip can be facilitated by collapsing the sac with a needle puncture [33], shrinking it by coagulation, or, when it is thrombosed [123], by prior thrombectomy. Parkinson mentions the possibility of airgun retraction [78].

Most anterior communicating aneurysms are managed using the pterional approach through a frontotemporal craniotomy. Drilling the orbital roof can offer additional space in which to handle the instruments. However, this approach cannot

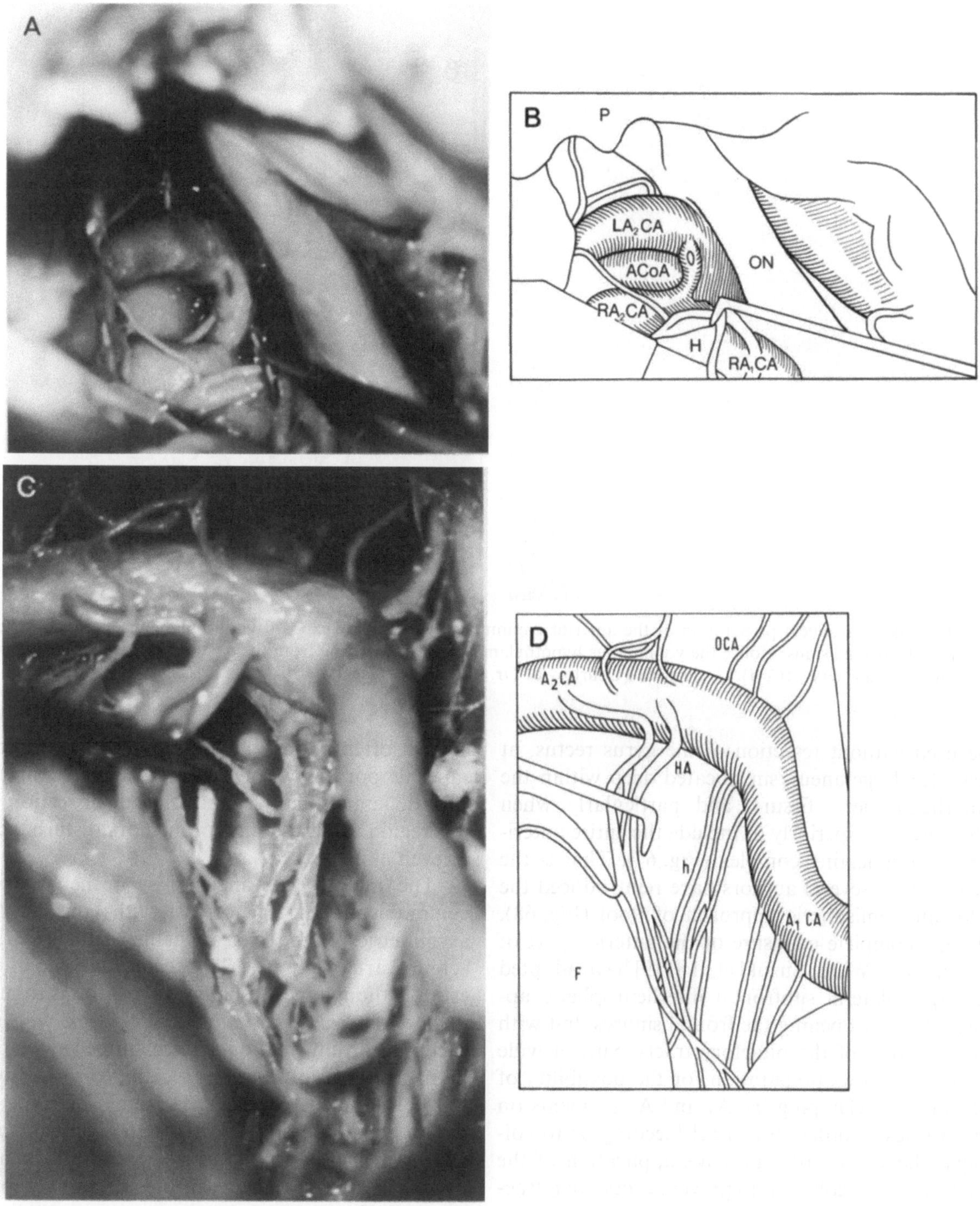

Fig. 67 A–D. Anatomical preparation of the anterior communicating artery through a right pterional approach. **A, B** Anterior communicating complex (*ACoA*) exposed after resection of the right gyrus rectus. LA_2CA, left A_2 cerebral artery; RA_2CA, right A_2 cerebral artery; RA_1CA, right A_1 cerebral artery; *H*, right Heubner artery retracted with the hook; *ON*, right optic nerve. **C, D** right aspect of the anterior communicating complex, exposed after resection of the right gyrus rectus. A_1CA, right A_1 cerebral artery; A_2CA, right A_2 cerebral artery; *HA*, Heubner artery retracted by a hook. Notice the hypothalamic arteries (*h*) arising posteriorly from the anterior communicating artery. *OCA*, optic-chiasmatic artery arising anteriorly from the anterior communicating artery. *F*, retractor on the right frontal lobe. (Courtesy of Dr. P. Mercier, Angers)

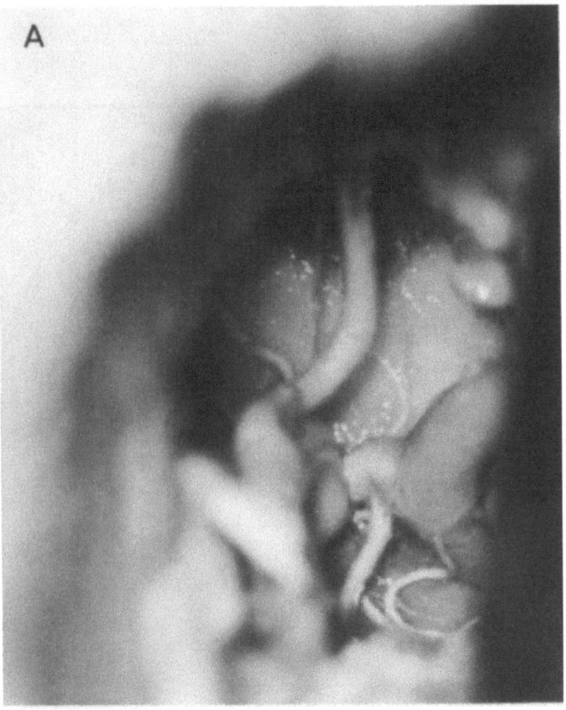

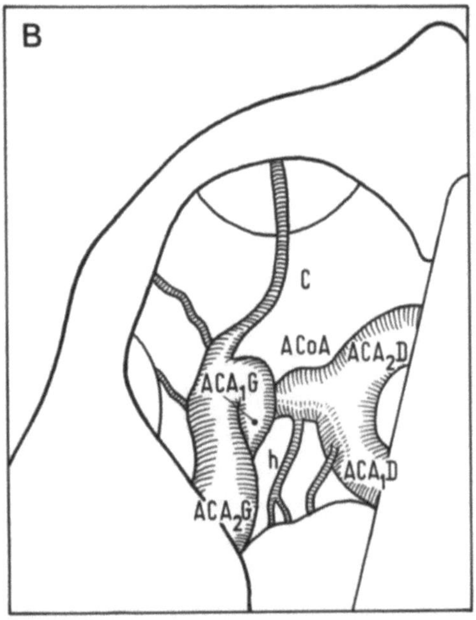

Fig. 68 A, B. Anatomical preparation of the anterior communicating complex exposed via a interhemispheric approach, through the frontal sinus. Notice the voluminous hypothalamic artery (*h*), arising from the posterior aspect of the anterior communicating artery (*ACoA*). *C*, chiasma. (Courtesy of Dr. P. Mercier, Angers)

be used without resection of the gyrus rectus, at least for large aneurysms located deep within the interhemispheric fissure, and particularly when they project superiorly or include the entire anterior communicating complex (Fig. 67). That is the reason why several authors have reintroduced the old interhemispheric approach of Pool (Fig. 68). To get complete exposure of the anterior part of the circle of Willis, Suzuki et al. [119] have adopted a large bilateral subfrontal interhemispheric approach, after opening the frontal sinuses, but with preservation of the olfactory tracts. Such a wide exposure allows preparation for the possibility of temporarily clamping the A_1 and A_2 segments on both sides in order to control bleeding or to collapse the sac in order to make application of the cup easier. By contrast, to prevent excessive retraction of the frontal lobes and dangerous manipulation of the anterior cerebral arteries, Ito [50, 51], Fukushima, Watanabe and Yeh and Tew [142] prefer a trephination craniotomy performed just above the frontal sinuses, through a small transverse linear skin incision in a wrinkle of the lower forehead.

Results are given in Table 4. Giant aneurysms of the anterior communicating artery are unsuitable for wrapping as complete exposure of the sac is most often impossible, notably in its posterior-superior portion when this is invaginated in the hypothalamic-septal region. Indeed, dissection of this region can lead to major memory disturbances or even akinetic mutism.

The majority of aneurysms of the anterior communicating artery coexist with considerable asymmetries of the first segments of the anterior cerebral artery [13, 62, 128]. Accordingly, an interesting although merely palliative method is to produce *occlusion of the dominant A_1 segment* with a clip according to Logue's technique or, better, by means of a tourniquet, in order to slow down the development of the aneurysm. This type of method could be more widely used – even bilaterally – when performing a prior extra-intracranial bypass in a cortical artery of the anterior cerebral system [49].

Recent microvascular techniques may be of help in some complicated cases. Thus, Yasargil [137] has carried out a *complete resection of the sac with reconstruction* of the anterior communicating artery by suturing its attachment site. Furthermore, although this is beyond the scope of aneurysm surgery, it is interesting to mention that in two cases of occlusion of the anterior cerebral artery on one side, Ito performed a terminolateral

Table 4. Aneurysms of the anterior communicating and pericallosal arteries managed by neck occlusion

	No. of cases	Mortality	Morbidity	Good results or identical to preoperative condition
Anterior communicating artery aneurysms				
Ito et al.	1			1
Maxwell and Chou	2			2
Drake	2	1		1
Hosobuchi	1			1
Onuma and Suzuki	10	1	2	7
Sundt and Piepgras	2		2	
Sato et al.	1			1
Cooperative series SNCLF	19	8	3	8
Total	38	10(26%)	7(19%)	21(55%)
Pericallosal artery aneurysms				
Drake, Pia et al., O'Neill et al., Pozzati et al., Smith and Parent	5	1	1	3

reimplantation of segment A_2 on the occluded side into segments A_2 and A_3 on the patent side [52].

Aneurysms of the Pericallosal Artery

Five cases of giant aneurysms developing on the pericallosal artery have been reported in the literature. These were managed by neck occlusion [26], resection of the thrombosed aneurysm [74, 94], clipping of the parent artery with resection of the aneurysm [89], and resection of the aneurysm with reestablishment of vascular continuity by means of an end-to-end bypass [109]. Results are shown in Table 4.

Aneurysms in the Vertebrobasilar System

A large number of papers dealing with vertebrobasilar aneurysms do not distinguish giant aneurysms from other aneurysms in the series [1, 16, 24, 35, 41, 46, 63, 65, 84, 87, 112, 120, 132, 138]. Therefore, the following study is based only on papers devoted specifically to the giant types.

The following analysis of the therapeutic modalities and corresponding results will only take into account cases reported before the end of 1983. Unfortunately, the lack of precise data concerning the numerous cases operated upon by Drake and Sundt since then made it impossible to include them in this study. However it may be of interest to mention that by the beginning of 1986 Drake's series of giant aneurysms of the posterior circulation amounted to 300 cases out of a total of 1300 located in the posterior fossa; 132 of these were treated by proximal ligation of the vertebral or the basilar artery. Sundt's series consisted of 73 cases out of 200.

Aneurysms of the Posterior Cerebral Artery

Classification

According to Drake [26], aneurysms of the posterior cerebral artery must be divided in two categories:

1. Those which arise from P_1, which are almost always *fusiform*. Having little room to develop, they are revealed by compressive syndromes of the brainstem and of the surrounding cranial nerves.

2. Those which arise from P_2, which are essentially *saccular* and are often revealed by hemorrhagic rupture.

Management

In Drake's series [26], aneurysms of the first group, not being clippable, were managed by *proximal occlusion* as close as possible to the neck, in order to preserve the posterior perforating branches. This was practicable because there was enough room between the neck and the perforators. When the posterior communicating artery refilled the aneurysmal sac (this was verified by puncture of the sac or angiography), proximal occlusion was completed by trapping. In the nine cases of occlusion of P_1 or P_2, the operation was well tolerated (except in one case, when the patient developed a deficit), owing to the good collateral circulation of the posterior cerebral artery.

Five out of seven cases of aneurysms of the second group were occluded at the neck by *clipping* (Fig. 69), with good results in four cases (Table 5).

Table 5. Giant aneurysms of the vertebrobasilar system

	No. operated/ total no.	Technique	Mortality	Morbidity	Good results or identical to preoperative condition
Posterior cerebral artery aneurysms					
Drake	5/12	5 Neck clippings Other cases: 5 proximal occlusions 2 trappings, of which 1 preceded by a proximal clip		1	4
Sundt et al.	1			1	
Subtotal:	6			2(33%)	4(67%)
Superior cerebellar-basilar trunk junction aneurysms					
Drake	12/19	12 Neck clippings Other cases: 1 exploration 2 proximal occlusions 1 wrapping 3 trappings	5(42%)	2(16%)	5(42%)
Basilar trunk bifurcation and basilar trunk aneurysms					
Wilson et al.	3/4			1	2
Drake (basilar trunk bifurcation)	18/42		3	1	14
Drake (basilar trunk)	1/13	Neck clipping and removal of clots (after proximal ligation)			1
Onuma and Suzuki	3			2	1
Sundt and Piepgras	14/15		1	5	8
Ganti et al.	1/8			1	
Cooperative series SNCLF	1/4		1		
Subtotal:	41		5(12%)	10(24%)	26(64%)
Vertebrobasilar junction aneurysms and vertebral artery aneurysms					
Drake (vertebrobasilar)	0/12				
(vertebral)	3/8		1		2
Beck et al. (vertebrobasilar)	1	Neck clipping and removal of clots (after proximal ligation)			1
Sugita et al. (vertebral)	2				2
Cooperative series SNCLF	1/3				1
Subtotal:	7		1(14%)		6(86%)
Total:	66		11(17%)	14(21%)	41(62%)
Aneurysms of the posterior-inferior cerebellar artery and the anterior-inferior cerebellar artery					
PICA	5	One case of excision with reestablishment of circulation with termino-terminal bypass (Dolenc). Good result (most were managed by trapping-excision).			
AICA	2				

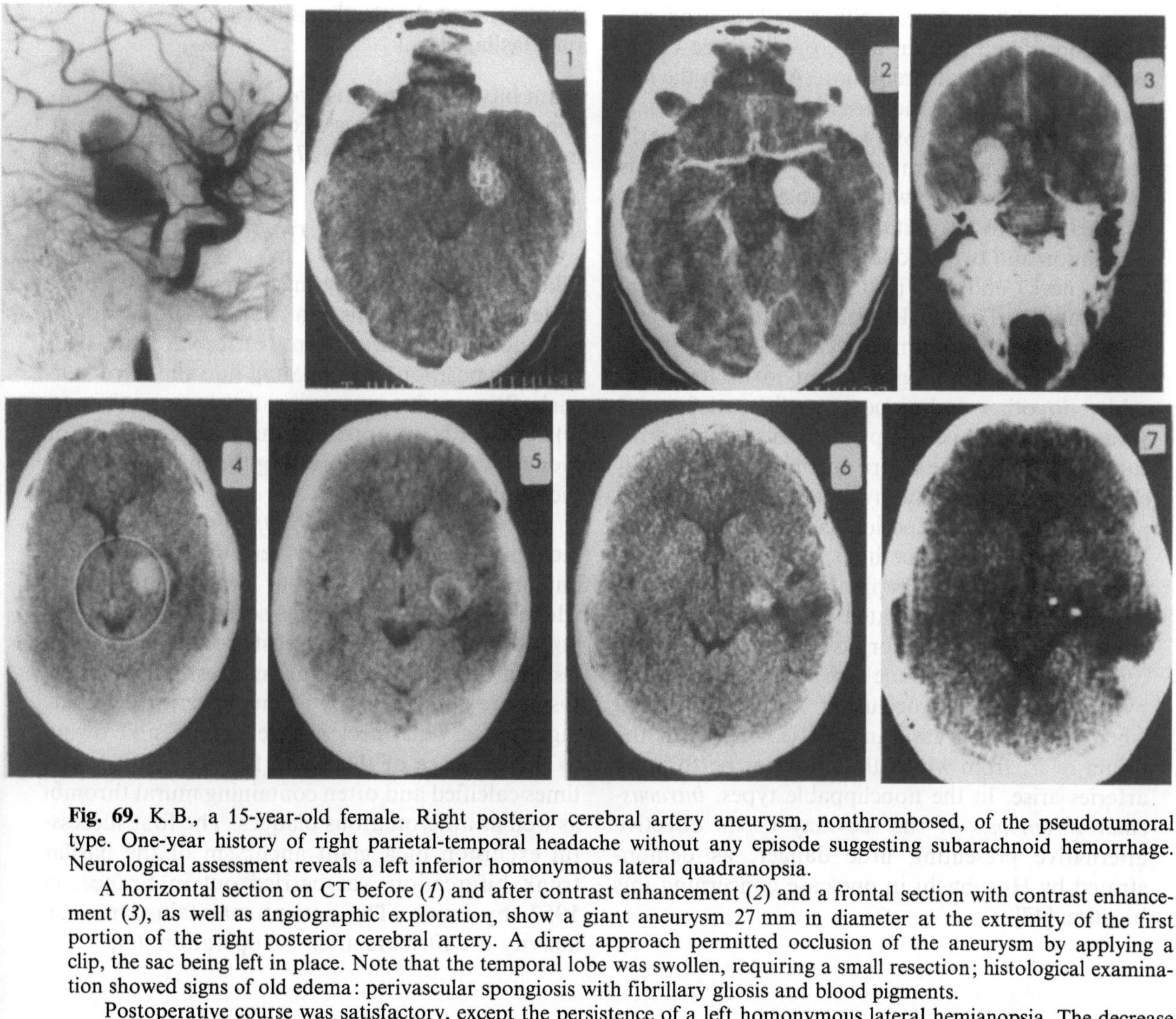

Fig. 69. K.B., a 15-year-old female. Right posterior cerebral artery aneurysm, nonthrombosed, of the pseudotumoral type. One-year history of right parietal-temporal headache without any episode suggesting subarachnoid hemorrhage. Neurological assessment reveals a left inferior homonymous lateral quadranopsia.

A horizontal section on CT before (*1*) and after contrast enhancement (*2*) and a frontal section with contrast enhancement (*3*), as well as angiographic exploration, show a giant aneurysm 27 mm in diameter at the extremity of the first portion of the right posterior cerebral artery. A direct approach permitted occlusion of the aneurysm by applying a clip, the sac being left in place. Note that the temporal lobe was swollen, requiring a small resection; histological examination showed signs of old edema: perivascular spongiosis with fibrillary gliosis and blood pigments.

Postoperative course was satisfactory, except the persistence of a left homonymous lateral hemianopsia. The decrease in volume of the sac was followed by successful CTs without contrast enhancement. At the 2nd week, CT showed hyperdensity of the sac corresponding to the recent thrombus (*4*); at the 6th week, decrease in density corresponding to maturation of the thrombus (*5*); at the 5th month, a decrease in size of the sac (*6*), and at the 13th month, only a little scarred spot located external to the clip opacity (*7*). (Photographs by courtesy of Professor G. Stroobandt, Catholic University of Louvain)

Aneurysms of the Cerebellar-Basilar Trunk Junction

Individualized as an entity by Drake [26], aneurysms of the junction between the basilar trunk and the superior cerebellar artery in fact arise at the origin itself of the latter, but in close proximity to the basilar trunk. In general, they project laterally to the basilar trunk and displace P_1 upwards. These vascular relationships make surgical approach to them extremely difficult. In three quarters of all cases, these aneurysms manifest as space-occupying lesions, especially Weber's syndrome; in half the cases they bleed.

A direct approach to these aneurysms is considered by most authors to be difficult; but Drake's determination led to his finding or artifically making a clippable neck in 12 out of his 19 cases. The application of the clip was made possible in the most favorable cases by reducing the neck with a ligature, and in the cases with a mural thrombus by performing a prior thrombectomy during circulatory arrest, either with a proximal occlusion of the basilar trunk or, in three cases, using extracorporeal circulation. Although the latter greatly facilitated the procedure, heparinotherapy was responsible for two deaths due to early postoperative hemorrhage. The results of this 12-case group are shown in Table 5. There were five deaths (two attributable to the extracorporeal circulation and two secondary to operative tearing of the neck) and two postoperative neurological aggravations. The results were both clinically and angiographically good in five cases.

When neck clipping is found to be impracticable, no other technique is really satisfactory. Wrapping cannot be complete because of the difficulty of exposing the entire aneurysmal mass. Occlusion or trapping can give rise to ischemic complications in the superior cerebellar territory. However, these last methods can be justified in some special cases. Trapping may be indicated when there is an associated arteriovenous aneurysm on the distal territory of the of the superior cerebellar artery, as in one case successfully treated by Drake. Proximal occlusion can be performed when there is full assurance of leaving open the origin of P_1 from which the posterior perforating arteries arise. In the nonclippable types, *intravascular thrombosis* of the sac may be an effective alternative presenting little danger, as demonstrated by Hosobuchi in one case concerning this location [47].

Aneurysms of the Basilar Bifurcation and Basilar Trunk

Giant basilar aneurysms are located at the bifurcation in about two thirds of cases and on the basilar trunk itself in one third [27, 91, 95, 126].

Aneurysms of the Basilar Trunk Bifurcation

Like the saccular aneurysms from which they originate, giant aneurysms can project (a) upwards in the interpeduncular cistern, (b) forwards in a suprasellar position, invaginating into the third ventricle floor and compressing the optic pathways, (c) backwards, compressing the mesencephalon, or even (d) laterally, compressing the third nerve and the cerebral peduncle.

Their *extreme surgical difficulty* is due to the fact that the neck, usually very wide, is not only implanted onto the basilar trunk bifurcation, which is itself ectasic, but also most often incorporates the origin of both posterior cerebral arteries and superior cerebellar arteries. These aneurysms are adhere closely to the posterior perforating arteries. Their neck is barely depressible owing to the presence of thick and fibrous walls, sometimes calcified and often containing mural thrombi as well as atheromatous plaques. The first successful exclusion of a giant aneurysm of the basilar trunk bifurcation was carried out in France, in 1957, by Laine. The patient maintained normal activity for 10 years after the operation [63].

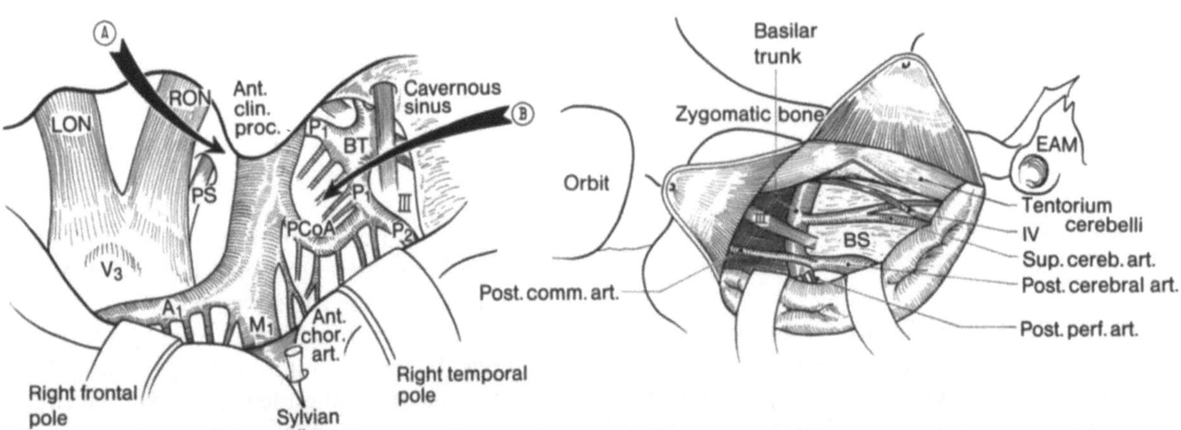

Fig. 70. Surgical approach to the basilar trunk. *Right:* right subtemporal approach. *Left:* right pterional approach, with its two variants: interoptic-carotid (*A*) and retrocarotid (*B*) (cf. microsurgical anatomy of the surgical approaches). *LON*, left optic nerve; *RON*, right optic nerve; *PS*, pituitary stalk; *PCoA*, post. comm. artery; *BT*, basilar trunk; *BS*, brain stem; *EAM*, external auditory meatus

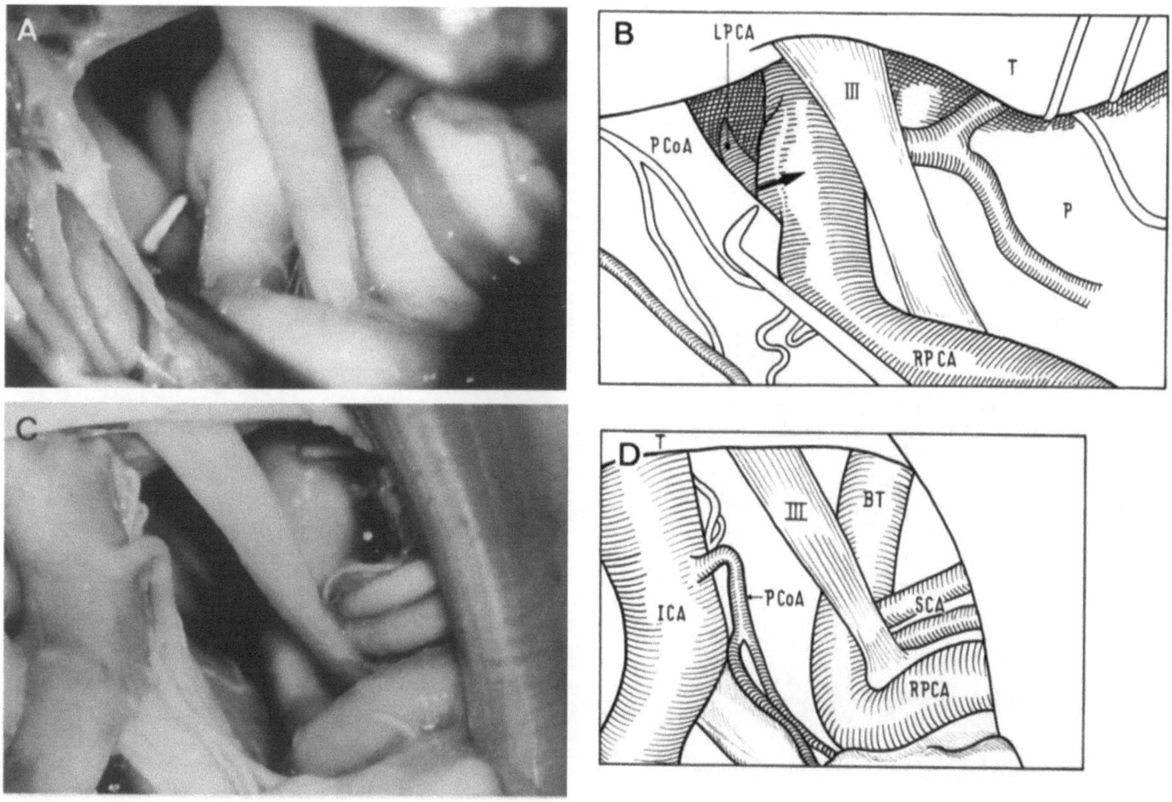

Fig. 71. A, B Anatomical preparation of the basilar bifurcation (*arrow*) through a right lateral subtemporal approach. *T*, edge of the tentorium; *P*, pons; *III*, right third oculomotor nerve; *RPCA*, right posterior cerebral artery; *LPCA* left posterior cerebral artery; *PCoA*, right posterior communicating artery. **C, D** The lateral subtemporal approach allows access to the junction between the basilar trunk and the right posterior cerebral artery (*SCA*), early duplicated in this case, and also to the upper third of the basilar trunk (*BT*). (Courtesy of Dr. P. Mercier, Angers)

Tip basilar aneurysms [38, 98] can be approached by several routes. The lateral subtemporal approach as described by Drake [25, 27] (Fig. 70, right; Fig. 71), is the most classical one. Caution is necessary to avoid excessive retraction of the temporal lobe as well as tearing of the posterior temporal veins. The subtemporal approach can be enlarged by removal of the zygomatic arch (Sano et al.), especially for basilar aneurysms situated on the bifurcation or basilar trunk. These aneurysms can also be managed using the pterional route popularized by Yasargil [138] (Fig. 70, left) passing either through the interoptic-carotid triangle or the retrocarotid space (Fig. 72). The interoptic-carotid triangle may be enlarged by unroofing the optic canal so that the optic nerve can be displaced medially, and by drilling the anterior clinoid process to get more space on the medial side of the internal carotid artery. When the approach is retrocarotid, the access to the basilar bifurcation is generally done inferiorly to the posterior communicating artery. This is easy when the posterior communicating artery is flexible enough to be retracted upwards, but difficult and, moreover, dangerous when it is short. In the latter eventuality, the basilar bifurcation may be approached – although dangerously – going superiorly to the posterior communicating artery through the network of its tributaries (Sugita). Dividing the posterior communicating artery itself is only admissible if it is thin and provided that PC_2 be correctly fed by the PC_1 segment. A large opening of the sylvian fissure, as proposed by Sugita et al. [113] under the name of transsylvian approach, allows better retraction of the temporal lobe and provides wider exposure of the operative area. The pterional approach can be enlarged by removal of the orbitofrontomalar bone structure (Lesoin et al.), especially for basilar and cavernous aneurysms. Whatever the route, lateral subtemporal or pterional or transsylvian, the approach must preferentially be made on the right side (at least in right-handed patients) unless there are neurological deficits corresponding to the left hemisphere.

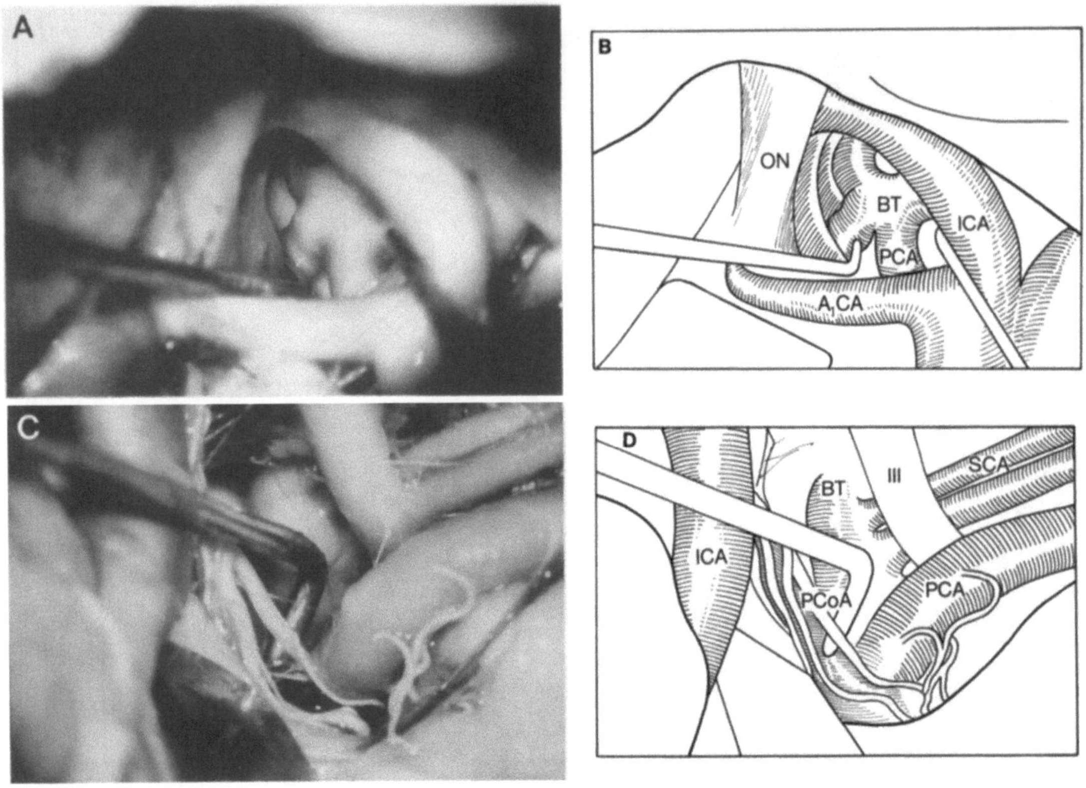

Fig. 72. A, B Anatomical preparation of the basilar trunk (*BT*) via right pterional approach, through the interoptic-carotid space. *ICA*, supraclinoid carotid artery; *ON*, right optic nerve; A_1CA, right A_1 cerebral artery; *PCA*, posterior communicating artery. **C, D** Anatomical preparation of the basilar trunk via a right pterional approach through the retrocarotid space

The choice of approach depends on the one hand upon the anatomical configuration of the carotid artery and its tributary system and of course upon the particular topography and spatial projection of the aneurysm on the other. Visibility of the perforating branches of the basilar bifurcation, on the controlateral side of the aneurysmal neck, is better when coming anteriorly through the pterional approach. But conversely, at least according to Drake, perforators can be better controlled posteriorly through the lateral subtemporal approach.

Aneurysms of the Basilar Trunk

These are aneurysms implanted in the middle third of the basilar trunk, between the vertebrobasilar confluence and the superior cerebellar arteries. They compress the pons on the midline and the surrounding cranial nerves laterally. The preferential approach to them is approximately the same as for basilar bifurcation aneurysms, but their lower location calls for technical adjuncts in order to provide deeper exposure of the basilar trunk. This may be achieved by incising the cerebellar tentorium along the fifth nerve, taking care not to injure the fourth nerve (Drake) drilling the upper ridge of the pyramid externally to the sixth nerve (Sugita) and/or the posterior clinoid process (Dolenc). It should be mentioned that the transclival approach [43, 45, 64] has not been used or at least reported for giant aneurysms of this location. When their neck is not clippable, a proximal occlusion by application of a clip, or better a tourniquet, on the basilar trunk can be done, but it requires a second operation through the cerebellopontine angle.

Results

The combined results of these two topographic groups are shown in Table 5.

For basilar trunk bifurcation aneurysms, Drake's results (18 neck occlusions in 42 patients, with 14 successes), and those of Sundt and Piepgras [117] (8 good results out of 14 clipped aneu-

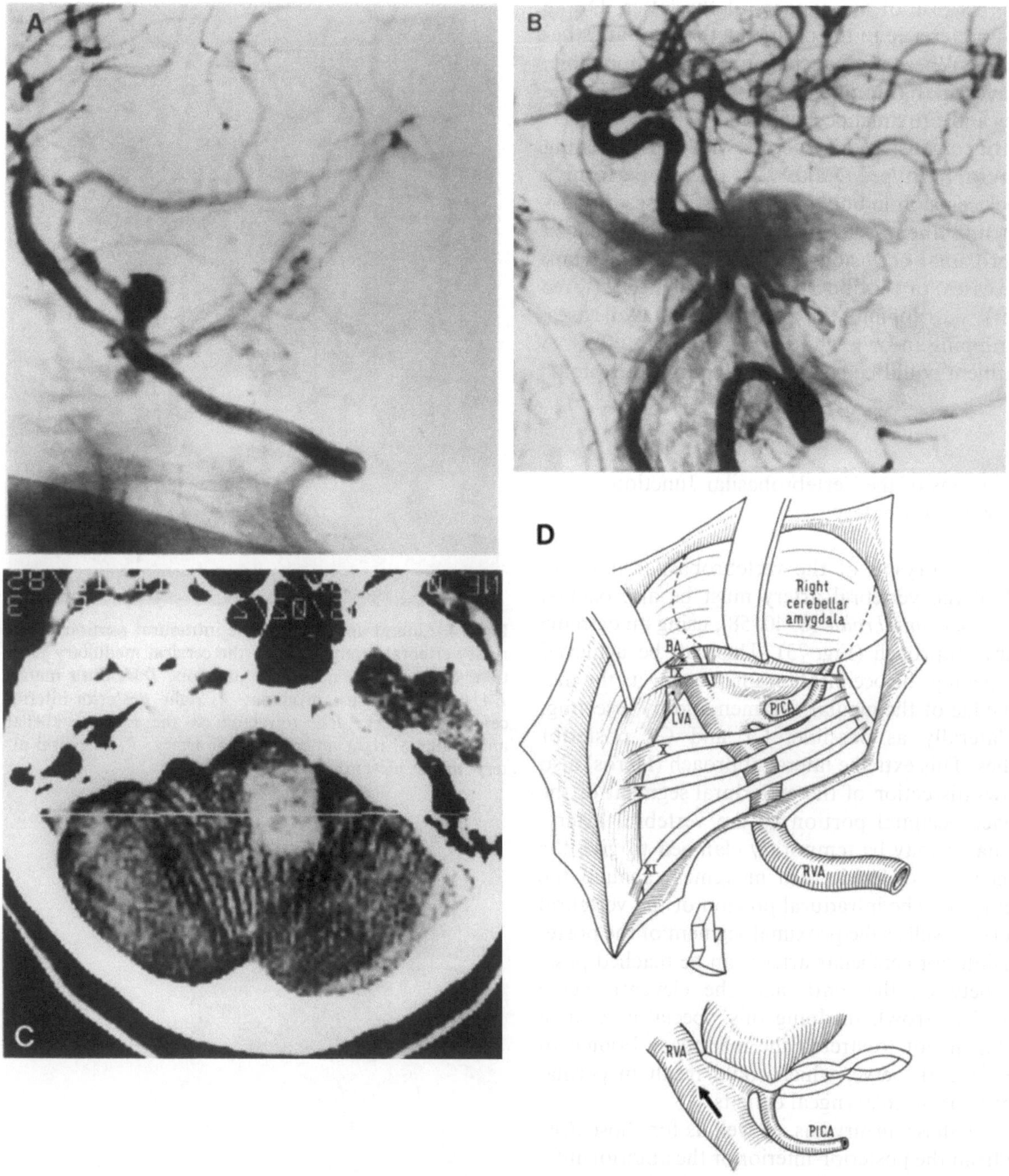

Fig. 73 A–D. G.P., a 66-year-old female, was referred in January 1986 for a subarachnoid hemorrhage associated with tetraparesia and medullary deficits. The CT scan (**C**) showed a hyperdense mass which the right vertebral angiogram (**A**) demonstrated to be a subtotally thrombosed giant aneurysm. The first-stage operation consisted of clipping the aneurysmal neck (**D**). Because of its rigidity and width, the ostium of the PICA could not be preserved (**B**); but this had no harmful consequence, thanks to the good collateral anastomotic supply of its distal territory. In the second stage, the sac was depressed using the CUSA. After shunting of the hydrocephalus, the outcome was favorable

rysms) demonstrates that in expert hands a number of these aneurysms can be clipped in a satisfactory way. In Drake's experience, although clipping was performed without any particular difficulty in seven cases because of the presence of a relatively narrow neck, it turned out to be difficult in the 11 other cases owing to a wide neck, despite the use of extracorporeal circulation. However, because of the dangers of the latter, Drake gives preference to the classic methods of anesthesiology. Where neck occlusion proved impossible, intravascular thrombosis was performed in three cases and proximal occlusion in 14.

By contrast to his success with the preceding topographic type, Drake was able to perform a neck occlusion in only one of the 13 cases of basilar trunk aneurysm. The majority were managed by proximal occlusion of either the basilar trunk (five cases) or the dominant vertebral artery (three cases); a trapping was performed in two cases, a wrapping in one, while in one case no effective treatment could be performed at surgical exploration.

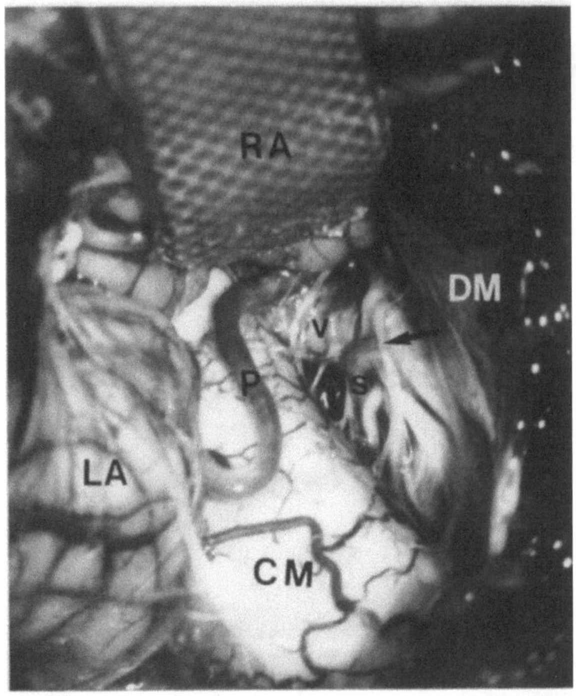

Fig. 74. Lateral approach of the intradural portion of the right vertebral artery through the cervical medullary junction. *CM*, cervical medullary junction; *DM*, dura mater; *LA*, left cerebellar amygdala; *P*, right posterior-inferior cerebellar artery; *RA*, retractor on the right cerebellar amygdala; *S*, right anterior spinal artery; *V*, vertebral artery; *arrow*, eleventh nerve

Aneurysms of the Vertebrobasilar Junction and Vertebral Artery

Giant aneurysms of the vertebrobasilar junction and of the vertebral artery must be approached by a *suboccipital route* [8, 40, 58], using an extreme lateral approach (Fig. 73). This can be achieved by opening the occipital foramen as far as the medial edge of the jugular foramen and by resecting, as laterally as possible, C1 and C2 posterior arches. This extreme lateral approach (Heros) also allows dissection of the extradural segment of the cervico-occipital portion of the vertebral artery, so that it may be temporary clamped to give the surgeon more freedom of movement around the aneurysm. The intradural portion of the vertebral artery as well as the proximal segment of the posterior-inferior cerebellar artery can be reached passing between the tenth and the eleventh nerve (Fig. 74, arrow). In doing this, special care must be taken not to stretch the medullary branch of the eleventh nerve, which could result in permanent pharyngeolaryngeal deficits.

For these aneurysms, as well as for those arising from the posterior-inferior or the anterior-inferior cerebellar arteries, a translabyrinthine approach could be in some circumstances a useful alternative approach.

In Drake's experience, none of the 12 junction aneurysms turned out to be clippable. However, three of the eight cases located in the vertebral artery benefited from a neck occlusion, two of them with good results. Giant fusiform aneurysms of the vertebral artery, classically inaccessible to the direct approach, can be clipped with preservation of the parent artery by using the large fenestrated, angled Sugita clips [114] (Fig. 75).

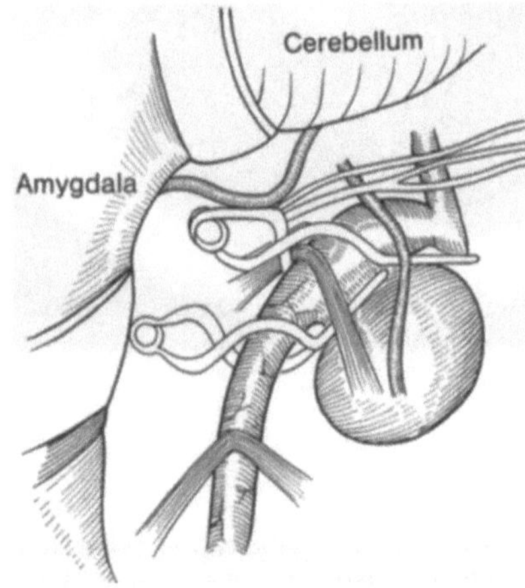

Fig. 75. Aneurysm of the right vertebral artery, approached through the right cerebellopontine angle and the right side of the cervical-medullary junction

Nonclippable cases can be managed quite easily by trapping or by proximal intracranial occlusion, taking care not to damage the origin of the posterior-inferior cerebellar artery, or even by vertebral occlusion at the cervical level. The method of intravascular thrombosis can also be an interesting option.

Aneurysms of the Posterior-Inferior and Anterior-Inferior Cerebellar Arteries

These aneurysms are rarities. For instance, posterior-inferior cerebellar artery aneurysms make up 1.2% of all intracranial aneurysms [58] and only one sixth of them are of the giant type. The present study was carried out on five cases located in the posterior-inferior cerebellar artery [17, 20, 54, 57, 143] and on two cases in the anterior-inferior cerebellar artery [14, 47].

They must be explored through a direct approach, since radical management by clipping, resection of the sac with reconstruction of the parent artery by microsurgical methods (Dolenc [20]), or even trapping-excision can lead to excellent results (four out of five operated cases).

Conclusions

An analysis of Table 5, which groups together the overall results in vertebrobasilar system aneurysms managed by selective neck occlusion (66 cases) shows that this surgical method has obtained good results in 62% of the cases, with a mortality of 17% and a morbidity of 21% (seven cases of aneurysms of the posterior- and anterior-inferior cerebellar arteries are omitted from this table as data concerning the results were not available). Any good impression one may have of the method, must, however, be balanced against remaining the fact that a considerable number of aneurysms of the vertebrobasilar system were managed by proximal occlusion or by trapping of the parent artery: these will be covered in the appropriate chapter.

Direct Surgical Treatment by Wrapping and Intravascular Thrombosis

Wrapping

Types of Wrapping

Certain types of aneurysms with a wide neck which incorporates a considerable part of the parent artery and the walls of which are hardened by atheroma cannot be clipped without danger. In such cases, *wrapping or coating of the neck and sac* can be a palliative treatment. The first attempts were carried out in 1933 by Dott [5]; the *autologous material* used was *muscle* and then *aponeurosis* or *dura mater*. However, experimental studies and clinical observations have shown that the degree of fibrosis obtained by these methods was not sufficient to provide adequate and lasting protection against hemorrhagic recurrence or enlargement of the sac. Therefore, Northfield in 1952 [18] and Gillingham in 1958 [10] respectively proposed wrapping by *cotton* fibers or *gauze*. With this material the fibrous reaction is almost always satisfactory, though its late onset offers no protection against an early hemorrhagic recurrence. Moreover, it can give rise to a secondary arachnoiditis responsible for irreversible lesions of the neighboring cranial nerves, at the base of the skull [4].

Over the last few years, wrapping with *plastic substances* has become widely used on the advice of Dutton [7] and Selverstone [19].

Results

The results of these three types of wrapping were carefully reviewed by Mount and Antunes in 1975 [15]. These authors, who personally managed 58 aneurysms of all sizes with muscle (8 cases), gauze (21 cases), and plastic substances (29 cases), consider that only the latter two are effective and attended by very low morbidity and mortality.

The results in giant aneurysms are summarized in Table 6. Mortality was nil and morbidity relatively low (two postoperative aggravations). The favorable impression given by this study must be moderated by the fact that the publications did not always mention the postoperative follow-up

Table 6. Results in giant aneurysms managed by wrapping

	No. of cases wrapped/ total no.	Cases in which topography is specified	Morbidity and mortality (†)	Good results or identical to preoperative condition
McMurtry et al.	1/12	1 Basilar trunk		1
Wilson and U	1/8	1 Basilar trunk bifurcation		1
Drake	6/50	3 Middle cerebral artery 1 Anterior communicating artery 1 Superior cerebellar artery 1 Basilar trunk	1 Hemorrhagic recurrence (10 years later) 1 Enlargement	4
Sonntag et al.	2/13	2 Basilar trunk bifurcation	1	1
Ganti et al.	4/8	4 Vertebrobasilar system	1	3
Cooperative series SNCLF	20/288 (Topography specified for 4)	2 Middle cerebral artery 2 Anterior communicating artery	1 (†) Hemorrhagic recurrence (1 month later)	3
Total	34/379 (9%)	18 cases	5/18 (28%)	13/18 (72%)

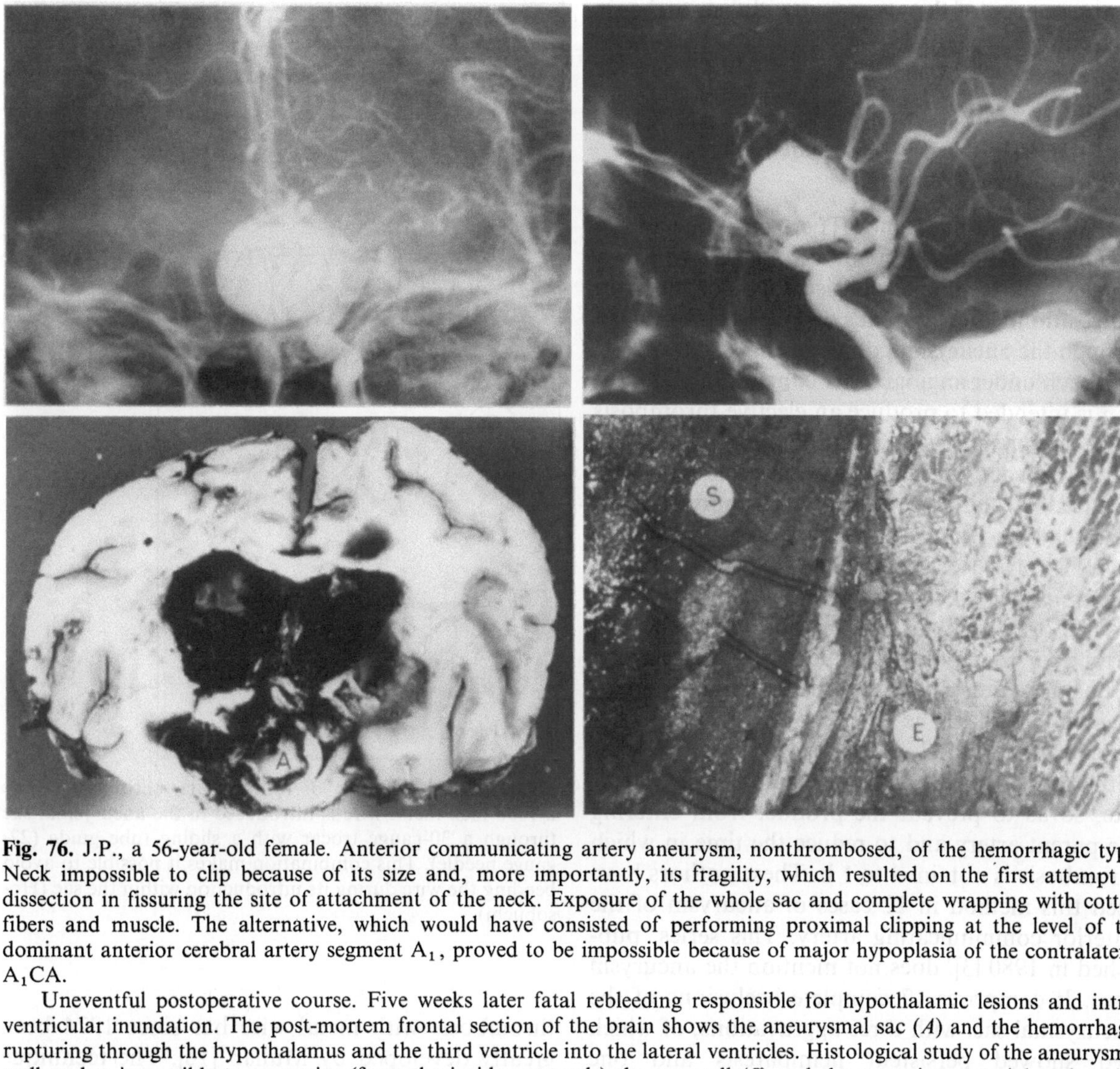

Fig. 76. J.P., a 56-year-old female. Anterior communicating artery aneurysm, nonthrombosed, of the hemorrhagic type. Neck impossible to clip because of its size and, more importantly, its fragility, which resulted on the first attempt at dissection in fissuring the site of attachment of the neck. Exposure of the whole sac and complete wrapping with cotton fibers and muscle. The alternative, which would have consisted of performing proximal clipping at the level of the dominant anterior cerebral artery segment A_1, proved to be impossible because of major hypoplasia of the contralateral A_1CA.

Uneventful postoperative course. Five weeks later fatal rebleeding responsible for hypothalamic lesions and intraventricular inundation. The post-mortem frontal section of the brain shows the aneurysmal sac (*A*) and the hemorrhagic rupturing through the hypothalamus and the third ventricle into the lateral ventricles. Histological study of the aneurysmal wall makes it possible to recognize (from the inside outwards) the sac wall (*S*) and the wrapping material undergoing fibrous organization (*E*)

and thus missed secondary hemorrhagic recurrence (Fig. 76).

The series presented in Table 6 [6, 9, 14, 21, 24] consist of ten cases of vertebrobasilar aneurysm, of which nine were situated at the basilar bifurcation, three cases of aneurysm on the anterior cerebral artery, and five of aneurysm on the middle cerebral artery. Drake [6] was the only one to supply details about the quality of the wrapping, which could be performed completely only in three cases of middle cerebral aneurysm. In the authors' view, only this topographic variety can be effectively managed by this method, and then only provided that the dome be completely dissected and wrapped.

Intravascular Thrombosis

This method permits treatment of nonclippable aneurysms by a minimal approach to the sac, without dissection or manipulation of the surrounding vascular and nervous structures and without interruption of the circulation in the parent artery.

The first material to be employed was *horsehair*, injected by an air compression gun within the aneurysmal sac [8]. This method has rarely been used since because of its low reliability. Introduced by Drake [6] in two cases of giant basilar trunk aneurysms, this technique led to a fatal extensive thrombosis in one case and was followed by a repatency of the aneurysm with hemorrhagic recurrence in the other. Current techniques make use of *metallic substances.*

Stereotactic Intrasaccular Thrombosis with Iron Filings

In 1962, Alksne and Rand [1] perfected the method of stereotactic intrasaccular thrombosis with iron filings. This technique consists of injecting iron filings into the sac by means of a needle introduced through the aneurysmal dome, using a stereotactic approach under angiographic control. Injection of iron is intended to produce an elective thrombosis of the aneurysmal sac. Retention of the iron filings within the sac is ensured by a magnetic probe introduced by the same stereotactic approach and maintained at 1 mm outside the dome of the aneurysm. To produce a thrombosis, the catheter must remain in place for 4 days.

The drawbacks of this method are the length of time for which the magnetic probe must remain in position and, especially, the risk of secondary fragmentation of the clot. To reduce this risk, Alksne and Smith [2, 20] used iron filings together with a polymerizable substance, methyl methacrylate, so as to prevent the product from entering the parent artery and to reduce the time in which thrombosis is obtained to 1 h. These authors have used this method in 22 cases of aneurysm of the anterior communicating artery. This series, published in 1980 [3], does not mention the aneurysm sizes. It comprises 17 complete occlusions of the aneurysmal sac, with three aggravations, of which two showed persistent hemiparesis and one showed cerebrospinal fluid fistula. There were no hemorrhagic recurrences, not did any deaths occur during operation. Sixteen patients returned to their original work.

These authors recommend that this exceptional method should be held in reserve for patients presenting a high operative risk who have aneurysms of the anterior communicating artery. The interest of this stereotactic method lies in the fact that it reduces cerebrovascular manipulations to a minimum. In aneurysms of the anterior communicating artery, it can be carried out by the transsphenoidal approach through the sphenoid planum.

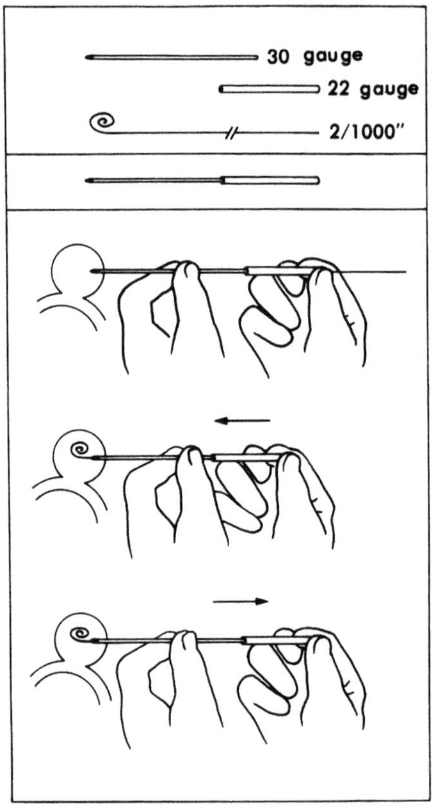

Fig. 77. The technique of intravascular thrombosis. The 2/1000-inch metal wire is introduced in the aneurysmal sac through a 30-gauge trocar with a sliding tube guide (22-gauge needle). This combination makes it possible to avoid bending the wire during its introduction within the sac (Hosobuchi)

Intrasaccular Thrombosis with Metal Wire

Performed for the first time on a giant aneurysm by Werner et al. [23] in 1941, and subsequently by Mazars [13], the method of intrasaccular thrombosis with metal wire has since 1974 been greatly developed by Mullan [16]. The technique consists of implanting in the sac, by direct approach, a metal wire of beryllium copper (of 2/1000-inch calibre) through a fine 33-gauge needle introduced within the sac wall (Fig. 77). The aneurysm lumen is packed with a combination of beryllium-copper alloy wire (two thirds of the total amount) and pure copper, wire (one third). These materials were chosen on the basis of experimentation performed on the femoral artery of the dog by Mullan. Beryllium copper which has the property of being neither too flexible (because of the beryllium) nor too brittle (because of the copper) has been found to be a good packing material, the more so as it can be performed in a spiral. As it has the disadvantage of not being very thrombogenic, it requires the additional use of pure copper wire which, because of its excellent thrombogenic properties, permits accelerated thrombosis of the sac. The copper wires are introduced only at the end of the operation, after packing the aneurysm with beryllium-copper wire which is a good support for the thrombus and prevents its entry into the parent artery. Complete occlusion of the aneurysmal sac most often requires several punctures of the sac in different areas. In some giant aneurysms, up to 18 m wire was introduced! The positioning of the wire and the development of intrasaccular thrombosis are followed by intraoperative angiography.

Other alloys have been recommended, especially phosphorus bronze, which is as thrombogenic as copper and has in addition the same elastic qualities as beryllium copper. It could have been the ideal material to induce intravascular thrombosis, but its excessive thrombogenicity presents the risk of extensive thrombosis in the parent artery. It is therefore only used for occlusions of the cavernous sinus in carotid-cavernous fistulas [17].

The thrombogenic properties of these different materials are linked to their positively charged metallic ions which favor the agglomeration of blood cells and fibrinogen, which at a normal pH of the blood are negatively charged, a phenomenon already noticed by Velpeau in 1831 [22].

The results of this method can only be evaluated from two series, few authors having experience of it. Mullan [16] in 1974 reported 15 cases of aneurysms managed by intravascular thrombosis, but without specifying their size. The method led to a complete thrombosis in 10 cases and a partial one in two cases. Two operative deaths occurred during operation and two secondary deaths by hemorrhagic recurrence.

Hosobuchi, using the technique he described in 1975 [11], reports 22 cases of giant aneurysms managed by this method, of which 16 were attended by good clinical and angiographic results (Fig. 78). The patients were followed up for several years [12]. Table 7 gives the results obtained, according to their topographic distribution.

The CT data being difficult to interpret, owing to the artefacts produced by the metallic material, the authors studied the development of the lesion by initial postoperative angiography which was followed by two others, one after 1 year and the other after 2 or 3 years. Of the 14 aneurysms presenting complete thrombosis on initial angiography, 11 remained totally thrombosed and 3 presented a partial secondary refilling. Three of the four aneurysms having an incomplete initial thrombosis became secondarily considerably enlarged.

Table 7. Results in giant aneurysms managed by intravascular thrombosis: 22 cases treated by Hosobuchi [12]

	Good	Aggravation	Mortality	Remarks
Carotid-ophthalmic (8 cases, of which 2 by the transsphenoidal approach)	5	2[a]	1	[a] Subsequent death by hemorrhagic recurrence
Posterior communicating (2 cases)	2			
Carotid bifurcation (1 case)	1			
Anterior communicating (5 cases)	3	1	1[b]	[b] Hemorrhagic recurrence
Basilar bifurcation (6 cases)	5		1	

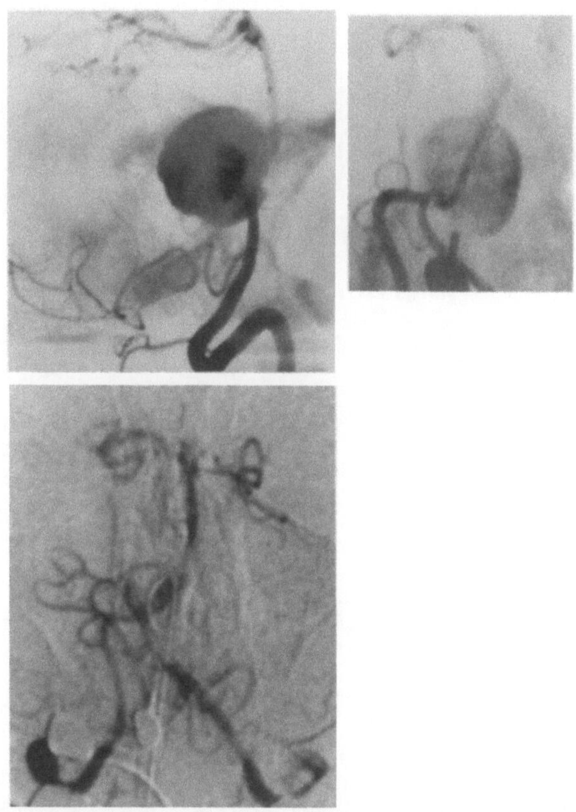

Fig. 78. Aneurysm of the vertebrobasilar junction managed by intravascular thrombosis. *Top left* intraoperative angiogram of the vertebral artery, lateral view. *Top right* intraoperative AP view. *Bottom* postoperative angiogram AP view, showing occlusion of the sac and patency of the parent arteries. (Courtesy of Professor Y. Hosobuchi, University of California, San Francisco)

Indications

With regard to the indications for these methods, Mullan and Hosobuchi advise against performing intravascular thrombosis in three circumstances: (a) when the sac already contains a thrombus; (b) when the contrast medium enters the sac too early and in too large amounts, before injecting the distal branches; and (c) in general, when the neck is wide. This anatomical configuration can lead to a protrusion of the metal material into the lumen of the parent artery and to a spreading thrombosis or the migration of emboli into the distal territory. Furthermore, when the neck is large, there is a risk of intravascular thrombosis leaving part of the latter patent, thereby leading to the re-formation of a new growing aneurysm, with a secondary risk of hemorrhagic rupture, as it occurred in the only case treated by Drake.

According to Hosobuchi, this method is particularly indicated in giant aneurysms located on the basilar trunk bifurcation (five good clinical and angiographic results out of six cases) and on the internal carotid artery bifurcation (one good result out of one case). In his view, the carotid-ophthalmic types are unsuitable for intravascular thrombosis which, moreover, may by dangerous because of the risks of massive thrombosis in the parent artery and embolism into the distal territory.

Extracorporeal Circulation

The preceding review of the different techniques used in the direct surgical approach shows that a number of giant aneurysms can satisfactorily be managed using current techniques of anesthesiology (induced hypotension and moderate hypothermia with neuroanesthesiological protection) and by having recourse to temporary clamping of short duration.

However, the surgical approach in specific types of giant aneurysms would be greatly facilitated "if there were a simple way to achieve prolonged regional or general exclusion of the cerebral circulation" [12]. We accordingly deemed it of interest to ask the team of Rennes, France, in view of their personal experience [6] to review the present status of the methods of inducing hypotension by extracorporeal circulation, stressing the technical problems created by their application in the surgical treatment of giant aneurysms.

Closed-Thorax Extracorporeal Circulation with Deep Hypothermia and Circulatory Arrest in Giant Aneurysms

Historical

The literature on this technique divides naturally into three periods, which can be reviewed as follows:

1. Prior to 1970, extracorporeal circulation (ECC) with hypothermia, with or without circulatory arrest, is described in several articles [2, 3, 4, 5, 8, 10, 11, 17, 19, 20]. In France, in particular, Guiot reported one case in 1960 [7] and Lepoire reported three cases in 1963 [1]. These observations deal with aneurysms of all types, including in particular giant aneurysms as well as aneurysms of the vertebrobasilar area.

2. Between 1970 and 1980, despite the good results that had been obtained and the advantages that the authors had clearly described, the technique fell increasingly into disuse for several reasons: (a) two surgical teams were required and the procedure was time-consuming; (b) the risk of postoperative complications was greater since thoracotomy was necessary (several teams, however, reported cases of closed-thorax surgery [10, 19]); (c) many factors, especially coagulation factors, were not fully understood.

Drake wrote, as early as 1964, "The use of cardiopulmonary bypass and deep hypothermia in the surgical treatment of ruptured intracranial aneurysms creates enough additional hazards so that it is probably not warranted in cases in which the aneurysms can be obliterated by more conventional means," and clearly confined the use of this technique and its specific risks to very difficult cases, in particular to giant aneurysms. However, the severity of the clinical condition and risks involved in preoperative angiography (spasm) should be borne in mind in analyzing the results of this period.

3. Silverberg reintroduced the technique in 1980 [14] and in 1981 published a report on a remarkable series of nine patients (one case of medullar hemangioblastoma and eight giant aneurysms) operated on with extracorporeal circulation and deep hypothermia [15]. His series is the most important of recent years and shows that great progress had been made in the use of extracorporeal circulation and hypothermia with closed-thorax surgery. Of the eight giant aneurysms, five originated from the middle cerebral artery, two from the basilar artery and one from the internal carotid artery. The outcome in five cases was excellent, with no postoperative neurologic deficit. In three cases the results were good: two patients had transient neurologic deficit and in one case the aneurysm clip had slipped with occipital ischemia probably due to thrombosis 6 months after the operation. The advantages of the technique seem to outweigh the hypothetical difficulties, particularly hemostasis. This point will be discussed again.

Riemens [13] has also recently reported a patient operated on successfully by this technique.

The main reason for the interest that neurosurgeons are now showing in the procedure is the great progress that has been made by cardiovascular surgeons in extracorporeal circulation, in improved modalities for the treatment of complex congenital heart defects and aortic arch replacement, and in the possibility of extracorporeal circulation without thoracotomy. Coagulation disorders are better understood and controlled. Comprehension of the physiopathology of hypothermia and its consequences has also progressed.

Now that the risks inherent in the cardiovascular technique itself have been reduced to a minimum, neurosurgeons can reconsider its application to their discipline.

The use of the technique of closed-thorax extracorporeal circulation by femoral cannulations appears a particularly adequate answer to the imperatives of neurosurgery.

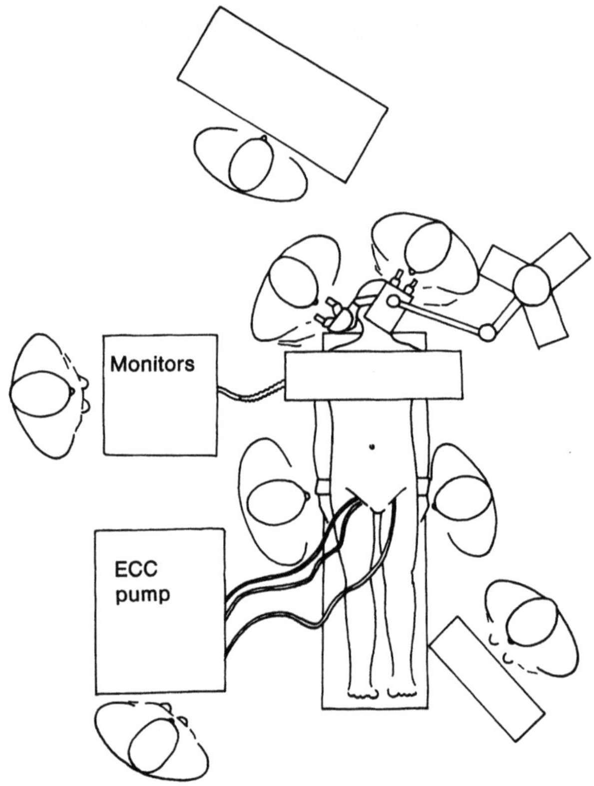

Fig. 79. Organization of the surgical teams. *ECC*, extracorporeal circulation

Surgical Technique

The authors have always used femoral cannulation for extracorporeal circulation during closed-thorax surgery. The technique is routine practice in our department of cardiac surgery and for this reason we have preferred to operate on our patients in that department with postoperative follow-up in the neurosurgery intensive care unit. The immediate proximity of the two departments is an undeniable advantage.

Surgery requires the close collaboration of two operating teams, one neurosurgical and the other cardiovascular, each composed of two surgeons and one theatre nurse. Including two anesthetists, the pump operator, and one or two theatre nurses, the entire team should not exceed 10 persons. Figure 79 shows the organization of the surgical teams and Fig. 80 shows the surgery timetable. The thorax must be easily accessible in case defibrillation by external shock is necessary during rewarming.

Extracorporeal Circulation

Cannulations

The femoral vessels are approached bilaterally by oblique incisions in the fold of the groin. The vessels are dissected along their vertical axes. A good dissection must respect the main lymphatic system and afford closure without drainage. This surgical approach has long had our preference over the conventional, more destructive vertical incision which does not always heal well.

Heparin (90 mg/m^2 body area) is administered intravenously. Venous cannulation, which is the most delicate, is performed first, beginning on the right. The common femoral vein is opened transversally between two clamps. A multiperforated no. 28 French catheter is inserted and pushed through the inferior vena cava to the right atrium. The catheter often comes up against the iliac bifurcation. Gently manipulation and a rotating movement combined with Vasalva's maneuver usually make continuation possible. In one of five cases, this was not possible and the catheter was left in the iliac position. A normal venous return was obtained, however.

Next, cannulation of the left common iliac vein is performed (no. 26 or 28 French catheter) and the venous line is connected. The right femoral artery is then cannulated (no. 16 or 18 French catheter). As venous cannulation is occlusive, the left femoral artery must be clamped to prevent edema of the lower limb (Fig. 81).

Temperature	Anesthetic	Neurosurgery	ECC
37° C	Induction Variables monitored: – Arterial pressure (radial A) – Central venous pressure – ECG – Cardiac output – Nasal temp. – Rectal temp. – Esophag. temp.		Priming cooled to 15° C
		Skin incision Bone flap Dura suspended Dissection begun HEMOSTASIS	Femoral vessels approached
34/32° C	HEPARIN ventilation + 5% CO_2		
24/28° C	Ventricular fibrillation Ventilation stopped	Aneurysm approached – Neck dissected – Nearby dissected arteries Clip or aneurysm opened and sutured Aneurysm phase ended	Cannulation femoral Vx ECC full flow (2.5 to 3 L/min) Cooling to 20° C (Maximum duration 50–60 min) ECC FULL FLOW REWARMING
24/28° C	Heart defibrillation Ventilation restarted		
37° C	PROTAMINE	HEMOSTASIS	ECC STOPPED DECANNULATION Hemostasis
		CLOSURE	CLOSURE

Fig. 80. Timetable for surgery

Extracorporeal Circulation Circuit

The unit comprises a conventional bubble-type oxygenator with a good heat exchanger (Bentley Bos. 10). The solution used to prime the extracorporeal circuit (priming) is the same as for routine cardiac surgery. For an adult of 60 kg, dosage is as follows:

Ringer's lactate	1000 ml
Isoglucose 5%	500 ml
Dextran	500 ml
$NaHCO_3$	50 mEq
Cefazolin (Cefacidal)	750 mg
Heparin	0 mg

The priming solution is cooled to a temperature of 15° C, as is usual in cardiac surgery. Due to hemodilution, hematocrit drops to about 25%. Unless there is a heavy loss of blood, transfusions are rarely necessary, whether in extracorporeal circulation or postoperatively.

We no longer use heparin in the priming solution if no blood is lost. Activated clotting time is regularly monitored during extracorporeal circulation. Heparin is little used during hypothermia and is therefore only reinjected as needed and at a minimum.

This anticoagulant protocol has proved itself in about 1500 cases of heart surgery using extracorporeal circulation, resulting in a drastic reduction in postoperative hemorrhage and in all inherent complications (late diagnosis of hemorrhage directly due to surgery, reoperation for hemostasis, postoperative infections, and complications due to multiple blood transfusions).

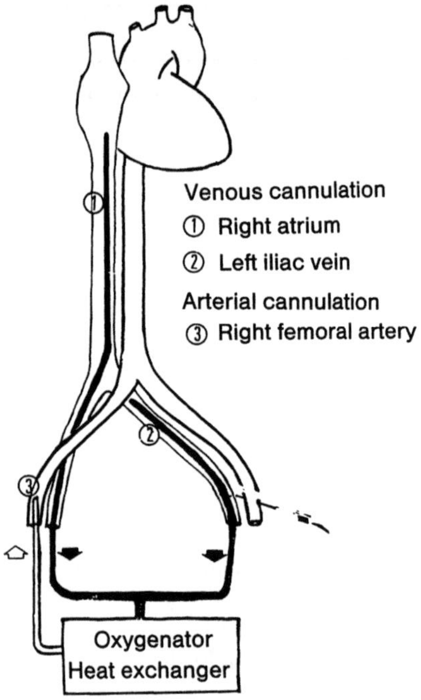

Fig. 81. Extracorporeal circulation

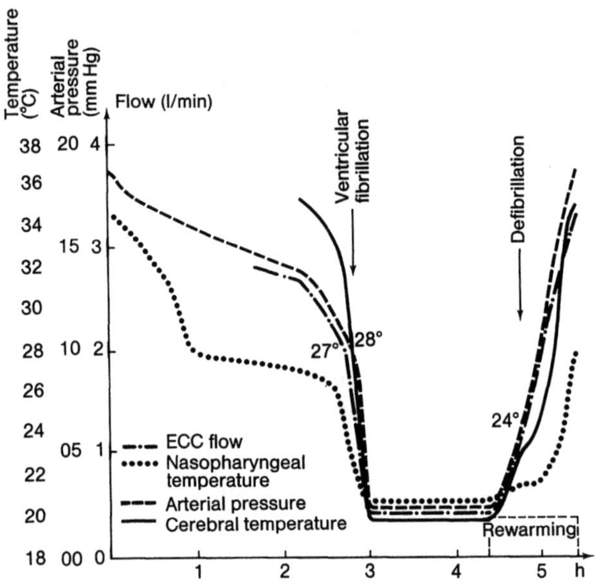

Fig. 82. Course of hypothermia

Hypothermia

The timing of hypothermia is shown in Fig. 82. The target nasopharyngeal temperature is 20° C. The temperature of the oxygenator priming solution is fixed at 10° C above that of the venous blood return. The extracorporeal circulation flow based on that the venous return is 2.5–3 l/min. This is obtained by different maneuvers: positioning the patient higher than the oxygenator with his feet as low as possible, and filling the vascular bed with Ringer's solution to increase central venous pressure. When ventricular fibrillation occurs, an appreciable increase in the venous return is observed together with an increase in the central venous pressure. Ventilation is stopped as soon as extracorporeal circulation has reached a satisfactory flow rate.

When the nasopharyngeal temperature is 20° C, the low extracorporeal circulation flow rate is 600–900 ml/min with an arterial pressure of approximately 20 mmHg. If circulatory arrest is performed, its length must not exceed 50–60 min. Arrest can be extended, if necessary by one or several recirculations. During rewarming, the oxygenator priming must not exceed the vein temperature on entry by more than 10° C and at the end of rewarming must not exceed 40° C.

Defibrillation of the heart was in all cases spontaneous. However, if it is not, electric shock can be given when the body temperature is 28° C, or earlier if important ventricular tachycardia is seen on the ECG tracking. Ventilation is restarted after defibrillation. It should be prolonged if rectal temperature is too low.

After decannulation, heparin is neutralized in the usual way: total protamine = heparin [initial dose + reinjection(s)] × 1.3–1.4.

Neurosurgery

The neurosurgical protocol can and must be the same as that of any conventional operation on an intracranial arterial aneurysm. The operative site is exposed at the same time as the femoral vessels are approached. The cardiovascular team always finishes first and waits for an indication from the neurosurgeons before initiating extracorporeal circulation. Hemostasis must be perfect throughout the exposure. This precaution is of great importance as it determines the conditions in which the teams will have to work for the rest of the operation. In particular, the dura mater must be very carefully suspended; otherwise epidural venous oozing can make surgery very awkward. If this is correctly carried out, hemorrhage should not be greater than in conventional surgery.

One important point open to discussion is the

way to approach the aneurysm itself. Two methods have been used in our department: (a) before the start of extracorporeal circulation and (b) after the start (and therefore during heparin therapy). In one case, a resection of the anterior part of the temporal lobe was performed during heparin therapy without any difficulty. In our opinion, however, a safe approach to the aneurysm prior to extracorporeal circulation is important. This permits dissection with hemostasis under normal conditions of perfusion and arterial pressure.

During extracorporeal circulation, several local alterations take place. The brain becomes firm and, in particular, the color of the vessels (veins and arteries) becomes uniform. They must therefore be precisely localized during dissection and possible vascular lesions must be well visualized in case immediate hemostasis is necessary (particular attention must be paid to the veins). It must be emphasized at this point that a low circulatory flow rate is important. This ensures that a permanent check can be kept on any possible vascular tears.

Neurosurgery is concluded during rewarming, which depends on the hemodynamic conditions and is therefore variable in duration. It is essential that hemostasis be checked during the rewarming period. Return to a perfusion flow rate and arterial pressure must be spontaneous. In our experience, external electric shock has never been necessary. This procedure is perfectly feasible provided access to the thorax is kept free.

Closure with perfect hemostasis can only be considered after protamine sulfate has been injected and decannulation performed. We have never encountered any serious problems at this point. In particular, there have never been any signs of cerebral edema during the return to normal hemodynamic conditions. Immediate postoperative care is provided by both surgical teams in the neurosurgery department.

Clinical Study

Five patients were operated on according to the above protocol. All presented one or several aneurysms and one a giant aneurysm whose characteristics are detailed below.

The *patient* was a 62-year-old female, operated on in 1968 in another clinic, for a left carotid-ophthalmic aneurysm by partial clipping and wrapping. The postoperative course was marked by completely regressive dysphasia and right hemiplegia. The patient led a normal life until September 1981, when she had a new subarachnoid hemorrhage accompanied by blindness of the left eye and some langage disorders.

Angiography revealed a giant aneurysm on the left carotid artery, of which only one part was visualized, showing partial thrombosis of a spheroidal pouch about 3 cm in diameter. This aneurysm was in the midline position, probably infra- and interchiasmatic. The neck seemed to be attached to the initial part of the last segment of the internal carotid artery from its exit out of the cavernous sinus. Clips from the first operation were visible above and inside the aneurysm.

Surgery on 6 October 1981. Left frontopterional flap and simultaneous opening of the two femoral vessels by the cardiovascular team. After opening of the sylvian fissure, a calcified and fibrotic mass was visualized at the level of the anterior clinoid process, which obstructed the way and was a remnant of bone dust introduced during the first operation. Extracorporeal circulation started. Ventricular fibrillation at 20.5° C nasopharyngeal temperature. Brain temperature 20° C. Pump output 900 ml/min. Arterial pressure 20 mmHg.

The bone fragments were progressively removed. The removal of the most voluminous of them covering the anterior clinoid process, the optic foramen, and the whole internal portion of the aneurysm was greatly facilitated by the hemodynamic conditions which made it possible to depress the aneurysmal sac. Thus the third nerve, the internal edge of the optic nerve, which was scarcely visible in the fibrous tissue that envelops it, and the internal part of the aneurysm under the optic nerve were visualized. The neck appeared between the carotid artery and the optic nerve. During the removal of the two old clips, a small tear of the aneurysmal sac was produced at the junction with the neck. The consequent hemorrhage was not massive and did not hinder the course of the operation. Exclusion of the neck was carried out with silk thread and finished with a Yasargil clip. The aneurysm was opened wide, and the presence of clots and completeness of the exclusion confirmed.

Duration of the low blood flow: 65 min.

Spontaneous defibrillation at 32° C nasopharyngeal temperature. Throughout the rewarming and the return to normal hemodynamic conditions, hemostasis was rigorously monitored and controlled as necessary.

Postoperative course uneventful. Rapid awakening. Some language disorders regressed within a few days. Barbiturate protection and preventive anticoagulation from the 48th hour. Check-up at 6 months: normal life being led; definite blindness in the left eye.

Comments. Giant left carotid-ophthalmic aneurysm with a neck difficult to see. Dissection very difficult because of the tightly packed organization of the bone dust into a block around the aneurysm. Hemodynamic conditions allowed the release and exclusion of the aneurysm without massive hemorrhage and vascular sacrifice.

Discussion

Complete extracorporeal circulation by simple peripheral cannulation has the advantage of avoiding opening the thorax and the straightforwardness of the bilateral Scarpa's triangle approach, which means that cannulations are situated well outside the neurosurgical operating field, must be emphasized. The difficulty lies in obtaining an adequate venous return to ensure its efficacy.

The authors decided on a hypothermia temperature of 20° C. This affords sufficient protection for the brain and makes complete circulatory arrest lasting 50–60 min feasible.

In practice, complete circulatory arrest was not undertaken in any of our cases. Protecting the brain was not the only reason for this; a very low flow was selected to maintain a certain amount of intravascular pressure. One of the reasons for this was to prevent air from passing through the vessels. Another reason was to obtain better intraoperative control of hemostasis. Monitoring possible vascular tears can also be carried out as necessary. In the event of massive bleeding, complete circulatory arrest is possible.

It follows easily from this that the combination of extracorporeal circulation and deep hypothermia, compared to other more conventional techniques, such as controlled hypotension or moderate surface cooling, affords unrivaled flexibility and therefore greater security. In fact, controlled hypotension [using trimethaphan camsylate (Arfonad) or sodium nitroprusside] means that a mean pressure of 20–40 mmHg is possible. This greatly facilitates surgical procedure but allows an important circulatory flow to be maintained. When hemorrhage occurs intraoperatively, it considerably hinders the exact localization of the aneurysm site. If the position of the aneurysm, or bleeding due to rupture, necessitates vascular clamping, then cerebral protection becomes indispensable. This protection may be insufficient when using conventional techniques. Extracorporeal circulation, on the other hand, allows regulation of temperature conditions, output and arterial pressure as required.

Conclusion

Surgery of this type requires time and personnel and must be limited at present. In the opinion of the authors, giant aneurysms and vertebrobasilar aneurysms can best benefit from the use of this technique. Aneurysms that are difficult of access, whose features are hard to assess on the arteriogram, and which seem at great risk of rupture or vascular sacrifice, should benefit from the best operative technique available. It is often the neurosurgeon's personal assessment of the risks involved that leads to the extracorporeal circulation-hypothermia option being considered. The use of this modality is particularly justified in the case of giant aneurysms where the risk of rupture and the need to monitor the collateral branches are permanent worries.

Surgical Occlusion of the Carotid Axis (Cervical Common Carotid Artery and Cervical Internal Carotid Artery)

Cervical occlusion of the carotid arteries was widely used as a definitive treatment for intracranial aneurysms regardless of their size, from 1885 untill microsurgery was introduced in the 1970s. Initially used on an empirical basis, the method achieved wide recognition after hemodynamic studies established that it was possible to reduce pressure in the artery distal to the occlusion. In order to evaluate its clinical results, we have conducted a literature review including the main series published during the period when carotid occlusion was regarded by many as the least dangerous treatment for intracranial aneurysms.

Effects of Carotid Occlusion

Hemodynamic Effects of Carotid Occlusions

Methods of Evaluation

The hemodynamic effects of carotid ligation have been evaluated essentially from direct measurements of distal intravascular pressure. These were carried out at the level of the cervical internal carotid artery or at the level of the arteries of the circle of Willis and their cortical branches. In a few cases, measurements were taken within the aneurysmal sacs [2, 3, 7, 14, 48, 49, 67, 68, 69, 71]. These as well as other studies have also confirmed that ophthalmodynamometric measurements quite faithfully reflect pressure in the distal internal carotid artery [10, 20, 57, 61, 62, 70]. More recently, supplementary information has been provided by measurements of cerebral blood flow [6].

Results

Progressive occlusion of the carotid artery leads to a fall in pressure and distal flow only after a 70% reduction of the caliber of the vessel. Beyond that point, pressure and flow decrease rapidly in proportion to the reduction of the diameter [61].

In normal conditions the systolic pressure in the distal artery will have the same value as the internal carotid artery if the outside diameter is more than 0.4 mm. Following carotid artery ligation, the same decrease in pressure occurs in the trunk of the anterior cerebral artery and middle cerebral artery as occurs in the intracranial carotid artery; but in the cortical arteries, pressure is only 86% of that measured in the intracranial carotid artery [2, 3, 7, 58, 67].

Most authors agree that there is little difference between the reductions in distal pressure produced by ligation of the internal carotid artery and of the common carotid artery or even of the common carotid artery and the external carotid artery combined. In fact, some authors [20, 60, 61, 62] consider that, after ligation of the common carotid artery, one quarter of the residual pressure in the distal internal carotid artery depends on the collateral tributary circulation of the homolateral external carotid artery. Others hold that, following ligation of the common carotid artery, there is an inversion of the direction of flow from the internal to the external carotid arteries [57, 62]. However, the inversion is said to be always transitory [74].

Repeated tests of temporary occlusion of the internal carotid artery show that, in a given patient, the same reduction in pressure is produced in the intracranial carotid artery as in the middle cerebral artery [68].

Carotid ligation, whether performed at the level of the internal carotid artery or at the level of the common internal carotid artery, leads immediately to a drop in distal pressure, followed in the ensuing weeks by a slow rise and stabilization of pressure, as has been demonstrated by measurements carried out 16–19 weeks after ligation [20, 59, 70].

The reduction in pressure produced by carotid artery ligation varies to some extent from one subject to another. Thus, Tindall et al. [59] have observed, after progressive occlusion of the common carotid artery in 42 patients, an initial reduction in the mean distal carotid artery pressure of more than 60% in four patients, from 60% to 40% (average 50%) in 28 patients, and less than 40% (average 31%) in 10 patients. Pressure was again measured after periods of 1–48 months (average 13 months) and was found to have dropped to 45% in the first group, to 28% in the second and to 30% in the third group. From this study, as well as from other clinical studies [60] and other experimentation on the monkey [43, 49], it is evident that a reduction of 25% of distal mean pressure persists for several years after ligation.

Reductions in flow distal to an extracranial carotid occlusion have been confirmed by measurements of cerebral blood flow which show that an internal carotid artery accounts for approximately 26% of the total cerebral blood flow and that its occlusion leads to a persistent 18% reduction of the flow and lasting hypoperfusion.

Clinical Effects of Carotid Artery Occlusion in the Management of Aneurysms of All Sizes

We have attempted to evaluate the clinical effects of carotid ligation from several series in the literature, the first of which is the cooperative series analyzed by Nishioka [38]. This study covers approximately 2000 cases of carotid artery ligation performed not only for giant aneurysms but also for small saccular aneurysms, at a time when the direct surgical approach was not as safe as it is today.

A detailed analysis of the content of Nishioka's cooperative series gives an idea of the range of indication for carotid ligation:

– This study groups together 814 cases managed by carotid artery ligation (most often of the common carotid artery: 90% of the cases) out of a total of 3265 aneurysms operated on between 1957 and 1965.

– Six hundred and eighty-five patients had a ruptured aneurysm, and 129 a nonruptured aneurysm.

– Five hundred and twenty-one had an aneurysm of the intracranial internal carotid artery, 51 of the middle cerebral artery, and 106 of the anterior communicating artery; 106 had multiple localizations.

– An occlusion of the common and of the internal carotid artery was performed in 89% and in 9% of the cases respectively. A combination of the common carotid artery or the internal carotid artery and the external carotid artery was performed in 2% of cases.

– Fifty-five per cent of the patients had a "sudden" occlusion and 45% a "gradual" one.

Throughout this study – despite considerable difficulty in interpreting the data collected – we have endeavored to *evaluate the efficacy of carotid artery ligation* as a treatment for intracranial aneurysms, by considering the frequency of hemorrhagic recurrence and the anatomical status of the aneurysm after ligation, and to assess its risks, especially those of ischemia.

Frequency of Hemorrhagic Recurrence

The frequency of *early hemorrhagic recurrence* is very difficult to establish. In Nishioka's cooperative study, for instance, it is impossible, in the overall early mortality figures (30% for ruptured aneurysms, 2.7% for nonruptured aneurysms), to distinguish the deaths related to a hemorrhagic recurrence from those associated with the development of vasospasm or ischemic complications.

The frequency of occurrence of a *hemorrhagic incident during the first 2 years* (excluding the initial period) is easier to interpret. In the cooperative study for example, the frequency amounted to 8% for the ruptured types and 3.5% for the nonruptured types. It was 3% for internal carotid artery aneurysms, 19% for those of the middle cerebral artery, 9.6% for the anterior communicating artery, and 10.4% in the cases of multiple aneurysms. It will be seen, therefore, that the best results have been obtained – as may be felt to be logical – in internal carotid artery aneurysms; this confirms the study of Kak et al. [26] on 1298 patients, where a recurrence rate of 4.4% is mentioned for internal carotid artery localizations.

Evaluation of the rate of *long-term hemorrhagic recurrence* is rendered difficult by the paucity of follow-ups longer than 2 years. In the Nishioka's cooperative study, only 10% of the cases were followed up for more than 2 years. However, two other papers give an idea of their frequency. Winn et al. [66], reporting on 60 cases of supraclinoid aneurysms managed by ligation of the common internal carotid artery, followed up for more than 1 year (average 8 years), found a rate of 14% of hemorrhagic recurrence (against 30% in the nonmanaged types). Roski et al. [45] give a recurrence rate of 7.5% in a series of 39 cases followed up for more than 10 years after ligation.

Status of the Aneurysm After Ligation

The status of the aneurysmal sac after ligation was studied from data in the literature giving the results of postoperative follow-up angiography [31,

32, 34, 38, 39, 52, 59]. However, our study was complicated by difficulties due to (a) the small number of cases with follow-up angiography (only 168 cases out of 814 in the cooperative series); (b) the frequent lack of indications concerning the angiographic method used; (c) the fact that the topography of the aneurysm and the ligation site were not always specified.

Our study shows – if it can be admitted that nonvisualization of the lesion means a thrombosis of the sac – that *thrombosis of the aneurysm occurs in 20%–35% of cases after ligation of the common carotid artery and in 65% of cases after ligation of the internal carotid artery.*

As regards the site of the aneurysm, all authors reviewed agree that the efficacy of ligation (as judged by nonvisualization or reduction in the size of the aneurysm) is greatest in aneurysms of the internal carotid artery, less in those of the anterior communicating artery, and least in middle cerebral artery aneurysms.

Early Ischemic Complications

Early ischemic complications associated with therapeutic occlusion of the carotid artery can be attributed to cerebral hypoperfusion, extensive thrombosis, emboli, or, more rarely, reflexes of carotid sinus origin. The time occurrence of these events is difficult to extract from the published series, because other factors presenting as ischemic-like complications, including preexisting neurological problems leading to intracerebral arterial spasm, were not fully ruled out.

Ischemic complications reached an overall rate of 22%–28% depending on the series [26, 29, 30, 37, 39, 42, 45]. They appeared in 80% of the cases within the first 48 h and in 95% of the cases before the end of the 1st week after ligation. The possible interaction of factors other than occlusion in the development of postligation ischemic complications can be appreciated when we consider the following facts:

– When occlusion was performed later than the 15th day following the hemorrhage, the rate of ischemic complications was 20% (versus 44% during the 1st week and 27% during the 2nd week).

– The mortality rate (whatever the cause) was 8.8% when the patients were operated on at Botterell grade I or II (versus 25% at grade III, 45% at grade IV, and 90% at grade V).

– The percentage of ischemic complications was only 12% for nonruptured aneurysms (versus 33% for ruptured types), with a mortality (whatever the cause) of 2.7% for the first group (against 30% for the second).

Only the rate encountered in the group of nonruptured aneurysms reveals real risk associated with carotid artery ligation itself. Furthermore, the frequency of ischemic complications in ruptured aneurysms tends to approach that observed in the nonruptured types when ligation is made in Botterell grade I or II patients who are operated on late after the initial hemorrhagic episode: this is an important argument against performing early ligation in these cases.

The *previous state of the cerebral circulation and the age* of the patient play an important role as risk factors. In nonruptured aneurysms, 9.3% of patients under 50 and 15.3% of those over 50 years old presented ischemic complications.

The incidence of ischemic complications may also differ according to the site and mode of occlusion. Concerning the *site of occlusion*, the results of the cooperative study show that these complications amount to 49% for the internal carotid artery and 28% for the common carotid artery. These results are confirmed by Kak et al. [26] who reported rates of 35% and 10% respectively, and Scott and Skwarok [48], who showed rates of 22% and 11%.

The *mode of occlusion* also plays a role: 34% ischemic complications for "sudden" occlusion and 25% for "progressive" occlusion. Table 8 summarizes the data. Table 8 shows that progressive occlusion is followed by a lower rate of ischemic complications than sudden occlusion. However, it offers no protection against the risk of sudden thrombosis during closure and probably carries a greater risk of embolism should the necessity arise to reopen the clamp.

Table 8. Manner of carotid artery occlusion

Manner of occlusion	Percentage of ischemic complications
Sudden: internal carotid artery (34 cases)	59
Progressive: internal carotid artery (37 cases)	41
Sudden: common carotid artery (393 cases)	32
Progressive: common carotid artery (301 cases)	24

Late Complications

Carotid artery occlusion can cause late complications, including late ischemic complications, the onset of arterial hypertension, and the formation of aneurysms on the arterial intracranial collaterals to compensate for the loss of one of the axes of cerebral circulation.

The incidence of *late ischemic complications* linked with hypoperfusion by carotid artery ligation is difficult to quantify [5, 26, 30, 40, 45, 63, 65]. The complications are reported to occur in 5%–20% of the cases, depending on the series, and are revealed in two thirds of the cases by transient ischemic attacks and in one third by infarcts.

The risk of developing *arterial hypertension* by ligation of one carotid artery was pointed out in 1977 by Winn et al. [66] on the basis of a study covering a series of 64 supraclinoid aneurysms managed by the authors and followed up for 8 years on average. These authors separated the cases observed into two groups: one managed by ligation of the common carotid artery (22 cases) and a control group (27 cases) left untreated. The results, summarized in Table 9, seem to implicate carotid artery ligation in the induction of arterial hypertension.

Finally, some clinical observations published in the literature [21, 22] and one case seen by the present authors, as well as two experimental studies [16, 18, 19], suggest that occlusion of a carotid artery is liable to favor the *development of aneurysms by increased flow* on the anastomotic intracranial collaterals, especially when arterial hypertension is associated. At any rate, this potential risk calls for caution in assessing the indication for carotid artery ligation in all patients with multiple aneurysms (rate estimated at 12–23% depending on the statistics).

Table 9. Frequency of secondary arterial hypertension following carotid artery ligation

Mode of treatment	Arterial hypertension
Group 1: managed by carotid artery ligation (22 cases)	13/22
Group 2: (control) conservative treatment (27 cases)	6/27

Conclusions

In spite of their disparity, analysis of the preceding results permits the following conclusions:

1. As has been shown by hemodynamic studies, carotid artery ligations generally have *clear and lasting effects on pressure (minus 25%) and on flow (minus 18%) in the distal territory*, up to the distal branches of the carotid system. Although there are few studies dealing with long-term results, most authors are united in recognizing that carotid ligations reduce the frequency of hemorrhagic recurrences by almost 50%, especially in aneurysms of the internal carotid artery.

2. *The choice of the ideal site for ligation* was for a long time an object of controversy. Until now, most authors gave preference to ligation of the common carotid artery because it was considered substantially less dangerous that of the internal carotid artery, although this method is less capable of producing a rapid thrombosis of the sac (30% of cases versus 65% for the internal carotid artery). At the present time, the majority prefer the internal carotid occlusion [33], since it is more effective and its ischemic complications can be reduced if a prior extra-intracranial bypass is performed.

3. *As regards the mode of occlusion* some authors, including Murphey [36], give preference to an "acute" occlusion, especially when distal intra-arterial pressure after clamping remains above 60% of its initial value. However, the majority [33, 38, 42, 43, 60] prefer a "gradual" occlusion by means of a progressive occluding clamp because of its lower rate of ischemic complications (25% versus 34%).

Practical Considerations

These notions lead to the following practical considerations:

1. *Cervical carotid artery occlusion*, by diminishing intrasaccular pressure and/or favoring sac thrombosis, may be useful for *diminishing the risks of hemorrhage and reducing the mass effect* of aneurysms considered to be too dangerous to manage by the direct surgical approach, especially for aneurysms located on the internal carotid artery.

2. The preferential choice of the *internal carotid artery* as the site of occlusion, which is more effective than that of the common carotid artery in the production of sac thrombosis, can be strengthened by the possibility of *performing a prior extra-*

intracranial bypass [51]. Such a bypass is of course obligatory when the test of tolerance to carotid compression demonstrates an insufficiency of the natural anastomotic collaterals. It could even be desirable to perform it systematically in order to prevent late complications associated with the loss of the carotid axis.

3. Finally, we feel that it is safer to perform *"gradual" occlusion* by a progressive occluding clamp, rather than "sudden" ligation. This method not only makes it possible to carry out occlusion during clinical and paraclinical monitoring, with the patient awake, but also facilitates the development of extra-intracranial anastomosis as well as natural anastomotic collaterals, thereby reducing the risk of immediate ischemic complications.

Carotid Artery Occlusion in Giant Aneurysms

When intracranial carotid artery giant aneurysms are judged to be too dangerous for direct surgery or when neck occlusion turns out to be impossible during the direct approach, proximal occlusion at the cervical level represents a good alternative, either completed by intracranial trapping or not. This method has been widely used by a large number of authors.

Results

The results from the most recent papers are shown in Table 10. The table, which sets forth 145 cases managed by occlusion of the common carotid ar-

Table 10. Surgical occlusion of cervical carotid arteries in giant aneurysms (excepting patients who had an associated extra-intracranial bypass – see Table 13)

	No. of occlusions/ total no.	Symptomatic types	Technique	Anatomical result	Good clinical result or identical to preop. condition	Complications	Mortality	Follow-up of cranial nerve compression	Remarks
Sundt and Piepgras [55]	13/51		1 CCL 6 ICL 3 Tr 3 CR		10				
Hosobuchi [23]	9/24	1 H 8 T	9 Tr	9 Th	8		1 GC		
Kak et al. [26]	22	22 T	14 CCL 8 ICL		19	2 IC	2 (1 HC) (1 GC)		
Drake [12]	18/45	4 H 14 T	13 ICL 3 Tr 2 CR	14 Th 1 N Th	12	2 IC 1 HC 1 GC	1 HC	9+ 4·	Cervical hemorrhage after clamp removal
Pozzati et al. [44]	5/5	5 T	5 CCL	4 Th 1 N Th	5			2+ 3·	
Sonntag et al. [53]	1/7		1 CCL		1				
Cooperative series SNCLF	77/191		70 (CCL ICL)[a] 7 Tr[a]		62	8	6		
Total	145/345 (42%)	5 H (9%) 49 T (91%)	21 CCL (33%) 27 ICL (43%) 15 Tr (24%)	27 Th (93%) 2 N Th (7%)	117 (83%)	14 (10%)	10 (7%)	11+ (60%) 7· (40%)	

GC, general complication; *HC*, hemorrhagic complication; *IC*, ischemic complication; *CR*, cervical clamp removed due to intolerance; *H*, hemorrhagic type; *ICL*, internal carotid artery ligation; *CCL*, common carotid artery ligation; *T*, tumoral type; *Th*, thrombosed; *N Th*, nonthrombosed; *Tr*, trapping; + improvement of cranial nerve compression signs; · cranial nerve compression signs unchanged

[a] Not included in total percentages due to lack of precision.

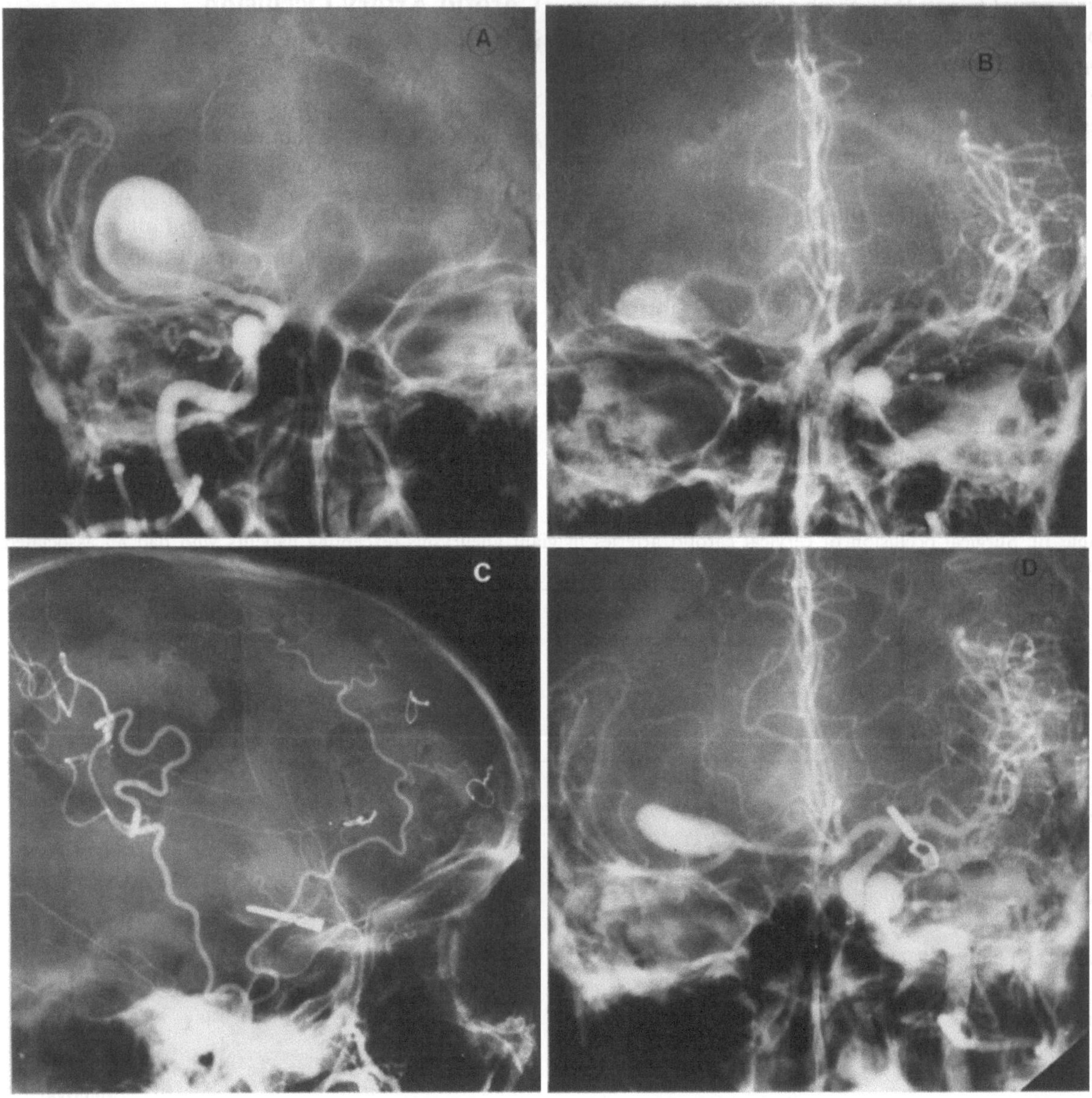

Fig. 83 A–D. G.P., a 44-year-old male presenting with a past history of chronic pulsatile headaches on the right side, was referred in September 1984 after the discovery, on the occasion of an insignificant traffic accident, of intracranial curved-shaped calcifications. The CT scan and the right carotid angiogram demonstrated a giant aneurysm located close to the internal carotid bifurcation (**A**), while the left carotid angiogram showed a symetrical berry malformation (**B**). As a first procedure, the left small aneurysm was clipped, in order to avoid its possible rupturing which could be favored by an excessive flow resulting from the right carotid occlusion. As a second procedure, a cervical internal carotid occlusion was made after performing an extra-intracranial bypass using the posterior branch of the superficial temporal artery (**C**).

The follow-up angiogram done 2 months later using a left carotid injection showed the satisfactory clipping of the left berry aneurysm and a only two-thirds reduction in size of the right giant aneurysm. Six months later, the patient was totally symptom-free and the CT scan demonstrated an almost complete thrombosis of the giant malformation

tery occlusion (33% of the cases), occlusion of the internal carotid artery (43% of the cases), or by extra- and intracranial trapping (24% of the cases), highlights the following facts:

– *Mortality and morbidity* rates were 7% and 10% respectively. Complications were due to ischemia in four cases (10%), hemorrhagic recurrences in three (4.5%), and general decompensations in

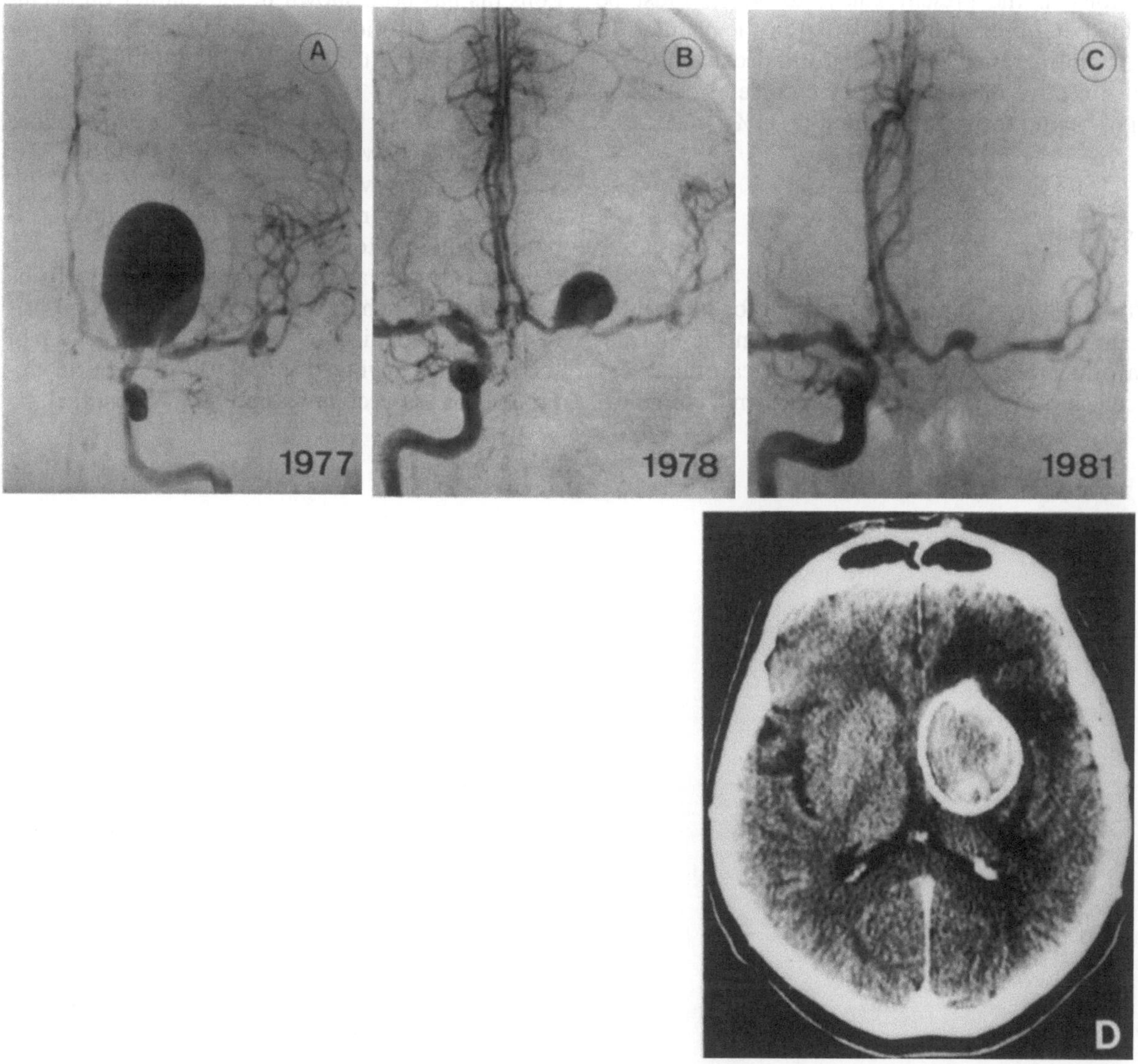

Fig. 84 A–D. S.R., a 45-year-old male, was referred for the first time in 1977 for transient right hemiparesis and aphasia. Bilateral carotid angiography showed a left carotid bifurcation giant aneurysm (**A**) with two associated small aneurysms: one on the bifurcation of the left middle cerebral artery and the other on the right carotid bifurcation. No direct or indirect treatment was performed at this time. In 1978, the patient was readmitted and the left giant aneurysm was treated by cervical common carotid occlusion after tolerance tests. The immediate follow-up was very good without neurological deficit and a decrease in size of the injected sac was observed on angiography (**B**). Three years later, examination showed the patient to be normal and the angiogram control showed only a minimal filling of the aneurysm (**C**). In 1985, follow-up pre- and postcontrast CT scans (**D**) demonstrated a thrombosed aneurysm without reduction of the volume of the sac. (Courtesy of Professor Vlahovitch, Montpellier [64])

others three (4.5%). In one case, removal of the Selverstone clamp produced a large cervical hematoma. Whatever the technique used, it yielded a good clinical result – i.e., stabilization or improvement of the patient's condition – in 83% of the cases.

– Occlusion led to *sac thrombosis* in 93% of patients reported. The thrombosis can be rapid or even acute, as demonstrated in Fig. 83, or progressive over several months or years, as shown in Fig. 84. When thrombosis was not obtained (7% of patients), the occlusion was generally performed at common carotid level.

– The *effects on the compressive phenomena* observed in the pseudotumoral types could satisfactorily be evaluated only from information provided by the authors on the evolution of cranial nerve palsies. This was available in only 18 observations in the present study, to which must be added 36 observations collected in the chapter on extra-intracranial bypass. Carotid occlusion led to an objective improvement or complete regression in 61% and mere stabilization in 35%.

Comments

Proximal ligation must be reserved for inoperable giant aneurysms arising directly from the internal carotid artery. Although common carotid artery occlusion is attended by fewer ischemic complications (as has been shown in the chapter on occlusions of the carotid artery), it cannot claim to produce aneurysmal thrombosis without fail [15]. The current tendency to give preference to definitive occlusion of the internal carotid artery is more effective in achieving total thrombosis of the sac. The use of a cervical progressive occluder is undoubtedly safer in preventing ischemic insults. If poor circulatory tolerance is suspected [17, 51, 73], a prior extra-intracranial bypass may have to be performed. When production of sac thrombosis is not accompanied by a sufficient reduction of the space-occupying effect, a direct surgical approach for sac decompression may be justified.

Surgical Occlusion of the Vertebrobasilar Axis (Vertebral Artery and Basilar Trunk)

First introduced for an aneurysm of the basilar trunk bifurcation by Mount and Taveras [35], occlusion of the vertebrobasilar axis proximal to the lesion has been frequently used by Drake in giant aneurysms of the vertebrobasilar system (39 out of 73 cases), either on the vertebral artery or on the basilar trunk itself. As in occlusion of the carotid axis, the aim is to produce a complete or, failing that, a partial thrombosis of the sac, or at least a decrease of intrasaccular pressure.

Hemodynamic Effects of Occlusion in the Vertebrobasilar System

These effects have not been studied as thoroughly in the vertebrobasilar system as in the carotid system. According to the studies consulted – Brunon [8], Brunon and Goutelle [9], Schott et al. [47] – the flow of the two vertebral arteries in the overall cerebral circulation averages around 30% (that is approximately 350 ml/min). Owing to the anastomotic supply in the circle of Willis, the reduction of overall cerebral flow produced by occlusion of the two vertebral arteries is 10% on average. However, these values vary widely from one subject to another.

Results in the Treatment of Giant Aneurysms

Occlusion of the Vertebral Artery

This study is based essentially on the experience of Drake [11, 12, 13] who performed an occlusion of the vertebral artery in 18 cases, out of a total of 28 patients with vertebrobasilar system aneurysms. This type of procedure was carried out on five of eight aneurysms of the vertebral artery, on all aneurysms of the junction of the vertebral artery-basilar trunk (10 cases), and on three of the 13 aneurysms of the basilar trunk. Of the 18 cases, proximal occlusion was twice performed extracranially and in 14 cases intracranially. Trapping was performed in two cases.

Results

The data from Drake's experience (18 cases) are shown in Table 11. They can be summarized as follows:

– Clinical results were considered excellent in eight cases, good in four, and bad in two. There were four fatal complications, of which one was by hemorrhagic recurrence and three were by ischemic complications.

– Of the 14 patients on whom postoperative angiography was carried out, the sac was totally thrombosed in eight, partly thrombosed in three, and identical with the preoperative condition in three.

Comments

The above results clearly show that *unilateral occlusion of the vertebral artery* is a method which is both reasonable in terms of ischemic complica-

Table 11. Surgical occlusion of the vertebral artery

Drake's series (18 cases): site of aneurysm	Extracranial unilateral vertebral artery occlusion	Intracranial unilateral vertebral artery occlusion	Trapping
Vertebral artery (5 cases)		Good: 2 Morbidity: 1	Good: 2
Junction of vertebral artery and basilar trunk (10 cases)	Good: 1 Mortality: 1	Good: 5 Morbidity: 1 Mortality: 2	
Basilar trunk (3 cases)		Good: 2 Mortality: 1	

tions and effective (with 12 partial or complete thromboses out of 14 cases followed up by angiography). However, there are two preconditions: (a) The aneurysms must be filled entirely, or at least to a great extent, by one of the vertebral arteries; (b) The controlateral vertebral artery must be sufficiently functional to supply the basilar trunk adequately.

Good results have also been found by other authors, including Hosobuchi [23] and Shibata et al. [50] as well as in the cooperative study of the SNCLF, which reports three patients operated on successfully; two by proximal occlusion and one by trapping of the vertebral artery.

On the other hand, it is ineffective to occlude one vertebral artery when the aneurysm is supplied equally by both vertebral arteries, as can happen in certain types located at the junction of the vertebral artery and the basilar trunk; in fact, in this particular case, thrombosis of the sac is unattainable.

Occlusion of both vertebral arteries is dangerous. Attempted by Drake on two patients, it led to ischemic disorders which required reopening of the clamp on one side. Despite this, the first patient died from extensive thrombosis spreading to the vessels of the pons. The second died secondarily from a hemorrhagic recurrence. However, in the literature [4] there is mention of a case of an aneurysm of the basilar trunk managed successfully by ligation of both vertebral arteries at the sulcus arteriosus of the atlas.

As regards the *definitive site of occlusion*, Drake gives preference to ligation performed intracranially, as close as possible to the aneurysm, in order to reduce the risk of ischemia in the territory of the posterior-inferior cerebellar artery and also in the anterior spinal artery.

When angiography and, even more, the operative findings reveal that there is not enough room between the origin of the posterior-inferior cerebellar artery and the site of attachment of the aneurysm to the vertebral artery, occlusion can be performed proximally to the emergence of the posterior-inferior cerebellar artery. In Drake's series, this type of ligation was well tolerated in all the cases, the territory of the posterior-inferior cerebellar artery being spontaneously supplied either by the vertebral stump by countercurrent or from the collateral cerebellar network.

When occlusion of the vertebral artery cannot be performed distally to the posterior-inferior cerebellar artery, it can be carried out intradurally or else at the sulcus arteriosus of the atlas, directly proximal to the entrance of the vertebral artery into the dural sac.

These sites should be preferred to low occlusion of the vertebral artery in the posterior triangle of neck. In fact, the anastomoses between the cervical vertebral artery and the deep cervical arteries are such that the intracranial vertebral artery can be revascularized from these supplies. Thus, Drake reports an aneurysm of the junction of the vertebral artery and basilar trunk treated by occlusion of the vertebral artery at its origin as having reopacified 5 years later due to supply from the deep anastomotic cervical branches.

In any case, when the therapeutic choice falls on unilateral occlusion of the vertebral artery, it is recommended that a prior *test of temporary occlusion* at the cervical level be performed, either with a progressively tightening clamp or a tourniquet or, even better, by an intravascular balloon introduced percutaneously.

Should the temporary occlusion not be tolerated, an *extra-intracranial bypass* might make possible a definitive secondary occlusion.

Occlusion of the Basilar Trunk

Rendered necessary by the frequent impossibility of ligating or clipping the necks of giant aneurysms of the basilar trunk, this method has been used by several authors, such as Mount and Taveras [34] in one case, Yasargil et al. [72] in one case. Rosario and Stein [46] in one case, Sundt and Piepgras [55] in one case, the cooperative study of the SNCLF in two cases, and, most importantly, Drake [11, 12, 13] in seven cases of aneurysms of the basilar trunk proper and 15 cases of aneurysms of the bifurcation in which angiography revealed functional posterior communicating arteries. In Drake's series, occlusion was achieved by clipping or trapping of the lesion in 12 cases and by progressive proximal occlusion of the basilar trunk with a tourniquet in 10.

Results

Drake's observations (22 cases), shown in Table 12, can be summarized as follows:

– The clinical results were considered excellent in 12 cases, good in two, and bad in five. There were three fatalities, of which one was by hemorrhagic recurrence and one by ischemic complications.

Table 12. Surgical occlusion of the basilar trunk (BT)

Drake's series (22 cases): site of aneurysm	Occlusion of BT by clipping or trapping	Occlusion of BT by tourniquet
BT bifurcation (15 cases)	Good: 6 Morbidity: 2	Good: 4 Morbidity: 2 Mortality: 1
BT (7 cases)	Good: 3 Mortality: 1	Good: 1 Morbidity: 1 Mortality: 1

– Postoperative angiographic follow-ups performed on 17 patients revealed complete thrombosis of the aneurysm in 16 and incomplete thrombosis in one.

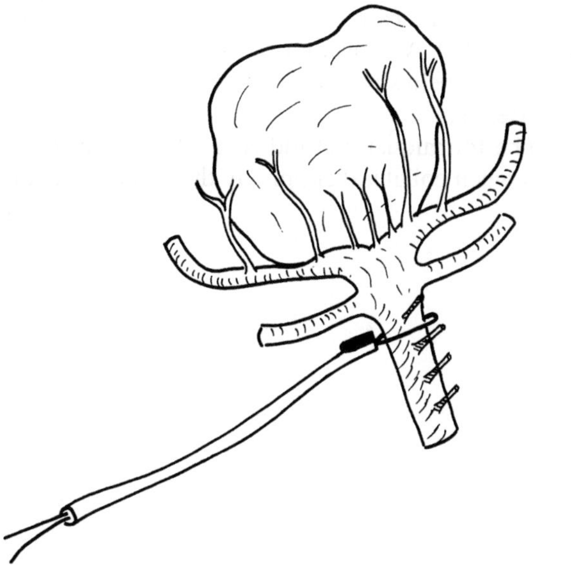

Fig. 85. Drake's tourniquet procedure. The tourniquet is prepared at the beginning of the operation so as to have it ready in case direct occlusion of the aneurysm neck proves impossible.

The thread (prolene Ethicon LTD 3-0; approx. 30 cm) is placed around the artery. Its two extremities are passed through a polyethylene tube (BE 190, approx. 10 cm), the internal extremity of which is marked with a small metallic clip to facilitate subsequent radiological location.

A careful attempt at temporary tightening by tourniquet intraoperatively is recommended in order to test its effectiveness and safety.

After closure of the dura mater, repositioning of the bone flap, and suture of the muscular layer (performed with due care to avoid bending of the tube), its outer extremity is passed through a stab incision of the skin flap and then protected by a sterile dressing.

Occlusion of the artery is generally carried out the day after placement of the tourniquet under angiographic guidance with the patient awake. If arterial occlusion leads to signs of ischemia, the tourniquet is at once loosened. Subsequently, new attempts are made to tighten up after artificially increasing systemic arterial pressure.

If ischemia does not develop, the tourniquet can be kept tight by means of vascular tweezers or a clip. Arterial occlusion is checked angiographically. Subsequently, under local anesthesia, the exit orifice of the tube is enlarged and a new clip placed in the tube in the subcutaneous space. The tube is then shortened in situ and the skin incision closed.

If the increase of systemic arterial pressure turns out to be insufficient for performing occlusion without danger of ischemia, the tourniquet can first be partially tightened in the hope of developing the anastomotic supply and of performing secondarily a complete occlusion of the artery

Comments

It is clear from the above results that proximal occlusion of the basilar trunk is a method which is both reasonable in terms of ischemic risks (one fatality out of 22 patients) and effective (16 complete and one incomplete thrombosis in 17 cases followed up angiographically).

The good results of Drake's series as well as those of other authors are attributable to its use only in the presence of *good anastomotic supply*, notably by the posterior communicating arteries. The supply can be tested during preoperative angiography by Allcock's procedure, which consists of the successive compression of each carotid artery during injection of the vertebral artery [41]. However, this procedure does not ensure that the basilar trunk occlusion will be well tolerated. Thus, in Drake's series, one case of mesencephalic infarct occurred despite the presence upon angiography of two posterior communicating arteries with good diameters.

For this reason, the author's current preference is for the positioning of a *progressive and reversible occlusion system by tourniquet* (Fig. 85). This technique, however, is not free from hazards. The tourniquet must be manipulated with care so as not to pull out the basilar trunk collaterals or even tear the intima or dissect the arterial wall.

The ideal site for occlusion, whether it is performed by immediate clipping of the basilar trunk or, which is better, by the tourniquet method, of course depends on the site of the aneurysm and on the position of the ostium of the collaterals on the basilar trunk. In basilar trunk aneurysms, the ideal procedure is to perform the occlusion between the posterior cerebral arteries and the origin of the superior cerebellar arteries. In practice, however, the space between these two groups of arteries is rarely sufficient (one case of Rosario and Stein, one case of Yasargil et al., two out of 16 of Drake). As a result, occlusions are most often performed below the origin of the superior cerebellar arteries.

The tourniquet method is satisfactory in most cases when collateral supply by the posterior communicating arteries is good. Thus Drake concludes: "It is remarkable how even one posterior communicating artery will perfuse the upper and even the lower basilar artery and its branches and how massive thrombosis begins to occur in the sac in a few minutes."

Intracranial Occlusion of the Parent Artery

When giant aneurysms cannot be occluded at the neck or if they rupture during surgery, proximal occlusion or trapping of their parent segment becomes the method of choice, provided that there is no great risk of ischemia in its distal territory.

Proximal Occlusion

This method is indicated only when there is sufficient evidence of a good collateral blood supply. According to Drake, if puncturing the sac causes relatively profuse bleeding during proximal temporary clamping, the retrograde distal circulation supply can be considered satisfactory enough to avoid irreversible ischemia. Although this test (if positive) generally justifies a definitive proximal occlusion, this author recommends, for safety, that it be carried out by the tourniquet method (see Fig. 85).

The results of this method, essentially evaluated from Drake's series, are set forth below according to the main topographic types of giant aneurysms.

Carotid Artery Bifurcation

(two cases both with good results)

Concerning the proximal occlusion procedure, in the group of giant aneurysms arising from the carotid artery itself, only two Drake's cases, of the bifurcation variety, were described in detail. In both cases the occlusion was made as close to the bifurcation as possible, in order to avoid ischemia in the anterior choroidal artery. Since complete thrombosis of the sac could not be achieved, an additional clipping at the origin of the A_1 segment of the anterior cerebral artery was performed, after an extra-intracranial bypass to protect the middle cerebral artery was made.

Middle Cerebral Artery

(four cases, all with good results)

In only four of Drake's giant aneurysms of the middle cerebral artery treated with a proximal occlusion were the operative technique and results detailed. The tourniquet was placed so as to preserve the perforating lenticulostriate arteries. All four cases achieved good results; three of them underwent a prior extra-intracranial bypass.

Anterior Communicating Artery

(one case, with good result)

In aneurysms in which the neck is not clippable, recourse may be had to occlusion of the dominant cerebral artery, immediately proximal to the ACA_1–ACA_2 junction (Fig. 86). This palliative technique, recommended by Logue in 1956, was quite widely used between 1950 and 1975 (review of the literature by Hockley [22] and by Karvounis et al. [27]) because of its effectiveness in preventing hemorrhagic recurrences as compared with more conservative treatment. The tourniquet procedure makes it possible to apply this method progressively and under clinical monitoring.

In the case of Drake, the tourniquet was placed in the A_1 segment of the dominant anterior cerebral artery, thus causing a partial thrombosis of the sac.

The indications for this method could be broadened by placing a tourniquet on both ACA_1s, after performing a bilateral extra-intracranial bypass on the cortical branches of the anterior cerebral arteries, as Ishii et al. [24] did in one case, or by developing an internal transposition of A_2 to contralateral A_2 and excise the aneurysm sac, as reported by Ausman and Diaz.

Posterior Cerebral Artery

(five cases, all with good results)

Proximal occlusion was performed in four cases by clipping and in one case by tourniquet, at the closest possible point to the aneurysm in order

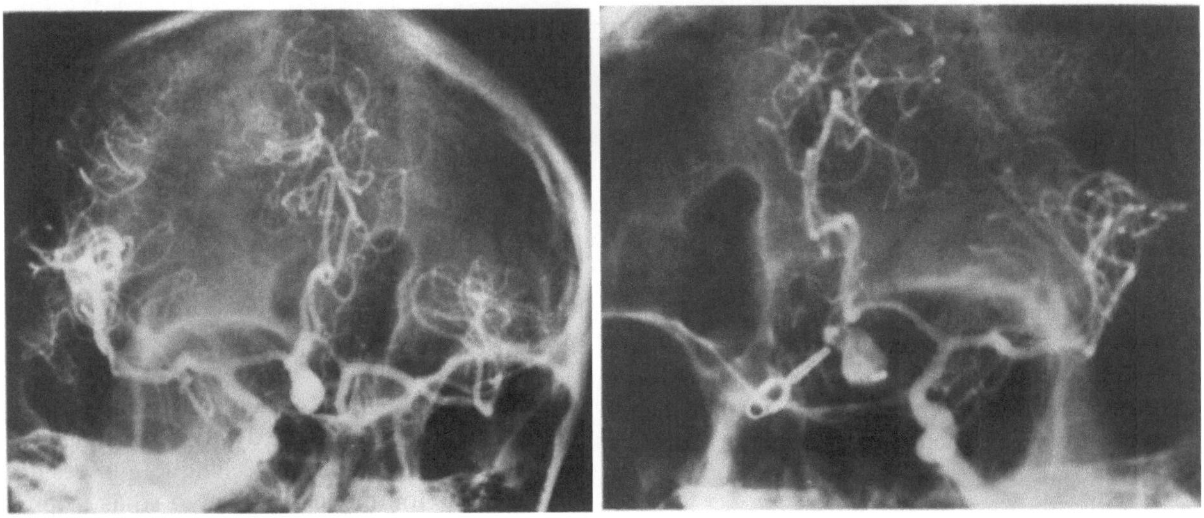

Fig. 86. G.B., a 58-year-old male. Giant aneurysm of the anterior communicating artery, partly thrombosed, of the pseudotumoral optic-chiasmatic type. As neck clipping was impracticable without running excessive risks, clipping of the dominant anterior cerebral artery was performed distal to the branches leading to the right anterior perforated substance. Postoperative course uneventful, with normalization of visual disturbances. Angiographic follow-up of the left carotid artery on the 20th day shows the persistence of injection of the aneurysmal sac by the left ACA_1 (*right*)

to protect the collaterals penetrating into the posterior perforated substance and the brainstem.

Kondo et al. [28] have also reported a case of posterior cerebral artery aneurysm managed by proximal clipping with clinical and radiological success.

Extra-intracranial bypass on the posterior cerebral artery can reduce the risk of ischemia [56].

Superior Cerebellar Artery
(two cases, with one good result)

In one of the cases treated by proximal clipping, the clip had occluded the origin of the posterior cerebral artery and of its surrounding branches, leading to an infarct of the posterior cerebral artery territory.

In these types, an extra-intracranial bypass can be performed between the superficial temporal artery and the superior cerebellar artery by the transtentorial subtemporal approach [1].

Trapping

Indications

When an aneurysm cannot be occluded at the neck, trapping is justified in three particular situations:

1. In an emergency, when the aneurysm ruptures during dissection and the neck cannot be successfully clipped.
2. As a rule, when the aneurysm has manifested through an embolic mechanism.
3. Secondarily, after proximal occlusion, when follow-up angiography shows the absence of sac thrombosis (Fig. 87).

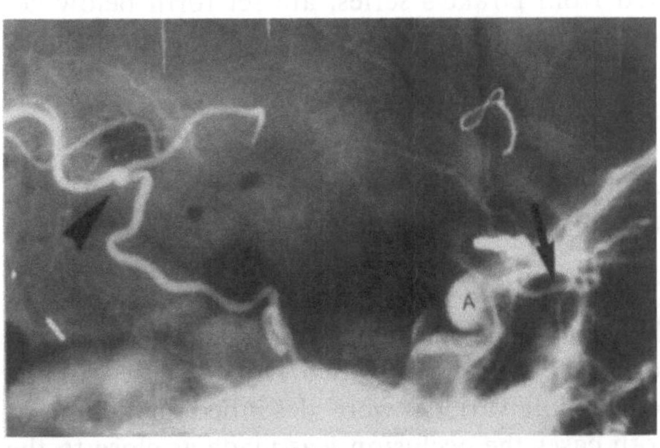

Fig. 87. M.V., a 31-year-old female. Asymptomatic aneurysm located astride the roof of the left cavernous sinus (in a patient operated on by neck clipping of an anterior communicating artery aneurysm of the hemorrhagic type. The aneurysm (*A*) was managed by a left cervical carotid artery ligation, preceded by an extra-intracranial bypass (*arrowhead*). Although this is not a case of a giant aneurysm, it is presented in order to demonstrate that *proximal occlusion does not always succeed in producing rapid thrombosis of the sac.* Follow-up angiography on the 12th postoperative day shows that the aneurysm is reinjected by the ophthalmic artery, which flows countercurrent (*arrow*)

In order to ascertain that the intrasaccular thrombosis is complete and stable, repeated CT examinations are indispensable [25], for the angiographic study after proximal occlusion of the parent artery may not be reliable enough. In some cases, thrombosis occurs within the 1st week of the proximal ligation, while in others it may gradually develop by successive layers of laminar thrombus formation and fibrosis of the aneurysm wall. In completely thrombosed aneurysms, CT examinations may demonstrate progressive reversal of the mass effect. On the other hand, it may show a remaining nonthrombosed stump at the neck level, which may lead – even if it is small – to a secondary rupture [31].

Method

Because it excludes the aneurysm, the trapping procedure is a generally effective method. Moreover, it allows excision of the sac, when this compresses the neighboring structures.

It carries the risk of ischemia through two mechanisms: (a) like for proximal occlusion, by producing ischemia in the distal territory; (b) by including some unexpected collaterals of the parent segment in the trapping.

This second eventuality could have serious consequences: ischemia in the territory of the collaterals and/or retrograde feeding of the aneurysm sac through peripheral anastomoses. This can be

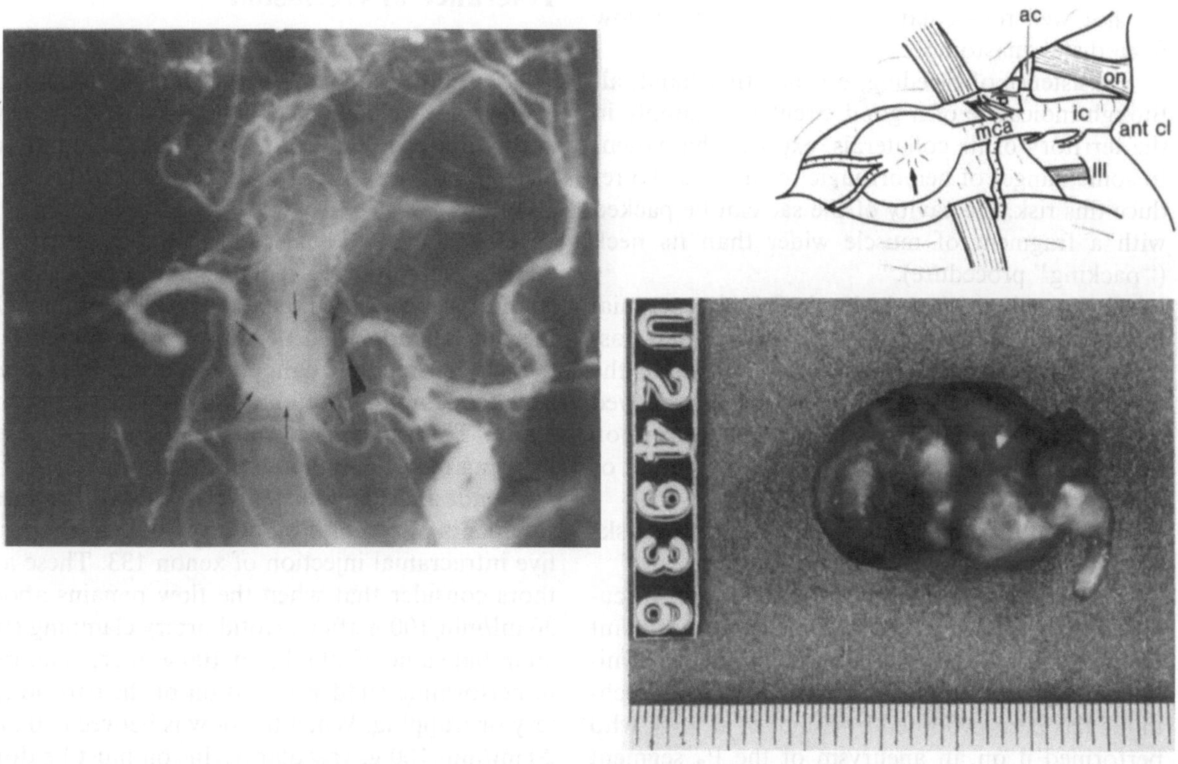

Fig. 88. R.B., a 56-year-old male. Right sylvian mycotic aneurysm, partly thrombosed, of the embolic and then hemorrhagic type. Endocarditis. Right sylvian embolism responsible for an infarct with left hemiplegia. Right carotid angiogram shows partial occlusion of the middle cerebral artery (*arrowhead*) and a mycotic aneurysm of the sylvian bifurcation (*small arrows*). The patient was treated with antibiotics and heparin; hemiplegia regressed partially. Two months later, digital venous subtraction angiography revealed considerable enlargement of the aneurysm. Heparin was stopped. However, 10 days later, the sudden onset of coma with hemiplegia from hemorrhagic rupture necessitated emergency surgery combining extra-intracranial bypass between the superficial temporal artery and the artery of the right angular gyrus, which remain patent; evacuation of the temporal hematoma; trapping of the aneurysm (30 mm long at its widest), which covered the entire sylvian bifurcation (*diagram*), and mass excision of the lesion, which was of friable consistency and was divided into numerous small chambers (operative specimen on *lower right*). Postoperative course: return to normal consciousness, but persistence of hemiplegia

Ant cl, anterior clinoid process; *ac*, anterior cerebral artery; *on*, optic nerve; *ic*, internal carotid artery; *mca*, M_1 cerebral artery

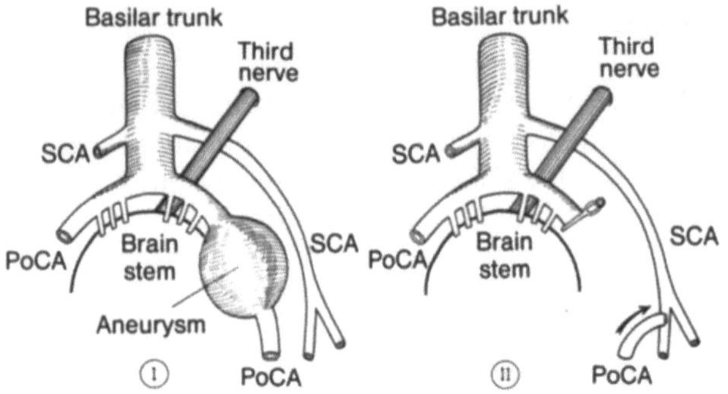

Fig. 89. Giant posterior cerebral artery (*PoCA*) aneurysm, managed by trapping and reimplantation of the distal segment (*arrow*) on the adjacent segment of the superior cerebellar artery (*SCA*). *III*, third nerve; *A*, aneurysm (after Sundt et al. [54])

screened by introducing a fine needle into the sac after trapping. Absence of bleeding does not, however, guarantee preservation of collaterals, if these are not well revascularized by a retrograde flow from distal anastomoses.

Persistence of bleeding, on the other hand, although indicative of a good circulatory supply in the territory of its collaterals, exposes the patient to some danger of hemorrhagic recurrence. To reduce this risk, the cavity of the sac can be packed with a fragment of muscle wider than its neck ("packing" procedure).

Commonly used at the level of the intracranial internal carotid artery when the anterior and posterior communicating arteries are functional, the trapping procedure has only rarely been employed in other aneurysmal locations, with the exception of certain sylvian aneurysms of the serpentine or the mycotic type.

Extra-intracranial bypass can reduce the risks of ischemia.

Occasionally, microsurgical intracranial vascular techniques can make it possible to reimplant the extremity of the distal arterial segment, terminolaterally, on a neighboring artery. This technique has been proposed by Sundt et al. [54], who performed it on an aneurysm of the P_2 segment of the posterior cerebral artery (Fig. 89, I) by reimplanting the distal segment of the posterior cerebral artery on the adjacent segment of the superior cerebellar artery (Fig. 89, II).

Other types of arterial repair can be performed, as in a 17-year-old patient seen by the authors with a partially thrombosed giant aneurysm (of the serpentine type) located at the peripeduncular portion of the left posterior cerebral artery, of which the aneurysmal mass and the parent segment were trapped and resected. The 4-cm gap was repaired using a graft harvested from the superficial temporal artery (April 1986). The graft, which was patent at the end of the surgery, was only slightly visible on the follow-up angiogram because of spasms at the origin of the posterior cerebral artery. A proposal of further angiography was rejected by the patient, whom outcome was normal with the exception of a single epileptic seizure.

Tolerance of Occlusion

Whatever the palliative method may be, it can be made more reliable and safer by a quantitative evaluation of tolerance of temporary clamping of the parent artery using measurements of pressure and flow.

Hosobuchi [23] has established that, when distal residual pressure remains above a mean of 50 mmHg, occlusion is generally well tolerated. On the other hand, when it is lower than 50 mmHg, there is considerable danger of ischemia, and tolerance to clamping should not be prolonged beyond 5 min. This time span can be slightly increased by using hypothermia and barbiturates.

Sundt and Piepgras [55] have carried out measurements of cerebral blood flow with intraoperative intracranial injection of xenon 133. These authors consider that when the flow remains above 30 ml/min/100 g after carotid artery clamping (for an initial value of 50 ml/min/100 g) there is no risk in performing sudden occlusion of the carotid artery or trapping. When the flow is between 30 and 20 ml/min/100 g, vascular occlusion must be done with a progressive clamping system. If the flow is less than 20 ml/min/100 g, occlusion is extremely dangerous and if done, must be preceded by an extra-intracranial bypass.

Implantable Vascular Occluder

A progressive and reversible system of occlusion of the parent arteries in giant aneurysms was designed especially for this report. It is applicable not only to cervical but also to intracranial arteries and affords a means of checking arterial flow by the study of the Doppler effect (M. Sindou, D. Cathignol, Y. Keravel, and J. Szapiro, unpublished experimental study; Fig. 90).

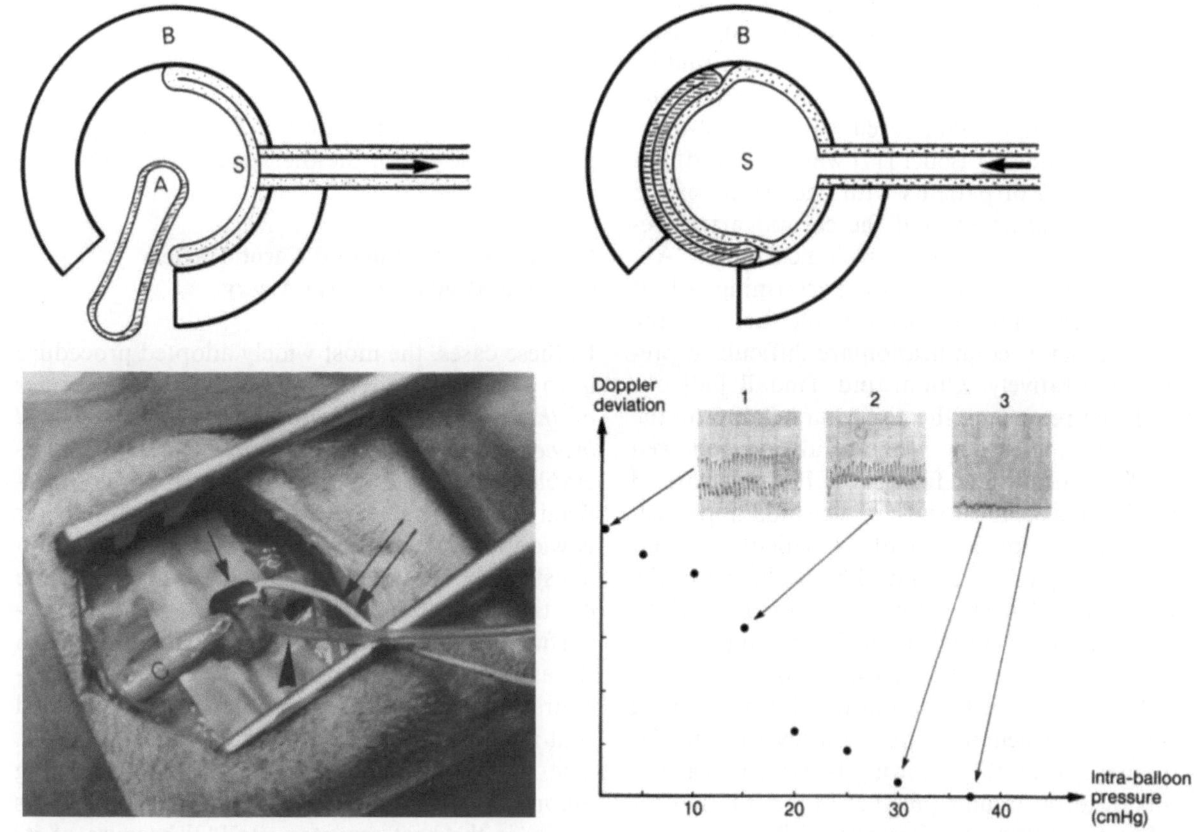

Fig. 90. Implantable vascular occluder.
Top Principle of the clamp, seen in transverse section. Incomplete ring (*B*) (7/8ths of a circle) made of rigid plastic with a 6-mm outer diameter and a 4-mm inner diameter to place round the artery (*A*, *hatched lines*) and equipped with an inflatable silicone balloon (*S*), connected to a catheter allowing inflation by saline with contrast medium (*arrow*). *Top left* Insertion of the artery (*A*) within the ring; *top right* artery occluded by the inflated balloon (*S*).
Lower left Clamp (*C*) in place on the common carotid artery in a dog. A Doppler microprobe (*arrow*), perfected by Cathignol et al. (CETAC, INSERM U 37, Lyon), is incorporated into the ring (*arrow*) and linked to a transducing cable (*double arrow*) satellite of the catheter (*arrowhead*). The clamp can be implanted on the parent artery proximally to the giant aneurysm in accordance with the technical requirements of the tourniquet and then, secondarily, inflated progressively under clinical, electroencephalographic, and where necessary angiographic guidance, with the subject awake. If occlusion is well tolerated, the proximal end of the catheter is closed with a clip or a polymerizable substance and is then introduced, together with the transmitting cable of the Doppler probe, in the subcutaneous tissue.
Lower right Doppler recording of the carotid artery in the dog before (*1*), during (*2*), and at the end (*3*) of balloon inflation, allowing evaluation of the degree of occlusion of the artery in relation to the pressure within the balloon. Clamps of varying diameters have been designed for performing occlusion of the cervical or intracranial internal carotid artery (large), vertebral artery, basilar trunk or sylvian artery (medium sized), and more distal arteries (small)

Extra-intracranial Bypass

Introduced in 1967 by Yasargil [64, 65] and Donaghy [13], the extra-intracranial bypass (EICB) can be useful before occlusion of the parent artery by reducing the risk of ischemia [50, 51] (Fig. 91).

As Miller et al. have demonstrated [39], carotid ligations are well tolerated, even after rigorous selection of the patients, in only 80% of cases. Thrombotic or embolic occlusions of the middle cerebral artery are tolerated at an even lower rate. These data should be compared with the post-mortem study made by Fischer [17] who observed that 90% and 67% of patients with occlusions of the middle cerebral artery and the carotid artery respectively had a history of neurological deficit. Another weighty argument for performing EICB prior to therapeutic occlusion is the fact that the risks of ischemic complication are difficult to predict preoperatively. Odom and Tindall [40] observed that reopening the temporary clamp on the internal carotid artery was not always followed by regression of the deficits, even if it was carried out as soon as clinical signs of ischemia appeared. This was true for 22 out of 34 patients in their series of 220 patients managed by occlusion of the internal carotid artery. Moreover, reopening of the clamp can lead to embolism of clots from the internal carotid artery to the middle cerebral artery.

These risks can be diminished by performing an EICB, the hemodynamic efficacy of which is demonstrated by the following facts: (a) measurements of intravascular pressure in the internal carotid and middle cerebral arteries, following occlusion, show that there is a considerable increase in residual pressure after the EICB; (b) flow measurements on the superficial temporal artery before and after clamping the parent artery [53, 54] show that an EICB is capable of contributing up to 200 ml/min to the cerebral flow in some extreme cases. This is particularly so when angiography reveals that the bypass feeds the whole sylvian territory (Fig. 92).

Besides these immediate hemodynamic benefits, EICB can ward off late complications, like: chronic circulatory insufficiency during development of the atheromatous involution [6, 34, 38, 41], onset of arterial hypertension secondary to the loss of a cerebral pedicle [63], and formation of aneurysms as a result of increased flow in the collateral circulation [19, 21, 22, 23, 27, 63].

Methods

The choice of a site for the EICB naturally depends on the site of the therapeutic occlusion.

Occlusion of the Internal Carotid Artery or of the Middle Cerebral Artery

In these cases, the most widely adopted procedure is to site the EICB *between one of the branches of the superficial temporal artery and a cortical branch of the middle cerebral artery* [20]. It is preferable to choose the posterior branch of the superficial temporal artery, provided that its diameter is wide enough, so as not to endanger the natural anastomoses between its anterior branch and the ophthalmic artery. When the diameter of the superficial temporary artery is too small, or when it has been impaired by a previous approach, recourse may be had to the occipital artery, provided that its diameter and length are large enough [61]. The choice of cortical artery varies according among the authors. Apparently the angular gyrus artery is the best receptor site [43] because of its constant topography (5–6 cm vertically from the external auditory meatus), its location prolonging the sylvian axis, its wide diameter, and its good tolerance to temporary clamping, including on the dominant side. Moreover, its posterior location renders the bypass safe for subsequent surgical manipulations during the direct surgical pterional approach for aneurysms of the carotid artery territory.

In certain cases where no artery of the scalp is usable, recourse may be had to a bypass with a *venous graft* after the principle of Lougheed et al. [37], who initially described this technique between

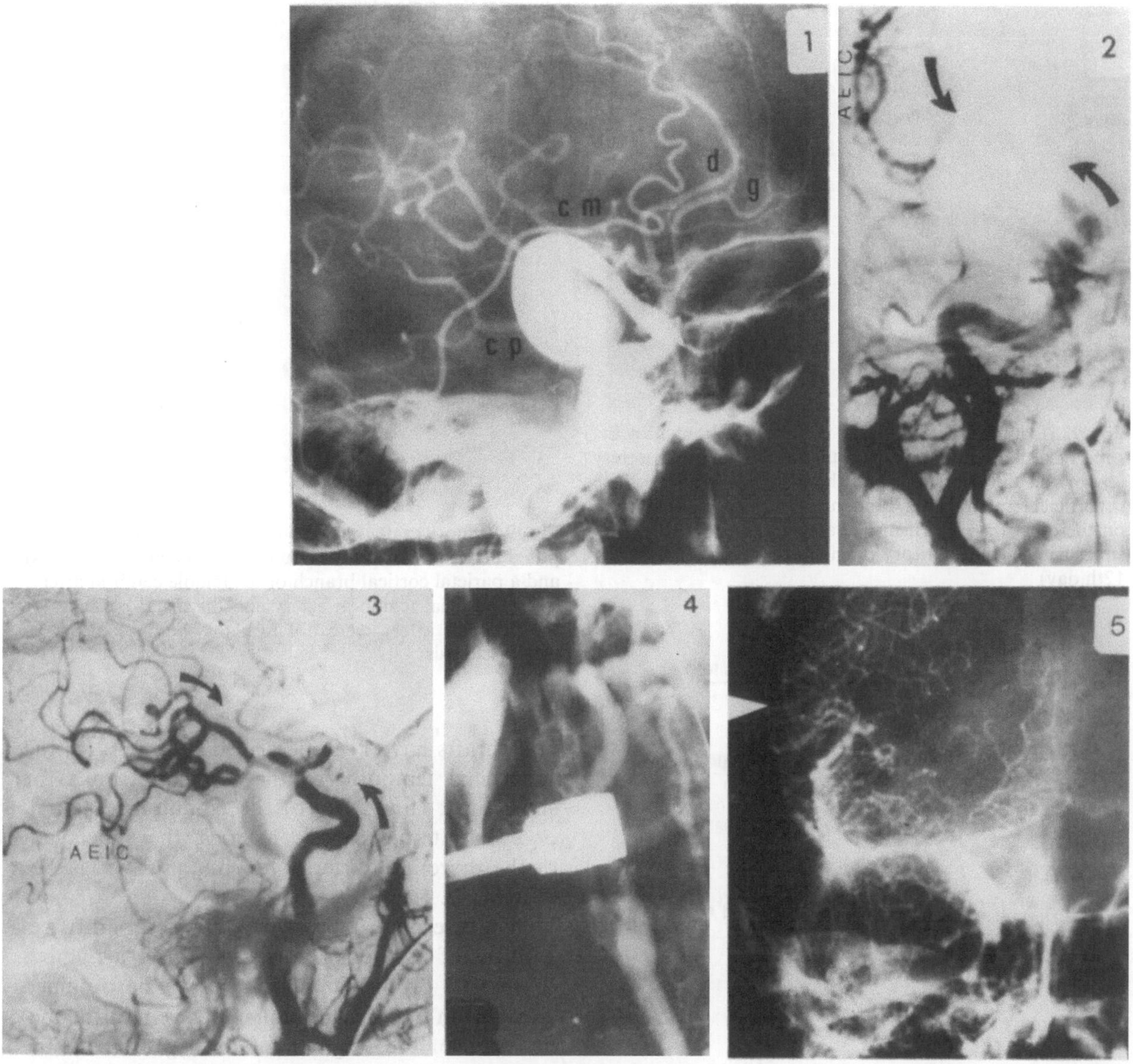

Fig. 91. J.R., a 54-year-old female. Aneurysm of the right posterior communicating artery, nonthrombosed, of the hemorrhagic type with left hemiparesis, managed by cervical occlusion and EICB. Angiographic assessment (*1*) reveals that the right carotid artery supplies not only the middle cerebral artery (*cm*) and the right anterior cerebral artery (*d*) but also the left anterior cerebral artery (*g*) and the right posterior cerebral artery (*cp*). Right cervical carotid artery compression leads within 3 min to loss of consciousness, totally reversible after removal of compression.

The operation was performed in several stages: first, EICB (*AEIC*) between the superficial temporal artery and the angular gyrus artery, together with positioning of a Selverstone clamp on the right cervical internal carotid artery; secondly, progressive tightening of the clamp over 15 days. Carotid angiogram performed on the 13th day of tightening – the carotid lumen being reduced by approximately on half (*4*) – shows on the frontal (*2*) as well as on the lateral view (*3*) that the flow arising from the internal carotid artery and the flow arising from the bypass (*arrows*) meet at the level of the aneurysm. Thirdly, replacement of the clamp by a ligation in the neck, after maximum tightening of the latter.

Four-vessel follow-up angiography shows no injection of the aneurysm. Right external carotid artery angiogram (*5*) reveals that the EICB (*arrowhead*) vascularizes the whole of the right hemisphere. Uneventful postoperative course, but persistence of slight left spastic hemiparesis of 5 years' duration

the common carotid artery and the supraclinoid internal carotid artery in case of thromboembolic occlusion of the internal carotid artery. Several variations of this type of bypass can be performed. They may be directed to the supraclinoid carotid artery, the middle cerebral trunk, or, more easily, to a sylvian cortical branch. Many different proximal sites of implantation for interposed ve-

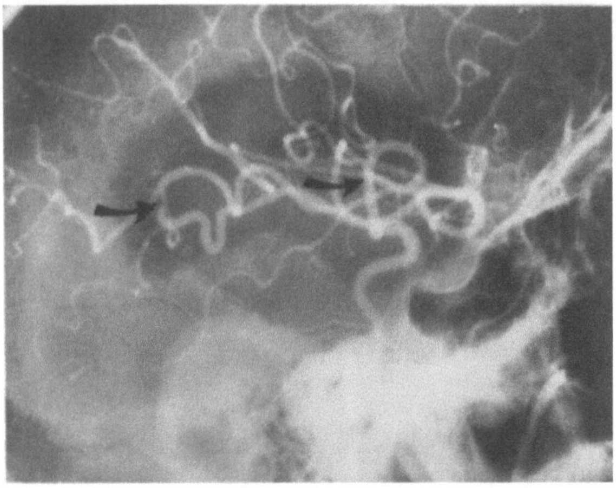

Fig. 92. Double EICB, between the anterior branch of the superficial temporal artery and the middle temporal artery (*arrow*) on the one hand, and the posterior branch of the superficial temporal artery and the posterior temporal artery on the other (*arrow*), ensuring vascularization of the entire superficial sylvian territory (angiographic follow-up on the 12th day)

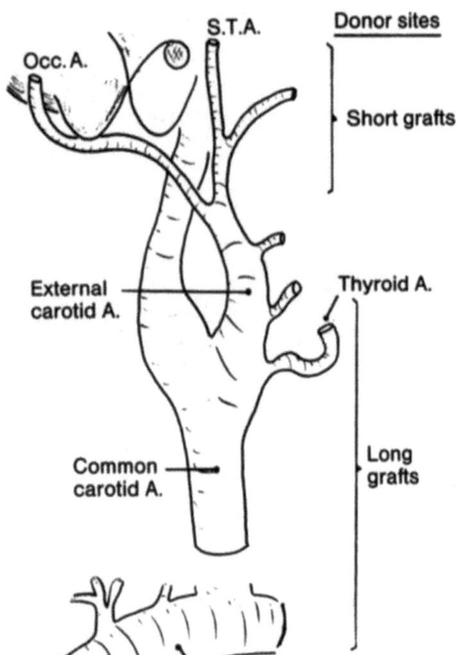

Fig. 93. Proximal sites for short and long interposed venous grafts. When the proximal implantation is made at the subclavian, the common, or the external carotid level, the anastomosis is of the end-to-side type. As these arteries are big and often arteriosclerotic, the arteriotomy must be performed doing a small resection of the wall and may sometimes benefit from a limited local endarteriectomy. When the graft is inserted in the thyroid, the superficial temporal, or the occipital arteries, and end-to-end anastomosis is generally preferred

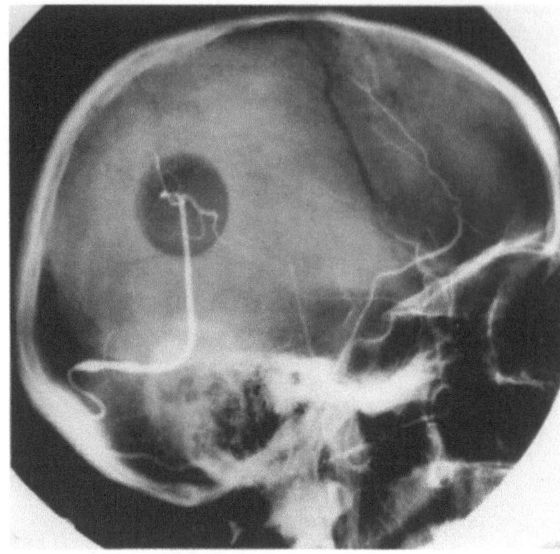

Fig. 94. Short graft, harvested from the sural vein, interposed between the occipital trunk (end-to-end anastomosis) and a parietal cortical branch of the middle cerebral artery. The superficial temporal artery and the distal branches of the occipital artery were not available because of severe arteriosclerosis

nous grafts have been described (Fig. 93): (a) the superficial temporal or the occipital trunks for short graft (Fig. 94); (b) the common, external, or even internal carotid arteries, the subclavian or the thyroidian arteries for long graft (Figs. 95, 96, 97) [52, 56, 60].

The use of a bypass with a venous graft, regardless of its topographic type, raises a number of specific problems. The graft can be obtained either from the internal saphenous vein in the medial side of the thigh or of the leg or from the external saphenous vein taken from the posterior aspect of the leg. The saphenous vein in the thigh, having a greater diameter, makes it possible in theory to obtain a better flow; but its connection to the cortical artery can give rise to specific technical problems linked with congruence defects, owing to the diameter of the lumen and the thickness of the walls (Fig. 98). Accordingly, the choice of the external saphenous vein or of the internal saphenous vein of the leg seems preferable when the receptor artery has a narrow diameter. The subcutaneous bed along the course of the graft must present no zone of compression, nor kinking, nor axial torsion or strangling by adventitial retraction, the more so as venous grafts carry a particular risk of wall collapse. Moreover, their great liability to thrombosis, heightened by the existence of two anastomotic sites, raises the problem of

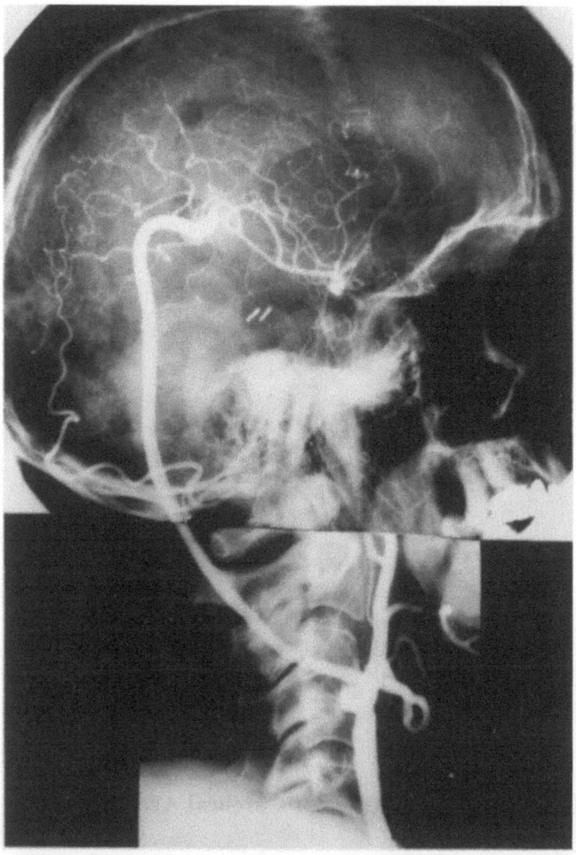

Fig. 95. Long graft, harvested from the saphenous vein, interposed between the thyroid artery (end-to-end anastomosis) and the gyrus angularis cortical branch of the middle cerebral artery. The superficial temporal artery was not available because of a previous frontotemporal approach

the advisability of associated anticoagulation, antiaggregation and/or antisludge therapy, which can be hazardous in the presence of an aneurysm. If rendered necessary because the branches of the external carotid artery are not usable, the bypass with venous grafts can be of help, as is evidenced by several observations, particularly as the measurements of flow at their level have shown that they are sometimes capable of contributing much more to arterial flow than does the arterial EICB.

Because of its higher flow, some authors, like Sundt and Piepgras (personal communication, 1986) prefer systematically to use interposed venous grafts rather than performing superficial temporal artery-middle cerebral artery (STA-MCA) anastomosis when acute occlusion of the carotid artery is needed.

Others, by contrast, give preference to STA-MCA anastomoses because of their higher patency rate (95% versus 50–91%), every time good circulation can be demonstrated in the external carotid system. In our group, we only consider interposed venous grafts to be indicated in patients with: (a) a thrombosed or stenotic external carotid artery, (b) excessively thin or short scalp branches, or (c) destruction of the STA due to previous cranial surgery. Provided technical faults can be avoided (Fig. 99) and the extra-intracranial pressure gradient is good, interposed venous graft can offer

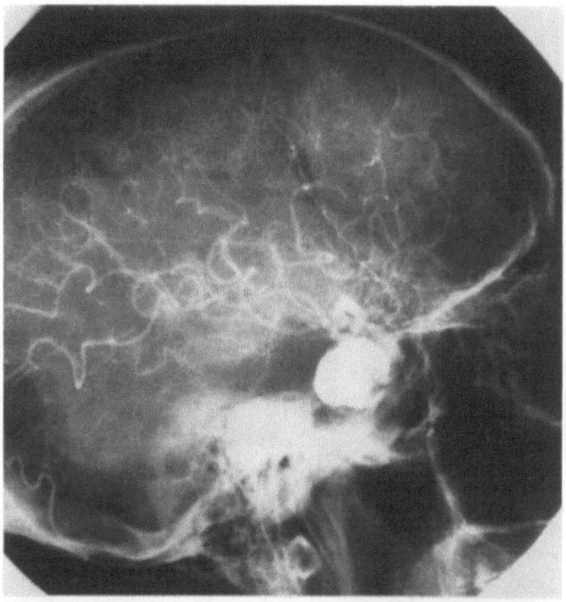

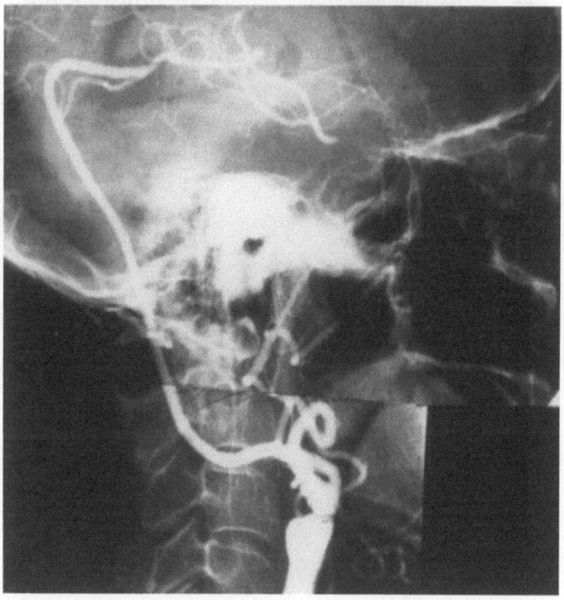

Fig. 96. Giant aneurysm of the right intracavernous carotid artery. Superficial temporal and occipital arteries not available because of inadequate size and length (*top*), long graft, harvested from the saphenous vein, interposed between the external carotid artery (end-to-side anastomosis) and the gyrus angularis cortical branch of the middle carotid artery before ligation of the internal carotid artery (*bottom*)

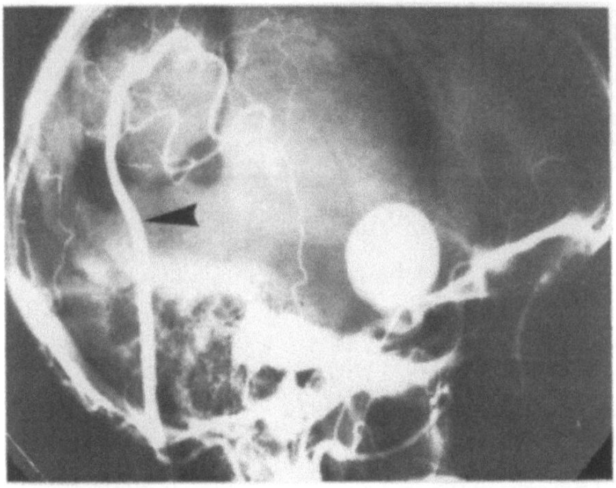

Fig. 97. G.M., a 50-year-old female. Right carotid-ophthalmic aneurysm, nonthrombosed, of the pseudotumoral type. Management by EICB between the external carotid artery and a parietal branch of the sylvian artery by means of a venous graft (*arrowhead*), which is followed by proximal occlusion of the intracavernous carotid artery with a Fogarty catheter. The postoperative course is uneventful, with improvement of visual disturbance

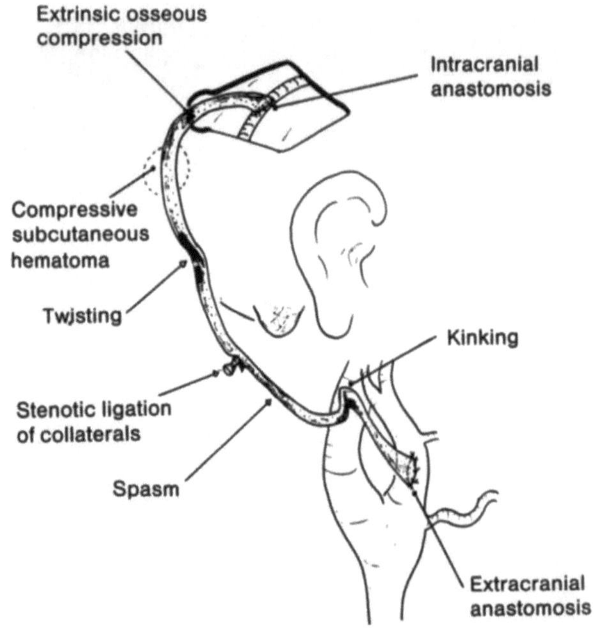

Fig. 99. Main technical causes of failure in graft patency (modified from [11a])

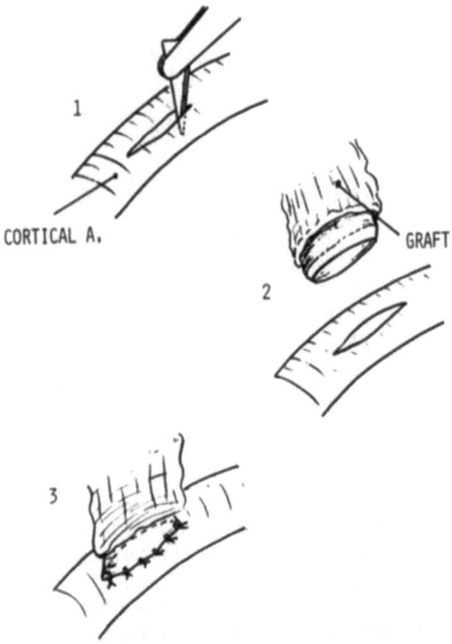

Fig. 98. The distal anastomosis on the cortical artery is of the end-to-side type. As the wall of the graft is most often thicker than the cortical wall, a total and partial coronal resection of the adventitial and the muscular layer of the vein, respectively, may be useful, in order to improve the congruence between the two vessels

valuable protection for therapeutic parent artery occlusion. Table 13 shows the authors' own experience, and Table 14 summarizes the literature review of extra-intracranial bypass using venous grafts.

Occlusion of the Anterior Cerebral Artery

In this case, a bypass can be performed between the superficial temporal artery and a distal branch of the anterior cerebral artery, where necessary with a venous graft in between: Ishii et al. [32].

Occlusion of the Vertebrobasilar System Arteries

Even though very few bypasses have been performed for the therapeutic occlusion of the arteries of the vertebrobasilar system, they can be of help [28, 57, 59]. Sundt et al. [59] were the first to treat a case of an aneurysm of the dominant vertebral artery operated on by the transtentorial subtemporal approach, by intracranial proximal occlusion preceded (during the same operation) by a bypass with an internal saphenous vein graft between the external carotid artery and the anterior segment of the second portion of the posterior cerebral artery. The publications dealing with the EICB document the possibility of successsfully performing several varieties of bypass in relation to the topography of arterial occlusion (Fig. 100). These are the bypass between: (a) occipital artery and posterior-inferior cerebellar artery (OA-PICA; Fig. 101): Khodadad et al. [35], Sundt and

Table 13. Extra-intracranial arterial bypasses using venous grafts (15 cases)

Etiologies	
Occlusive diseases	4
Cavernous sinus tumors	4
Giant aneurysms	7
Types of bypass (proximal sites)	
Common carotid artery (end/side)	2
External carotid artery (end/side, 5; end/end, 1)	6
Internal carotid artery (end/end)	1
Thyroid artery (end/end)	2
Occipital artery (end/side, 1; end/end, 3)	4
Causes of failure	
Technical difficulties	2
Poor extra-intracranial pressure gradient	4
Too early withdrawal of heparin	1
Necessity of venous graft	
External carotid artery occlusion	3
Scalp artery not available	7
Superficial temporal artery revascularizing ophthalmic artery	1
Destruction of scalp artery due to earlier surgery	4
Results	
No mortality, no morbidity	
Patency rate (overall)	
initial (2 weeks)	$^{9}/_{15}$ (60%)
later (>1 yr)	$^{8}/_{15}$ (53%)
Patency according to extra-intracranial pressure gradient	
good	$^{8}/_{10}$ (80%)
poor	$^{1}/_{5}$ (20%)

Source: Sindou M, Daher A, Goutelle A (1986) Autogenous vein grafts for arterial brain revascularization. Proceedings of the 8th international conference on anastomoses for cerebral ischemia, Florence, Sept 1986

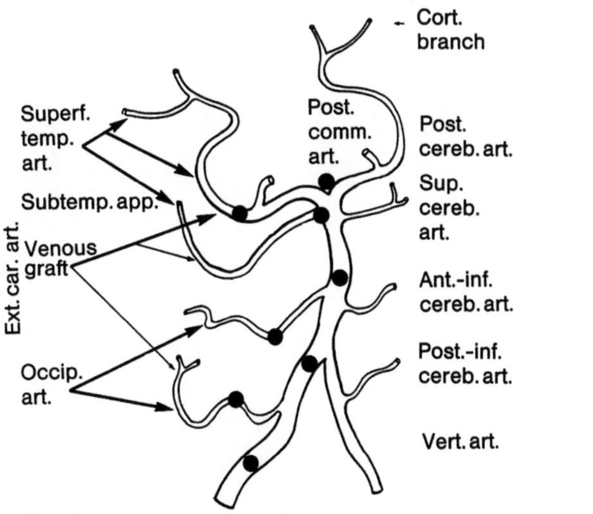

Fig. 100. Possible sites for EICB in the vertebrobasilar system in relation to aneurysmal locations

Piepgras [57]; (b) occipital artery and anterior inferior cerebellar artery (OA-AICA): Ausman et al. [3]; (c) superficial temporal artery and superior cerebellar artery (STA-SCA; Fig. 102): Ausman et al. [4, 5]; (d) superficial temporal artery and posterior cerebral artery (STA-PCA) or external carotid artery and posterior cerebral artery with a venous graft in between (VG (ECA-PCA): Sundt et al. [59]. These last authors have used such interposed venous graft on the posterior circulation in 73 occlusive diseases and 8 giant aneurysms.

Table 14. Extra-intracranial arterial bypasses using venous grafts (review of literature: 93 cases)

1. To:	Intracranial carotid artery (Lougheed [37], 1 case; Iwabuchi [33], 1)		
From:	Common carotid artery	1	Both patent
	Internal carotid artery	1	
2. To:	Middle cerebral artery (cortical branch) (Story [56], 1 case; Spetzler [52], 11; Samson [48], 25; Little [68], 21; Ausman [66], 1; Diaz [67], 17)		
From:	Subclavian artery	28	Patency rate 70%–90%
	Common or external carotid artery	17	Mortality 4%– 9%
	Superficial temporal or occipital artery	31	
3. To:	Anterior cerebral artery (cortical branch) (Ishii [32], 1 case)		
From:	Superficial temporal artery		Patent
4. To:	Posterior circulation (Sundt [59], 14 cases)		
From:	External carotid artery		Patency rate 79% Mortality 7%

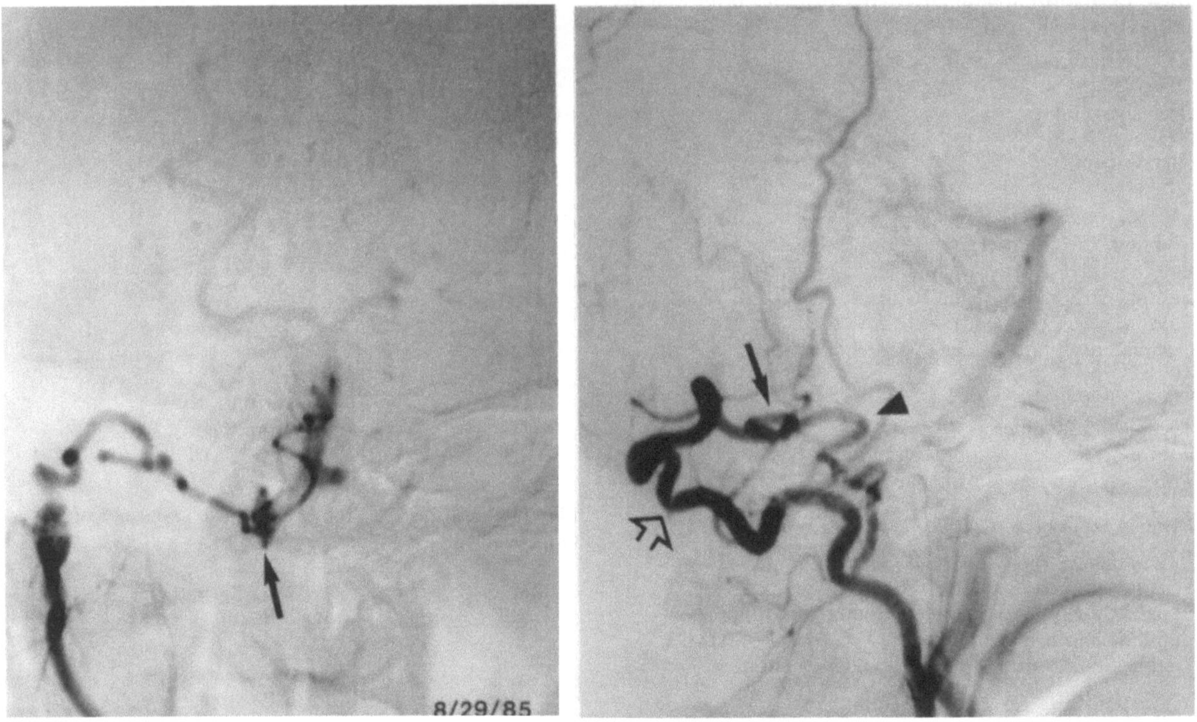

Fig. 101. Occipital artery to posterior-inferior cerebellar artery anastomosis. The AP (*left*) and lateral (*right*) angiographic views demonstrate patency of the anastomosis (*arrows*) between occipital artery (*open arrow*) and posterior-inferior cerebellar artery (*arrowhead*) (Photographs by courtesy of Professor F. Diaz, Henry Ford Hospital, University of Michigan)

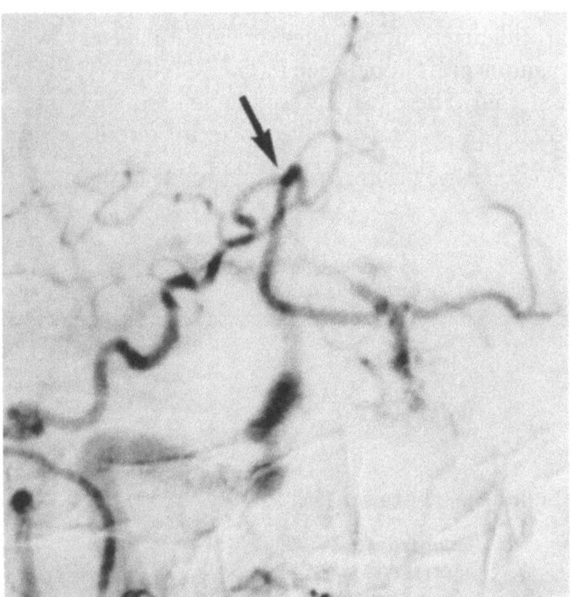

Fig. 102. Superficial temporal artery to superior cerebellar artery anastomosis. The AP angiographic view shows a good filling of the distal basilar artery through the patent anastomosis (*arrow*) (Photographs by courtesy of Professor F. Diaz, Henry Ford Hospital, University of Michigan)

Patency

The rate of patency of these cerebral revascularization methods applied to the anterior circulation is generally between 85% and 95%. Their risks can be evaluated from the cooperative studies by Reichmann [46], Samson and Boone [48] and Hopkins et al. [28]. The studies covered approximately 550 cases and were based essentially on series of atheromatous patients, with a mortality of 3%–4% and a morbidity with the following distribution: 2% local complications and 8% neurological deficits, of which 3% are permanent and generally secondary to hematomas [25, 36]. As far as we know, no study concerning the results of cerebral revascularization, methods applied to the posterior circulation has yet been carried out.

Applications in Giant Aneurysms

A bypass may be required in two different circumstances: during a direct surgical approach although not planned preoperatively, or planned, as a preliminary to therapeutic occlusion of the parent artery (Fig. 103).

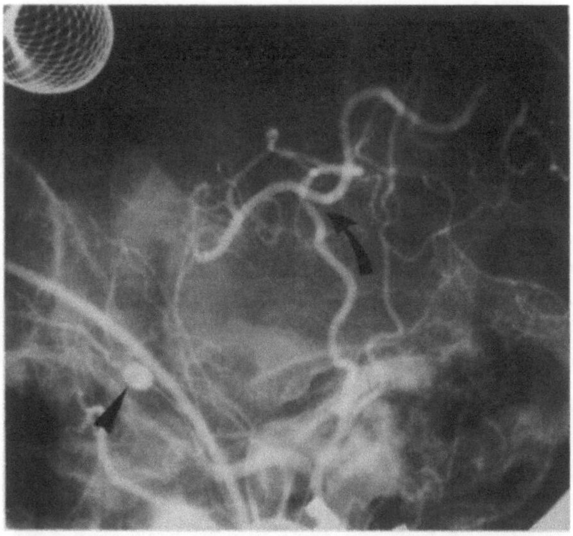

Fig. 103. Immediately postoperative angiogram of an EICB between the left superficial temporal artery and the left angular gyrus artery (*arrow*) performed prior to an occlusion of the intracranial internal carotid artery with a Fogarty catheter (*arrowhead*). Note the large area of the sylvian territory supplied the EICB from the time it is performed

Unplanned Bypass

The technical difficulties encountered during the direct surgical approach in attempting neck occlusion may be such that an EICB turns out to be necessary or at least useful during the operation. It is therefore safer to prepare in all cases both a skin flap to protect the branch of the corresponding external carotid artery and a craniotomy giving access to a receptor site. This can be useful in the case of obligatory occlusion of the parent artery owing to the impossibility of neck clipping or with rupture of the aneurysm at the attachment site requiring an emergency trapping. To a lesser degree, it can also be useful for improving tolerance to prolonged temporary clamping.

Middle cerebral artery territory can be revascularized by anastomosis of the superficial temporal artery or saphenous vein graft directly to one of the secondary trunks of the middle cerebral artery inside the sylvian fissure. This may be interesting in giant aneurysms of the middle cerebral trifurcation, especially when the parent artery or one of its branches has to be occluded or sacrificed as reported by Diaz et al. [12].

Planned Bypass

In programmed occlusions of the parent artery, the occlusion can be performed during the same procedure – immediately after the bypass – or at a later time. However, a prolonged delay to allow development of the bypass and to check its patency can expose the patient to two hazards. In the first place, the bypass may thrombose owing to a low pressure gradient between the extra- and intracranial areas [18]. The second hazard, by far the most dangerous, is that of the aneurysm rupturing, especially if it was first clinically revealed by a hemorrhage, as in one case of Drake's [14] and in another of Hosobuchi's [31]. Two accidents of this type even occurred in initially nonhemorrhagic aneurysms, one in the middle cerebral artery [49], the other in the upper basilar system [24]. Most authors therefore agree that the waiting time must be as short as possible, ending as soon as patency is proved by Doppler evaluation and/or angiography, the more so as the EICB may affect a large area relatively fast when the subject has nonatheromatous arteries, as shown in Fig. 103.

The case reported by Robbins et al. [47] provides an interesting illustration of possible consequences of flow augmentation through an EICB. As propagation of clot from a thrombosed middle cerebral artery produced transient ischemic attacks, an STA-MCA bypass was performed to augment cerebral blood flow. Postoperative angiography demonstrated filling of the aneurysm through improved collateral channels!

When the treatment of the aneurysm requires an *intracranial occlusion*, either by proximal occlusion (with clip or tourniquet) or by trapping, it can be performed during the same operative procedure as the bypass [15], immediately after the patency of the latter has been checked by micro-Doppler or electromagnetic flow measurements. Tolerance to clamping can be evaluated intraoperatively with electrocorticographic recordings and monitoring of cortical evoked potentials. Immediate occlusion is only justified when anastomotic conditions are good. The tourniquet procedure or a progressive implantable clamp closed at some interval from the operation, with clinical and electrophysiological monitoring, offers maximum safety.

When the treatment requires *cervical occlusion*, it is advantageous to perform it by means of a progressive clamping system put into position at the end of the bypass operation (Fig. 104). This allows immediate filling of the bypass by partial closure of the clamp, which favors the extra-intracranial pressure gradient. The degree of closure can be regulated on the basis of intravascular, Doppler, or electromagnetic flow measurements.

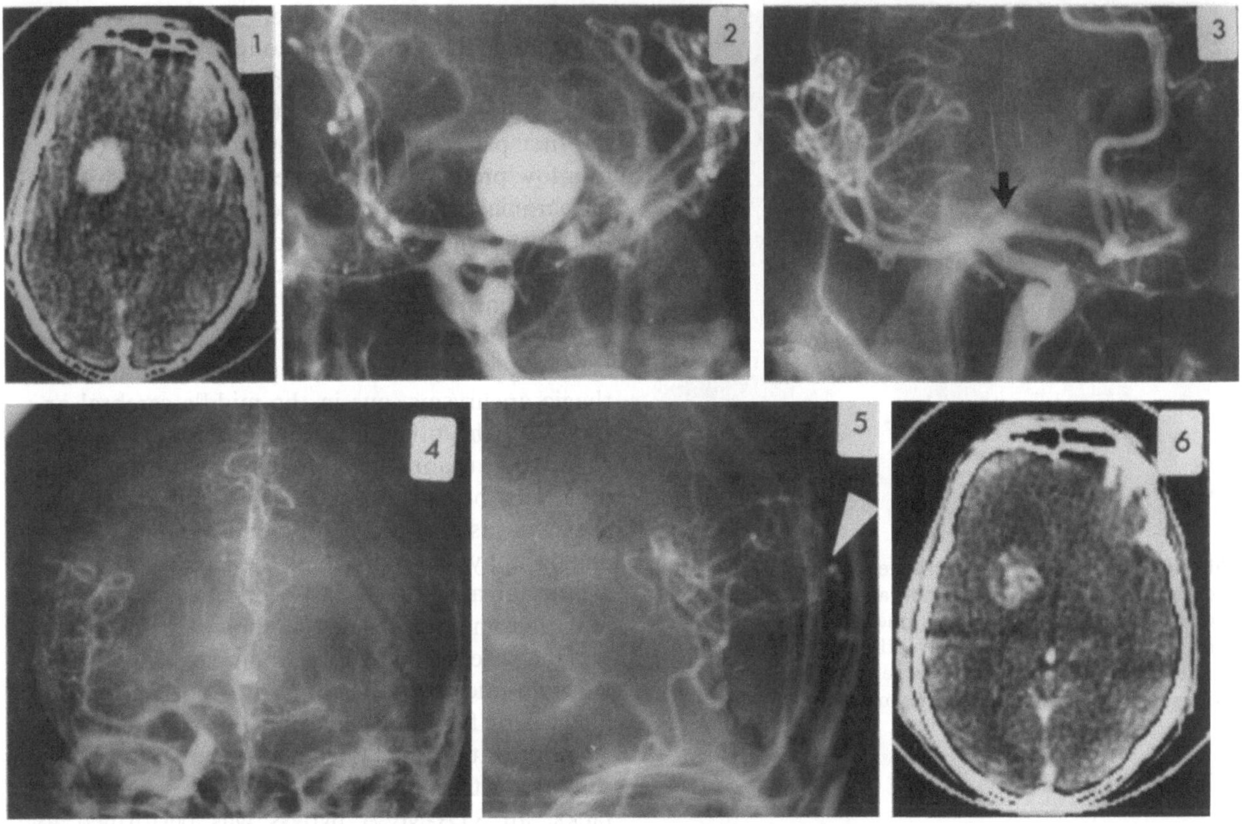

Fig. 104. J.L., a 40-year-old male. Aneurysm of the left carotid bifurcation, nonthrombosed, of the hemorrhagic type. Subarachnoid hemorrhage. CT scan shows the presence of blood at the base of the left basal ganglia, around a giant aneurysm located in front of the anterior perforated space (*1*). Four-vessel angiographic assessment reveals voluminous left carotid bifurcation aneurysm (*2*), as well as a small, symmetrical, saccular aneurysm (*arrow*) at the right carotid bifurcation (*3*). Operation one week later: first, EICB between the superficial temporal artery and a posterior branch of the sylvian artery; secondly, positioning of a Selverstone clamp on the left cervical internal carotid artery during the same operation. Tightening of the clamp 48 h later, after making sure of the patency of the bypass by Doppler sonography. The carotid artery can be occluded within 10 min and clinical assessment shows good tolerance to progressive tightening. Check-up on 12th day shows the absence of opacification of the giant aneurysm from either the right carotid artery (*4*) or from the vertebrobasilar axis. Left external carotid artery angiogram (*5*) shows the functional value of the EICB (*arrowhead*). Postoperative CT scan shows complete thrombosis of the sac (*6*)

The clamp is then occluded to a degree which induces an intravascular pressure intermediate between the values measured before and during the brief transient clamping. If an electromagnetic flowmeter is available and if there is enough space to take measurements distal to the clamp, the partial clamping may be carried out in accordance with flowmeter data. The clamp is then gradually tightened until the flow is reduced by 50%. The progressive tightening system is then occluded during the following few days, the patient being awake and under clinical and electrophysiological supervision, after checking the functionality of the bypass, at the very least using a Doppler flowmeter but preferably by angiography. Too slow tightening can be hazardous in that it favors clotting, with the risk of embolism into the distal circulation.

Location of the Bypass

The location must be chosen bearing in mind the possible necessity of performing subsequent surgery, either to carry out a trapping, if the proximal occlusion has failed to induce thrombosis of the sac, or to resect the aneurysmal mass, if it continues to manifest a space-occupying effect with clinical repercussions despite occlusion of the parent artery.

Results

Table 15 shows the results of 113 extra-intracranial bypasses for intracranial giant aneurysms. There was a 94% patency rate. Morbidity due to ischemic lesions secondary to the aneurysm sur-

Table 15. Results of 113 extra-intracranial bypasses for intracranial giant aneurysms

Authors	No. of cases	Type T H	Locali-zations ICA MCA	Type of bypass STA/MCA OA/MCA VB	Associated surgery ICA lig; Tr; To; Ex; Re; Wr; B	Patent bypass	Complications (when mentioned) I G	Oculomotor signs (when mentioned) – : aggravation ● : unchanged + : improvement
Ammerman and Smith	1	1 T	1 MCA	1 STA/MCA	1 Tr	1 +		
Drake	7	6 T 1 H	4 ICA 3 MCA	3 STA/MCA 2 OA/MCA 1 double STA/MCA + OA/MCA 1 VB	1 ICA lig 1 ICA lig + To 3 To (MI)	5 + 2 –	1 Death (hemorrhagic recurrence before ICA lig) 2 I (intolerance to definitive clamping + 1 hemiplegia)	
Hopkins and Grand	8	5 T 3 H	6 ICA 2 MCA	8 STA/MCA	6 ICA lig 1 Re 1 To + clipping + Ex.	7 + 1 –	2 Deaths G 3 I (2 hemiplegias, 1 hemiplegia + aphasia)	2 –
Hosobuchi	7		7 ICA	7 STA/MCA	6 ICA lig or Tr	6 +	1 Death (hemorrhagic recurrence before ICA lig)	
Iwabuchi et al.	1	1 T	1 ICA	1 VB	1 Tr + Ex	1 +	1 I (hemorrhagic infarct + hematoma)	
Sundt and Piepgras	13	13 H	11 ICA 2 MCA	13 STA/MCA	11 ICA lig 2 Tr + Ex	13 +	3 I (intolerance to definitive clamping)	3 ● 7+
Yonekawa and Yasargil	1		1 ICA	1 STA/MCA	1 ICA lig	1 +		
Bushe and Bockhorn	1	1 T	1 MCA	1 STA/MCA	Wr (1st operation) Re (2nd operation)	1 +	1 I (left hemiparesis)	
Césari et al.	1	1 T	1 ICA	1 STA/MCA	1 ICA lig	1 +		
Heros et al.	5		5 ICA	5 STA/MCA	5 ICA lig or Tr	No checkup	1 Death I 2 I	
Spetzler et al.	13	9 T 4 H	13 ICA	13 STA/MCA	13 ICA lig	13 +		5+ 5 ●
Brambilla et al.	1	1 T	1 ICA	1 STA/MCA	1 ICA lig	1 +	1 I (moderate aphasia)	1 +

Table 15 (continued)

Authors	No. of cases	Type T H	Locali-zations ICA MCA	Type of bypass STA/MCA OA/MCA VB	Associated surgery ICA lig; Tr; To; Ex; Re; Wr; B	Patent bypass	Complications (when mentioned) I G	Oculomotor signs (when mentioned) – : aggravation ● : unchanged + : improvement
Diaz et al.	6	5 T 1 H	6 ICA	5 STA/MCA 1 VB	6 ICA lig	6 +	3 I (regressive hemiparesis after clamp loosening)	2+ 2●
Scott et al.	1	1 T	1 MCA	1 STA/MCA	–	No checkup	1 Death (hemorrhagic recurrence before lig)	
Ouaknine	5	3 T 2 H	4 ICA 1 MCA	5 STA/MCA	5 ICA lig	5 +	3 I (TIA)	3 +
Debrun (Créteil, London, Boston)	6	6 T	6 ICA	6 STA/MCA	6 B	6 +	1 Death I	
Ferguson et al.	3		1 ICA 2 MCA	2 STA/MCA 1 STA + OA/MCA	3 To	3 +		
Albanese et al.	1	1 T	1 ICA	1 STA/MCA	1 Tr	1 +		1 +
Sindou	11	6 T 5 H	8 ICA 3 MCA	8 STA/MCA 2 OA/MCA 1 VB	9 ICA lig 2 Tr + Ex (MCA)	10 + 1 –	1 Death I (hemorrhagic infarct)	2 + 2●
Cooperative series SNCLF	21		20 ICA 1 MCA	21 STA/MCA	20 ICA lig 1 Tr + Ex (MCA)	19 + 2 –		
Total	113	47 T 29 H	96 ICA 17 MCA	103 STA/MCA 4 OA/MCA 2 double/MCA 4 VB	Occlusion of parent artery (except 3 cases)	100+/106 (94%) 6–/106 (6%)	1) Ischemic complications secondary to aneurysm surgery: 6 cases 2) Ischemic complications related to bypass insufficiency: 15 cases (16.8%)	

T, tumoral; *H*, hemorrhagic; *ICA*, inferior cerebellar artery; *MCA*, middle cerebral artery; *STA*, superficial temporal artery; *OA*, occipital artery; *VB*, venous bypass; *Tr*, trapping; *To*, tourniquet; *Ex*, excision; *Re*, resection; *Wr*, wrapping; *B*, carotid occlusion by balloon catheter; *I*, ischemic; *G*, general gery was 1%. Bypasses failed to prevent ischemia related to the occlusion of the parent artery in 15 cases (16.8%) including two deaths.

Comments

Even though the use of an EICB in conjunction with a therapeutic occlusion is a logical procedure, *its value in the prevention of ischemia is difficult to evaluate objectively.*

Comparison of the percentage of ischemic complications occurring in patients who had an EICB (17%) with the rate of intolerance to clamping in the group occluded without bypass (17%) does not argue in favor of the bypass. This lack of difference can be explained by the fact that occlusions without prior bypass were carried out after rigorous selection and in the majority with a progressive occluder, whereas most of the cases with a prior EICB were performed in patients considered intolerant to occlusion.

Although the effectiveness of the revascularization procedures remains statistically unproven in the fields of chronic cerebral circulatory insufficiency, most authors involved in the surgery of giant aneurysms estimate that EICB can be helpful when occlusion of a parent artery is needed.

If the benefit of EICB does not appear evident in patients with carotid artery aneurysms whose preoperative tests show good tolerance to compression (80% of cases according to Miller [39]), this does not hold when compression tests demonstrate intolerance to temporary occlusion. Recently (personal communication, 1986), Drake and Peerless reported 64 internal carotid occlusions in association with EICB, with 50 excellent results, 8 good results, 4 poor results, and 2 deaths.

However, while it is probably useful in reducing the risks of ischemia due to a decrease in blood flow after cervical carotid occlusions, EICB cannot, of course, totally protect the hemisphere from insults due to secondary embolic phenomena originating from the internal carotid clotting in the early period after its ligature [23].

On the other hand, EICB becomes definitely necessary for therapeutic occlusion of the middle cerebral artery, which is known to be attended by a very high rate of irreversible ischemic complications (90% according to Fischer's study [17]). This opinion, moreover, is shared by the team of Drake, Peerless, and Ferguson [16, 44], Hopkins and Spetzler [29, 30, 53, 54, 55], and Tognetti [62].

Even when the preoperative tests announce good tolerance of prolonged compression, EICB can ward off late complications like chronic circulatory insufficiency during the development of the atheromatous involution, onset of arterial hypertension secondary to the loss of a cerebral pedicle, and formation of aneurysms as a result of increased flow in the collateral circulation.

Finally, there are cases in which the indications for EICB is rarely discussed, as, for instance, in the presence of a preexisting carotid thrombosis in a different area from that of the aneurysm, or if there are multiple aneurysms [45], including one on the opposite side, which are liable to develop and rupture under the effect of a compensatory increased flow.

Whatever the field of application, the question of whether an EICB is indicated must be discussed with caution, according to rigorous selection criteria.

Tests for Tolerance of Therapeutic Occlusion

Evaluation of tolerance of occlusion is a precautionary measure to be taken prior to the management of any intracranial giant aneurysm, especially those located in the area perfused by the carotid artery.

Methods

Even though Matas' classic test, evaluating clinical and EEG effects of a 10-min digital compression of the cervical carotid artery, is considered somewhat unreliable, it nevertheless remains the only noninvasive means of reproducing preoperatively the effects of a subsequent therapeutic occlusion. To make it more valuable, it can be associated with a set of paraclinical explorations which evaluate as accurately as possible the anastomotic circulation and the capacity of the cerebral parenchyma to adapt to interruption of its proximal circulation.

Functional Exploration of Vascular Supply

Measurement of Flow by Doppler Flowmeter

When doing the Matas' test, placing an ultrasonic probe in the retromandibular space distal to the cervical digital compression makes it possible to ascertain whether the occlusion of the internal carotid artery is complete (Fig. 105). An increased flow in the contralateral carotid artery [6, 15, 27] reveals it to be involved in the supply of the hemisphere on the side of the compression via the anterior communicating artery. Recording flow in the angular artery of the orbit is of paramount importance in establishing whether or not compression leads to an inversion of the ophthalmic circulation. If this is combined with Strandness' test [13], which consists of compressing the superficial temporal artery, an indication is given of the functional value of the ophthalmic supply by the external carotid system. If the superficial temporal artery is substantially involved it is safer to keep its anterior branch intact and to use its posterior branch for performing the extra-intracranial anastomosis, or to undertake a bypass by means of an interposed venous graft branched onto the occipital trunk or the external carotid artery.

Cervical Intravascular Pressure

The pressure in the cervical internal carotid artery can be measured during four-vessel angiographic assessment not only morphologically but also dy-

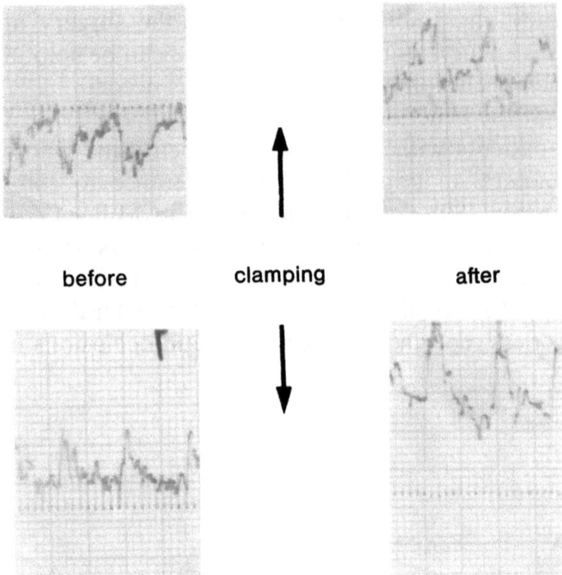

Fig. 105. Exploration by Doppler evaluation of the functional effectiveness of an extra-intracranial bypass during interruption of the internal carotid axis. *Top* Doppler recording of the ophthalmic artery before and after complete interruption of the cervical internal carotid artery with a Selverstone clamp. Note the inversion of the flow after clamping. *Bottom* Doppler recording of the superficial temporal artery before and after complete interruption of the internal carotid artery. Note the threefold increase of flow and its tendency to diastolic-like flow after clamping

namically. Carotid artery exploration must test the functional value of the anterior communicating artery by compression of the carotid artery on the side opposite to the axis undergoing angiography. Exploration of the vertebral axes must be accompanied by the Allcock procedure, i.e., successive compression of the two carotid arteries in order to bring the two posterior communicating arteries into function. Measurements of residual intravascular pressure can be carried out after digital cervical compression (in the knowledge that, although the latter affects only the common carotid artery, the internal carotid artery circulation can be stolen by the external carotid artery) or after introduction of an inflatable balloon catheter (see pp. 118–137).

Ophthalmodynamometry

A delicate but noninvasive examination, ophthalmodynamometry provides an indirect, but fairly reliable, reflection of pressure in the carotid-ophthalmic sector. If repeated during cervical carotid artery compression, it allows evaluation of residual pressure at that level.

Regional Cerebral Blood Flow Measurements

These can be carried out by means of xenon 133 (Fig. 106) either by intracarotid injection – if possible during angiographic exploration, in order not to repeat arterial punctures – or by inhalation,

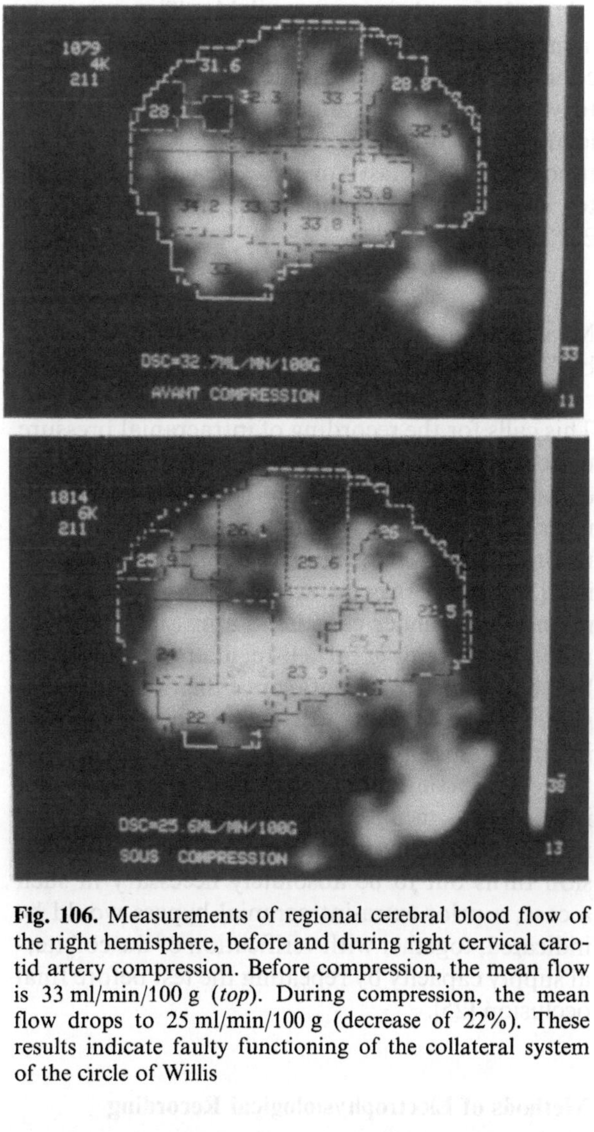

Fig. 106. Measurements of regional cerebral blood flow of the right hemisphere, before and during right cervical carotid artery compression. Before compression, the mean flow is 33 ml/min/100 g (*top*). During compression, the mean flow drops to 25 ml/min/100 g (decrease of 22%). These results indicate faulty functioning of the collateral system of the circle of Willis

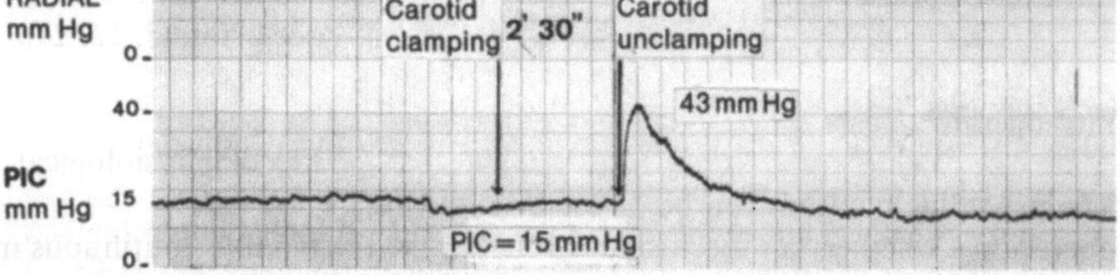

Fig. 107. Carotid clamping test, pathological, revealing an abnormal cerebral elastance with failing self-regulation. *PIC*, intracranial pressure measured with a frontal extradural receptor, homolateral to the clamping. Note the increase in PIC after unclamping. *PA*, mean systemic arterial pressure recorded in the radial artery. Time scale is in minutes. $FeCO_2 = CO_2$ fraction in expired air

this technique being now reliable. The measurements carried out after prolonged carotid artery compression make it possible to assess the circulatory reserves of anastomotic origin, as well as to identify low-flow zones with the aid of regional topography; this last can guide the choice of receptor site for the extra-intracranial bypass [5, 7, 9, 20, 21, 23].

Measurement of Cerebral Elastance by Recording of Intracranial Pressure

This calls for the recording of intracranial pressure under cervical compression after positioning of an extradural captor (Fig. 107). It should be held in reserve for exceptional cases for which preceding recordings suggest a high risk attendant on clamping [3, 18, 19]. An intracranial pressure that remains stable under carotid compression indicates the persistence of good self-regulation of the cerebral flow; this argues in favor of therapeutic occlusion. On the other hand, any substantial increase in intracranial pressure during compression – a fortiori if it continues to rise after the compression is released – means that there would be a major risk in performing therapeutic occlusion. If occlusion turns out to be absolutely necessary in such a case, a prior extra-intracranial bypass would be indicated, together with verification of the collateral supply capacity by repeating the test before final occlusion [25].

Methods of Electrophysiological Recording

Coupled with the vascular exploration tests, these methods are designed to evaluate the tolerance of the cerebral parenchyma to therapeutic occlusion. The sensitivity of *electroencephalography* can be improved by the techniques of automatic computerized analysis, which as a result make it more reliable. The recording of *cortical evoked potentials* can also be of use.

Intraoperative Tests

The preceding methods can be of use even during operation, whether an occlusion of a cervical carotid artery or of an intracranial artery is being performed. They are particularly useful during occlusion of the middle cerebral artery, the effects of which cannot be tested preoperatively.

Ultrasonographic Probes

The development of ultrasonographic probes of the Micro-Flotype [1, 2, 8], specially designed for vascular microsurgery, makes it possible at present to carry out Doppler study of intracranial arteries, including those of millimetric size [4, 8, 16].

Doppler study is of particular interest for intraoperative testing of the patency and functional value of an extra-intracranial bypass, with a view to performing proximal occlusion or trapping during the same operation. This also applies to the measurement of cerebral blood flow with electromagnetic probes, some of which are designed for recording the small cerebral vessels.

Electromagnetic Probes

Like the preceding methods, these probes can be useful for recordings in intracranial as well as cervical vessels.

Measurement of Intravascular Pressure

This measurement is easy to perform intraoperatively by means of thin epicranial-type needles connected to a pressure recorder. The measurement of mean residual pressure during a proximal temporary clamping test is of the greatest importance in evaluating the quality of the anastomotic collateral circulation. When the residual pressure is low there is a high risk of ischemia owing to final interruption of the vessel harboring the lesion [10].

Measurement of Regional Cerebral Blood Flow

Measurement of regional cerebral blood flow by injection of xenon 133 into the operated carotid artery, before and after clamping, can be of great help as an indicator of the circulatory adaptation capacity of the area corresponding to the vascular occlusion [5, 12, 24].

Electrophysiological Monitoring

Finally, continuous monitoring of the electroencephalographic behavior of the cerebral cortex can be performed on the side where the craniotomy has been performed by recording evoked potentials [25] and/or by electrocorticography [17, 22].

Table 16. Criteria for tolerance to carotid artery occlusion

	Doppler	CBF	Mean pressure	Elastance (ICP)	Electro-physio.
Normal	No inversion of ophthalmic flow	40 ml/100 g/min N 35 ml/100 g/min	≃70 mmHg	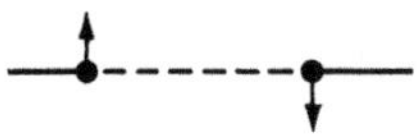	N
Safe		Less than 25% decrease (≃25 ml/100 g/min)	≥50 mmHg pulsatile	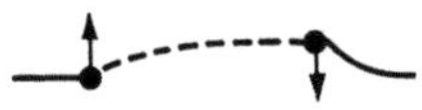	N
Unsafe	Inversion of ophthalmic flow	Less than 35% decrease (≃20 ml/100 g/min)	≥50 mmHg nonpulsatile	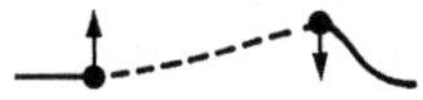	Transient anomalies
Ischemia certain		Neuronal necrosis if <17 ml/100 g/min	<50 mmHg	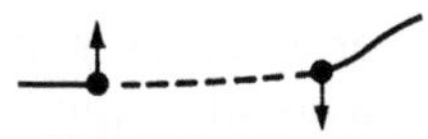	Increasing anomalies

CBF, cerebral blood flow; *ICP*, intracranial pressure

Selection of Patients

The use of these methods can help in as accurate as possible selection of patients with potentially difficult aneurysms. Table 16 shows schematically values given by the different functional exploration methods, below which there would be a possible risk (unsafe zone) or a near-certain risk (ischemic zone) in the performance of carotid artery occlusion, at least if performed without an extra-intracranial bypass. These selection criteria, developed on the basis of the authors' experience and from a review of the literature [11, 14, 20, 26], have only an indicative value and give no absolute guarantee against immediate or late complications.

When the recorded values are *above the safety limit*, carotid artery occlusion is basically practicable, without the necessity of an extra-intracranial bypass.

When these values are *below the safety zone*, occlusion is dangerous (Table 16). A prior extra-intracranial bypass can reduce the risks involved. However, caution makes it mandatory to repeat the tolerance tests after bypass before performing the therapeutic occlusion. This can be most advantageously carried out by a progressive occlusion with clinical and paraclinical monitoring.

Management by the Intravascular Approach

After a brief historical review, this chapter will discuss the experimental, technical, and clinical basis of intravascular occlusion. The experience of G. Debrun with a series of 21 giant aneurysms managed by the intravascular approach, with or without other neurosurgical procedures, will be presented, followed by a discussion of the present role of this rapidly developing method in the treatment of giant aneurysms.

Background

The management of intracranial lesions by the intravascular approach was conceived by Brooks [4] who, in 1930, introduced a fragment of muscle into the common carotid artery in order to embolize a carotid-cavernous fistula downstream. Since then, technological advances have made it possible to expand the indications for this tempting therapeutic approach. The percutaneous method of catheter insertion was introduced in 1963 by Straube and Dotter [33], and in 1964 Luessenhop et al. [24] passed a catheter beyond the carotid siphon. In subsequent years, this difficult maneuver was managed with catheters guided by flotation with the aid of an inflatable balloon (Serbinenko 1974 [32] and Pevsner [26] or by magnetic fields (Yodh et al. 1968 [39]). The balloon catheters, already in use in cardiac (Carlens et al. 1951 [5]), Swan et al. 1970 [34]) and vascular surgery (Fogarty et al. 1965 [16]), were used in neurosurgery in 1964 for the management of aneurysms by Luessenhop and Velasquez [24], who attempted catheterization of a carotid-ophthalmic aneurysm, and subsequently in 1970 by Wholey et al. [38].

The fundamental advance was made by the introduction of the detachable balloon catheter in 1974 by Serbinenko [32], refined by Debrun et al. [11, 12, 13] in 1975.

Materials Used

A number of intravascular techniques have been proposed for the management of arterial aneurysms. Some have remained at the experimental stage; only balloon catheters have had a clinical application. The principal technological features, advantages, drawbacks, attendant risks, and complications of the detachable balloon technique are discussed below.

Nondetachable Balloon Catheter

The Fogarty catheter is the most representative of this technique. The catheter is introduced into the neck by carotid artery puncture and has been successfully used in the management of carotid-cavernous fistulas [27, 28, 30]. This catheter can also be used in the treatment of certain aneurysms when the therapeutic decision is to perform an occlusion of the internal carotid artery.

The balloon being nondetachable, it is necessary to bury the carrier catheter in the soft tissues of the neck after making sure that it is permanently sealed by a clip.

Spontaneous deflation of the balloon occurs in a few weeks, but retrograde thrombosis of the proximal internal carotid artery segment ensures permanent occlusion. The advantage of this technique lies in its simplicity and reliability. Its major disadvantage is, of course, leaving a foreign body within the carotid lumen. Theron [36] has described three carotid-ophthalmic aneurysms managed by this method. In two of the cases, where the balloon of the Fogarty catheter was located in front of the aneurysmal neck, the carotid artery again became patent while the aneurysm remained thrombosed. This lead in one case to a transient paresthetic episode. Two and a half years later, the catheter perfectly tolerated and was probably endothelialized.

Detachable Balloons

Two basic types of balloon are currently available: latex balloons, the earlier and most commonly used, and, more recently, silastic balloons.

Latex Balloons

The first detachable balloons were developed by Serbinenko [32] in the USSR. The technique spread to Europe and, following a modification introduced by Debrun [10], to the United States of America. The technology and production of these balloons, as well as the technique of intra-arterial introduction, have been well described in the literature [7, 8, 9]. Some balloons have a small cavity in the tip where a radiopaque silver bead can be placed. This allows identification of the position of the balloon during fluoroscopy without the need to inflate the balloon with contrast medium.

The balloons may be attached to the catheters in different ways, usually with or without a ligature.

1. The balloons used by Serbinenko have no ligature at the neck. The catheter and the balloon are only held together by the squeezing of the neck of the elastic latex balloon on the end of the catheter. This technique has its advantages and disadvantages:

– Detachment is easily accomplished by gentle traction on the carrier catheter. Due to the ease of detachment, the diameter of the carrier catheter can be very small (0.3 mm internal diameter, 0.5 mm external diameter). It is thus possible to reach distal vessels owing to the flexibility of the catheter which is flow-guided by the balloon. Detachment is then possible without risk of the catheter breaking since it is not firmly attached to the balloon. However, this advantage is offset by the risk of untimely detachment of the balloon.

– The lack of permanent occlusion of the neck of the balloon makes it essential to replace the water-soluble contrast medium with a silicone polymer so that the balloon remains inflated after detachment. This entails a *risk of embolism* by silicone fragments. Furthermore, in the management of aneurysms, the traction transmitted by the catheter to the balloon during detachment may lead to trauma of the neck of the malformation.

2. The balloons developed by Debrun and Lacour have the addition of a latex thread ligature around the neck where it is joined to the carrier catheter. This technique also has its advantages and disadvantages:

– It confers greater safety with respect to untimely detachment.

– The ligature seals the neck of the balloon after removal of the catheter, so the latter can be detached without risk of rapid deflation, even if it is filled with a water-soluble contrast medium.

– If it is desired to fill the balloons with silicone, the existence of the ligature makes them leakproof. In that case, it is possible to detach the catheter before the silicone is completely polymerized. However, the use of this type of balloon requires a larger and therefore stiffer carrier catheter along with the addition of a coaxial catheter in order to avoid any displacement of the balloon during detachment (Fig. 108).

Whatever the type of latex detachable balloon used, its technological limits are quite apparent. First, there is the *secondary deflation of balloons filled with water-soluble contrast medium.* All latex balloons inflated with pure or diluted contrast medium end up deflating within a period of a few weeks. Unlike silastic balloons, this is not due to permeability of the wall but to leak at the ligature. This has been clearly demonstrated in an experiment by Debrun: two sets of balloons inflated with

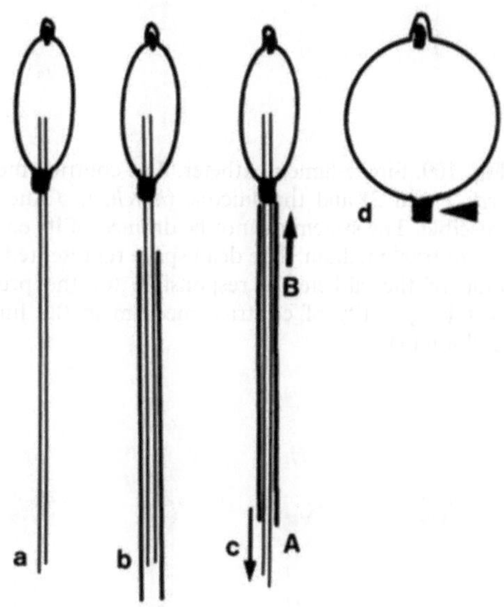

Fig. 108. Latex detachable balloon (Debrun type). The balloon is inflated by the central catheter (*a*) and detached by a coaxial catheter with a greater diameter (*b*) by the application of counter-pressure (*c*). This allows removal of the central catheter (*A*), without the traction effect which might cause movement of the balloon and trauma to the neck of the aneurysm (*B*). The occlusion of the balloon is ensured by the latex ligature, producing a sphincter system (*arrowhead*)

a contrast medium were detached in test tubes containing sterile plasma. The first set had normal ligatures such as are commonly used in clinical practice. The second set had larger ligatures, with three times as many strands of latex. The first set deflated after 1 month, whereas the second set was unchanged after 12 months.

To counteract the drawback of secondary deflation of the balloons filled with contrast medium, a rapidly polymerizing silicone can be injected into the balloon. Before using this product, the balloon should be drained of the water-soluble contrast medium which has been used during the positioning of the balloon. However, the cavity of the carrier catheter remains filled with water-soluble contrast medium which will precede the silicone column as it advances in the catheter toward the balloon (Fig. 109). The amount of *dead space* present can be considerable when the catheter is very long: this is the case when using the femoral approach in the management of intracranial lesions, or when dealing with small-sized balloons.

The only potential solution to this problem lies in the use of a polymerizable agent miscible with the contrast medium, or of a double-lumen catheter. Debrun has developed a double-lumen catheter (Ingenor Lab.) which allows positioning of the balloon and inflation tests with water-soluble contrast up to the moment of injection of an equal quantity of polymerizing substance. The contrast initially introduced into the balloon by one of these lumens can be aspirated by the other lumen until the balloon contains 100% polymerizing substance (the silicone used has a very low viscosity and solidifies within 15 min at 37°; (Fig. 110). The major drawback of a double-lumen catheter is its lack of flexibility due to the larger diameter, which in turn limits the possibilities of intravascular guiding.

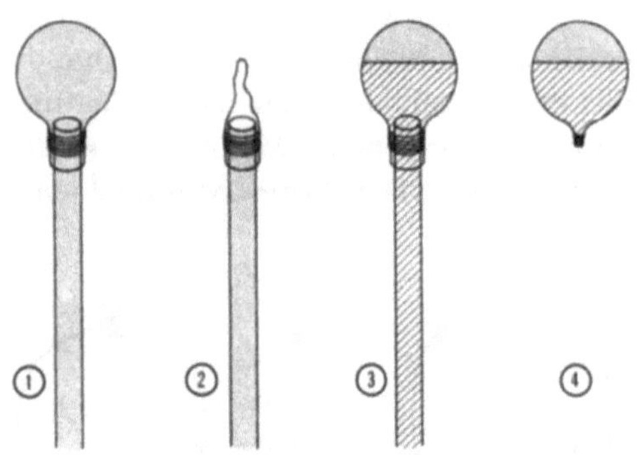

Fig. 109. Single-lumen catheter. The contrast medium (*dotted*; *1* and *2*) and the silicone (*hatched; 3* and *4*) are not miscible. The system cannot be drained of its entire content of contrast medium. The dead space represented by the volume of the catheter is responsible for the presence of a certain quantity of contrast medium in the lumen of the balloon (*4*)

Silastic Balloons

Of much more recent date, silastic balloons behave like the material from which they are made (B.D. Lab. and Heyer-Schulte) [14, 18, 37]. Silastic material does not have the elasticity, flexibility, or extensibility of latex. Latex balloons may be inflated to ten times their initial length, as compared with approximately three times for silastic balloons. This fact is of major importance if intravascular occlusion of a giant aneurysm is being planned. The walls of a silastic balloon behave like a simipermeable membrane, making it necessary to fill it with an isotonic water-soluble contrast medium. The silastic balloon has no ligature. Instead, small flaps in the neck of the balloon act like venous valves, occluding the orifice when the catheter is withdrawn. These balloons are carried by a flexible polyurethane catheter and do not require a coaxial

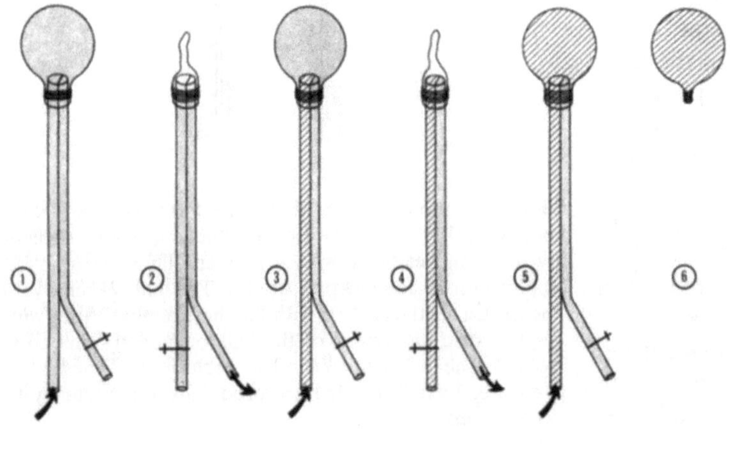

Fig. 110. Double-lumen catheter. This system allows replacement of all the contrast medium contained in the balloon (*dotted*) by silicone (*hatched; 6*)

catheter since detachment is obtained by simple traction on the carrier catheter. This ease of manipulation is offset by a greater risk of untimely detachment. Moreover, the balloons are not equipped with radiopaque clips at their extremity and are only visible when slightly inflated with contrast. When the balloon is maximally inflated, but not over-distended, progressive deflation can be expected to occur over a period of 30 days. However, the figures reported by White et al. [37] show considerable variations in the time for complete deflation, as noted on follow-up roentgenograms from 2 to 180 days.

Other Types of Balloon

Other types of balloon differ from the preceding ones mainly in their systems of release. Laitinen and Senvo [22] in 1978 proposed a latex balloon having a self-tightening neck which can be detached from the catheter, whose distal end is equipped with a metallic microtube. Taki et al. [35] published in 1979 an original system consisting of a latex balloon attached to a vector catheter by a very thin ethylene-vinyl-alcohol copolymer tube allowing detachment of the balloon by torsion of the small tube, induced by manipulation of the catheter itself. The use of these catheters has not, to our knowledge, had a wide clinical application.

Other Techniques of Intravascular Occlusion

Biological Glue

Some experimental publications mention the use of bucrylate injected within the lumen of the aneurysm while the neck is occluded [40]. The aim of this procedure is to selectively occlude the lumen of the aneurysm and to protect the flow of the parent artery. Unfortunately, this method entails considerable risks because it is almost impossible to prevent reflux of the embolisation medium into the artery. Only very rigid silicone balloons can guarantee real neck occlusion of the aneurysm, but their size and their lack of flexibility limit their use beyond the petrous portion of the internal carotid artery.

Intraluminal Exclusion of the Aneurysm

Some authors have proposed exclusion of the aneurysm from the circulation by experimentally performing what is in fact an internal angioplasty, by means of a tube or a balloon perforated in its middle portion and placed over the orifice of the aneurysm [17].

Use of Magnetic Fields

Since the first attempts of Montgomery and Hillal, advances in cryogenic technology have made it possible to develop a super-conducting coil by a joint team (Grenoble-Créteil) [20, 21, 25]. Experimental trials in the dog have produced solutions to certain problems of directing intravascular catheters by utilizing a clipped balloon catheter equipped with perforated magnets at the distal end. It has thus been possible to facilitate the intravascular guiding of catheters towards zones without preferential flow (experimental aneurysms). External direction by a superconducting coil has made it possible to enter arteriovenous fistulas against the direction of flow.

The use of ferromagnetic particles introduced and maintained in the aneurysmal lumen under the action of a strong magnetic field has proven to be more hazardous. The products tested were suspensions of particles of very small diameter. These are evidently not suited to the management of aneurysms owing to the ferromagnetic particles being set in motion by the swirling intra-aneurysmal flow and to re-release of the ferromagnetic particles by the catheter itself during its movements in the magnetic field. Advances may be expected in the near future with the use of more voluminous ferromagnetic particles introduced in microcapsules, which, it is hoped, will "fix" the particles within the aneurysmal sac under the action of the magnetic field.

Methods

The ideal treatment consists of occluding the aneurysm while protecting the arterial flow in the parent vessel.

Selective Occlusion of the Aneurysm

Selective occlusion of the aneurysm by balloon detachment, which allows flow in the parent vessel, seems especially tempting when surgical management is out of the question. The experimental

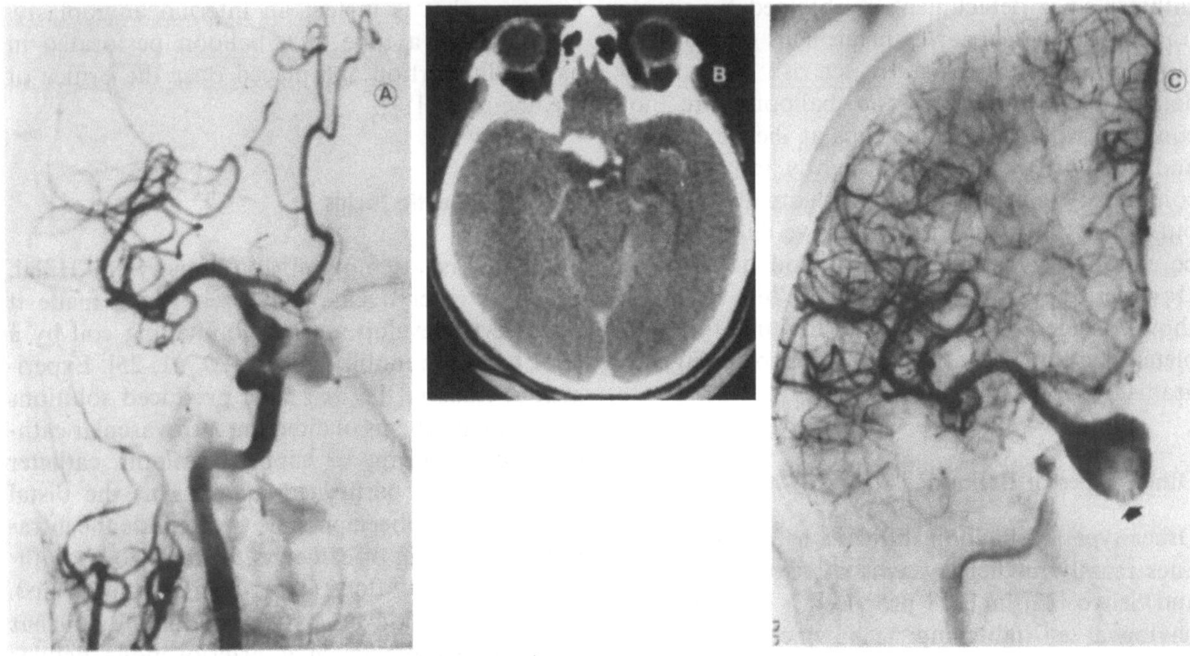

Fig. 111 A–C. Intravascular management of a subclinoid giant aneurysm. L., 58 years old. CT scan for suspected subarachnoid hemorrhage showed a right carotid artery aneurysm with intrasellar extension. **A** Selective occlusion of the aneurysm while preserving carotid artery flow. Uneventful postoperative course except for the secondary appearance of anterior pituitary insufficiency well controlled with substitutive medical treatment. **B** Routine CT scan 4 months later showed enhancement in the aneurysm, suggesting that it was again patent. **C** Angiography showed that the aneurysm had enlarged around the balloon, which remained visible as a radiolucent image (*arrow*). Definitive treatment included occlusion of the aneurysmal lumen with a second balloon combined with occlusion of the right internal carotid artery with two additional balloons. Uneventful postoperative course. Digital subtraction angiography performed one week later confirmed right internal carotid artery occlusion

study published in 1980 by Romodanov and Shcheglov [29] is impressive. It deals with 119 patients presenting with intracranial aneurysms, of whom 108 were managed by the intravascular approach alone. Ninety-three patients underwent selective occlusion of the aneurysm. For these authors, the treatment of choice for all intracranial aneurysms whose diameter is greater than 0.5 cm, and whose neck is smaller than the diameter of the balloon, is occlusion by the intravascular approach. Normally, intravascular treatment is carried out long after the revealing subarachnoid hemorrhage. In this series, 17 patients harbored giant aneurysms but, regrettably, their results are not individualized, and long term follow-up is unavailable. Immediate complications reported for the whole series are: one fatal ruptured aneurysm due to balloon overdistension, one ruptured balloon filled with nonpolymerized silicone which embolized the cerebrum causing death, three unwanted carotid artery occlusions causing fatal edematous infarcts, and, finally, two accidental displacements of the balloon into the sylvian artery causing transient neurological deficits.

This satisfactory experience is not shared by other authors. Debrun has reported the frequent occurrence of severe complications in attempts to occlude the aneurysmal sac while preserving flow in the parent artery. This led him to prefer permanent occlusion of the parent artery by detaching the balloon as near as possible to the aneurysmal neck. However, there are some special objections against this technique:

– Inflation of one or more balloons at the neck of an aneurysm carries a risk of rupture. This mishap was observed by Schialfa et al. [31] in one case of an intracavernous aneurysm, the rupture having led to the formation of a carotid-cavernous fistula.

– Complete occlusion of the giant aneurysm can lead to its over-distention, increasing the mass effect.

– When giant aneurysms are partly thrombosed, the introduction of the balloon into the lumen of the aneurysm can provoke a migration of clots to the distal territory.

– Intrasaccular thrombosis may be erratic because of poor adherence of the latex balloon to

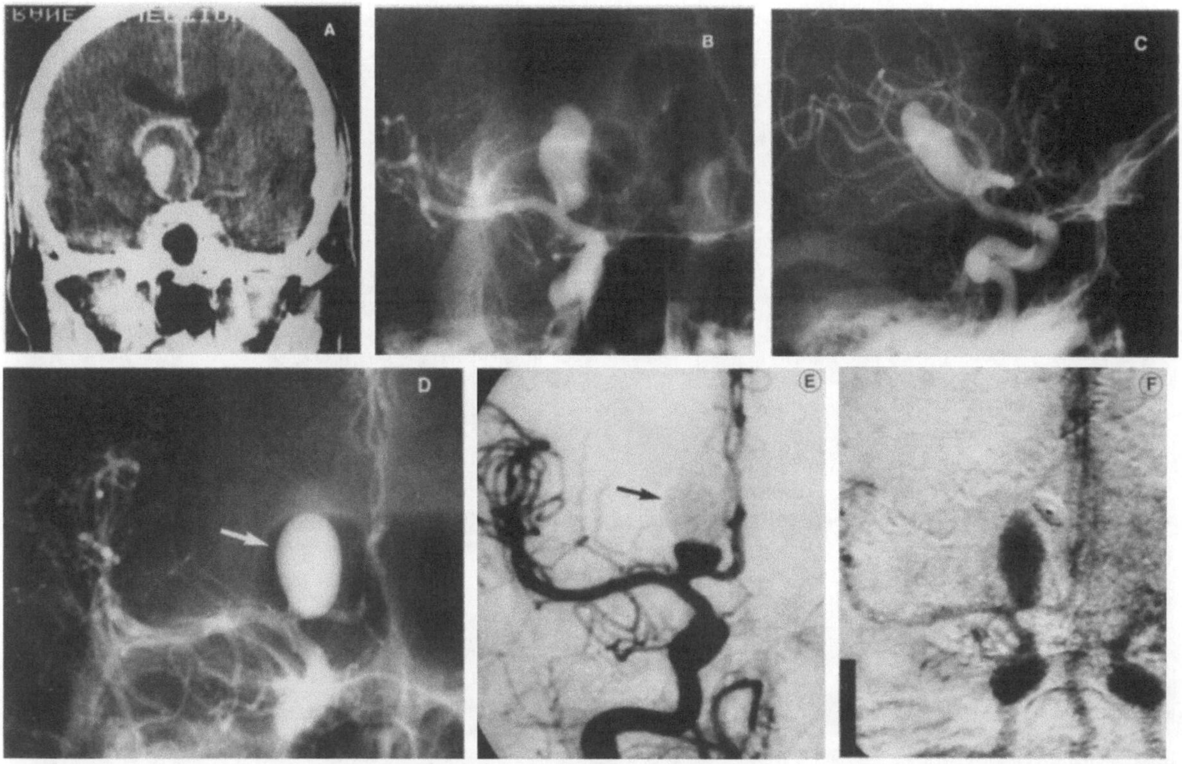

Fig. 112A–F. H.L., a 65-year-old male presenting with a long history of chronic headaches and behavioral disturbance, was referred in September 1985 for a recent loss of vision. The CT scan (**A**) and right carotid angiograms (**B**, **C**) showed a partially thrombosed giant aneurysm located in the right parasellar region. An inflatable balloon was detached inside the aneurysm, entirely occluding the patent lumen of the sac (**D**). Seventeen days later angiography showed a reduction in size of the balloon, resulting in a reopacification of the neck area (**E**). Six months later, IV digital angiography showed a deflated balloon pushed towards the dome of the sac with almost complete visualization of the sac (**F**). The patient underwent a second operation and the aneurysm neck was clipped with a fenestrated clip after removing the thrombus by thrombectomy so as to decompress the sac. Uneventful postoperative course

the walls of the aneurysm and to the newly-formed thrombus [20] (Fig. 111).

– In addition, the balloons have a marked tendency to a slow progressive deflation as shown in Fig. 112. This can result in their migration toward the dome of the sac, being pushed distally by blood pressure.

– On the other hand, when the balloon is blocked within the neck – which means that it extends inside the lumen of the parent artery – subsequent thrombosis of the parent artery may occur, as shown in Fig. 113.

Permanent Occlusion of the Parent Vessel

Tolerance of Occlusion

This method is principally concerned with aneurysms of the internal carotid (Figs. 114, 115), vertebral, basilar, and, to a lesser extent, certain intracranial arteries. It is presumed that occlusion of the artery in question is well tolerated. This can be tested by occluding the flow for 10–15 min with either a Fogarty catheter or a detachable balloon catheter while watching for clinical signs and symptoms of ischemia.

The purpose of the tests outlined here is (a) to assess clinical tolerance of acute and prolonged occlusion; (b) to evaluate the collateral supply from the circle of Willis by opacification of the other arteries; and (c) to study the other vessels that supply the lesion in question.

This method allows the occlusion test and definitive management by intravascular occlusion to be linked. The choice of the site for introduction of the catheter depends a great deal on the vascular condition of the patient and the preference of the angiographer. When a prior extra-intracranial bypass has been performed, it is imperative to avoid a direct carotid approach because of the risk of producing a traumatic occlusion of the external carotid artery during puncture.

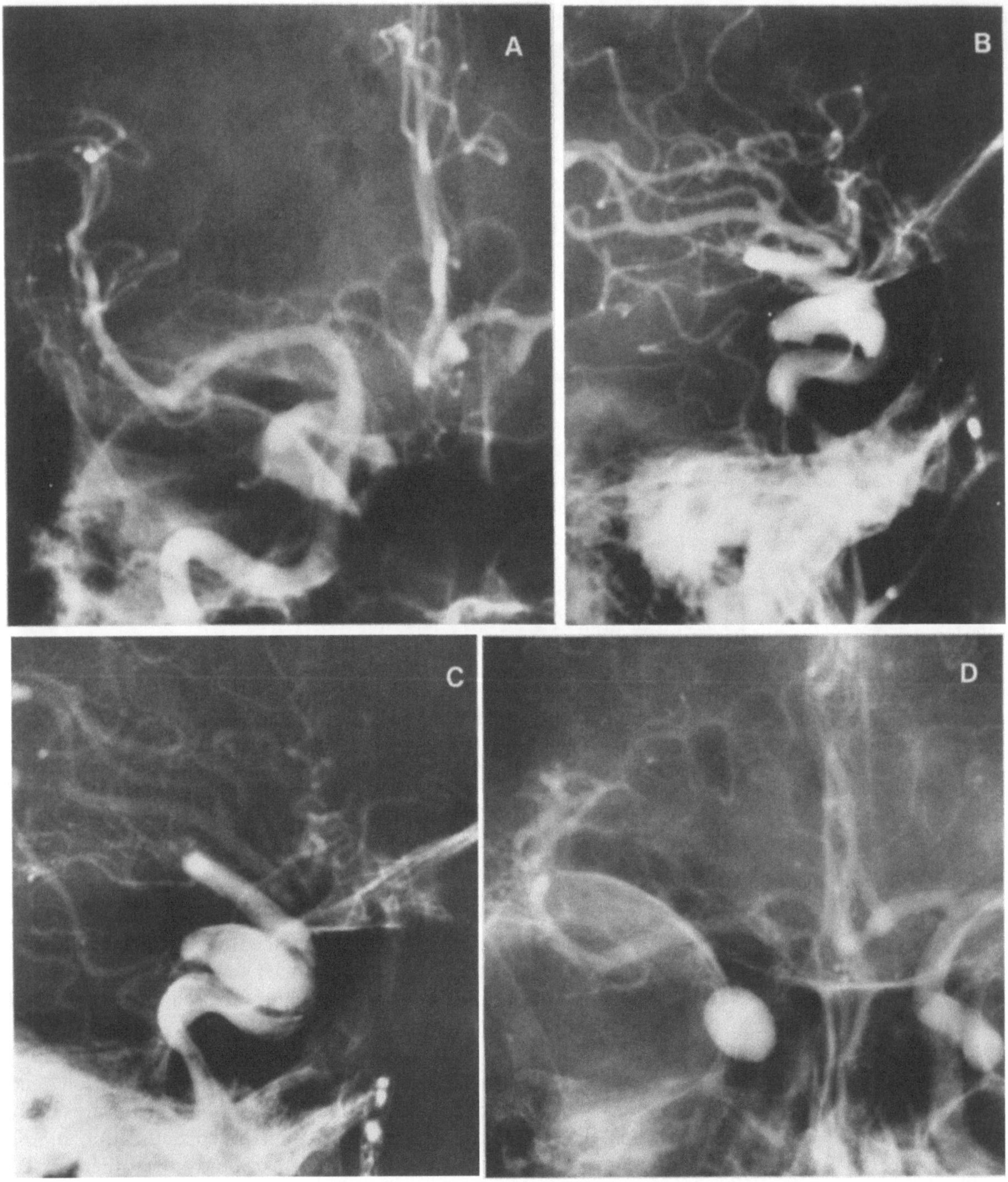

Fig. 113 A–D. M.R., a 64-year-old female, was referred in January 1986 for severe headaches associated with progressive oculomotor palsies on the right side. The CT scan and the angiogram showed a partially thrombosed cavernous sinus aneurysm (**A**, **B**). An inflatable balloon was detached inside the aneurysmal sac, but markedly reduced the carotid lumen (**C**). This resulted in rapid and complete occlusion of the parent artery (**D**), fortunately without any clinical complication

Whatever system is used (detachable balloon or other) and whatever the approach (femoral or carotid artery), the patient must be cooperative and wide awake so as to ensure the soundness of the neurological assessment. The occlusion must be removed within seconds of the appearance of the least sign of cerebral ischemia. The radiological set-up must allow immediate visualization of the balloon position and degree of occlusion (this can be ensured by leaving contrast medium in the

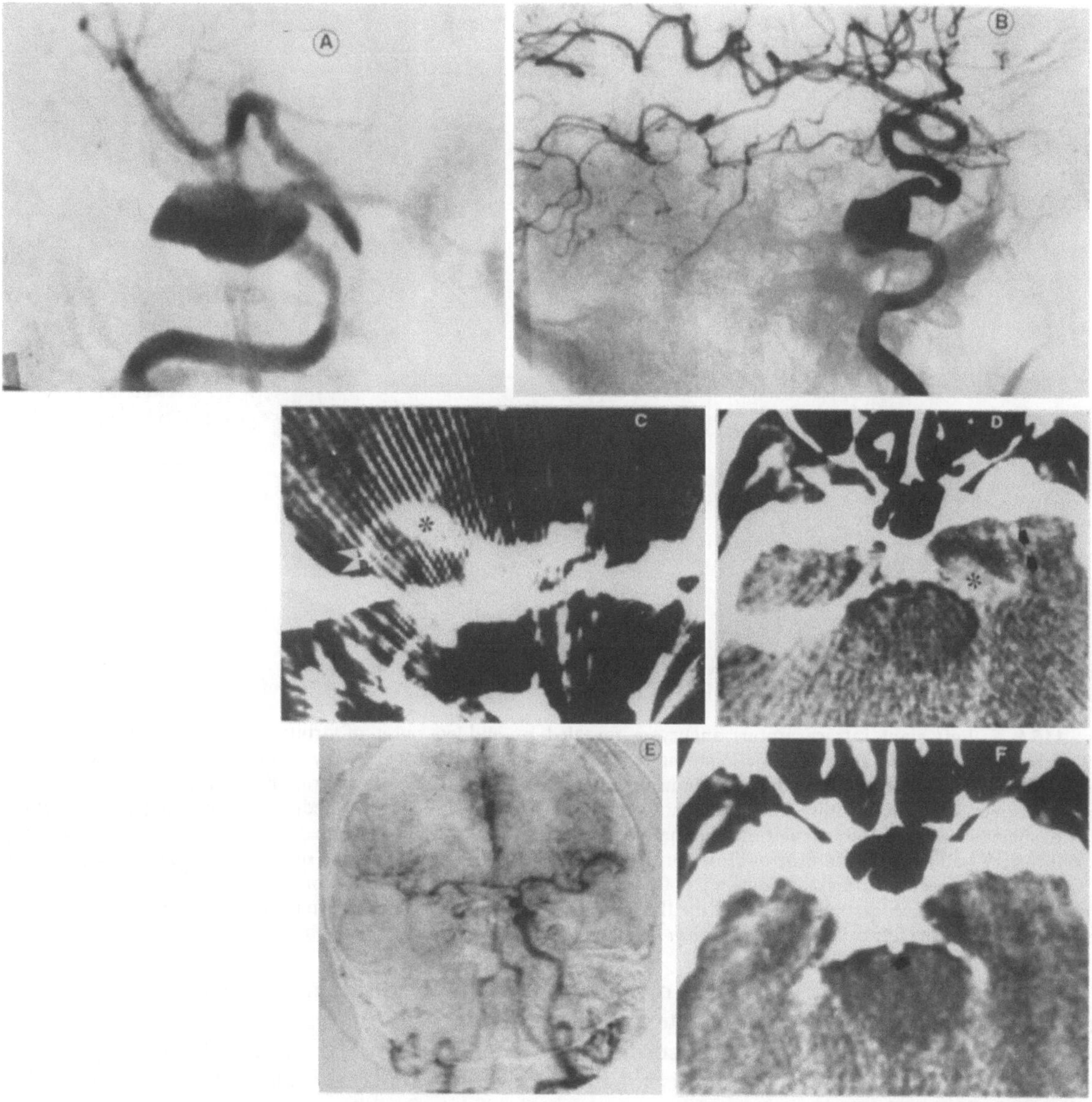

Fig. 114A–F. Intravascular management of a giant intracranial aneurysm. Patient P., 53 years old, with hypertension. Sudden onset of complete ophthalmoplegia with trigeminal anesthesia (V_1 and V_2). Right carotid artery angiogram: giant aneurysm of the right intracavernous carotid artery (**A**, **B**). CT scans during the first passage of an intravenous bolus of contrast medium. The axial view (**D**) shows a partly thrombosed aneurysm: there is a rim of peripheral enhancement (*arrows*), the circulating channel is visible in the posterior part of the lesion (*star*). **C** Coronal CT (the linear artifacts are from dental fillings); the thrombosed portion of the aneurysm (*arrow*) is below the circulating portion (*star*). Treatment was carried out 1 month later by intravascular occlusion of the right internal carotid artery with the aid of two occlusive balloons released proximally to the aneurysm, after clinical tolerance tests. **E** Digital subtraction angiography 10 months later showing persistent right carotid artery occlusion. **F** Dynamic CT scan showing the aneurysm is no longer visible. Opacification of the basilar artery (*arrow*). Clinically, the patient still has partial right ophthalmoplegia and partial right V_2 hypoesthesia

carotid lumen proximal to the occlusion). Serbinenko proposes positioning the balloon in front of the first, second, or third cervical vertebra where the low contrast of soft tissues makes the opacity of the balloon stand out in the lateral view. The clipped latex balloon (Ingenor Lab.) affords considerable flexibility for this technique and has been used in 18 cases of aneurysms of the internal carotid or vertebral arteries at the Henri Mondor Hospital, Créteil, without any mishaps.

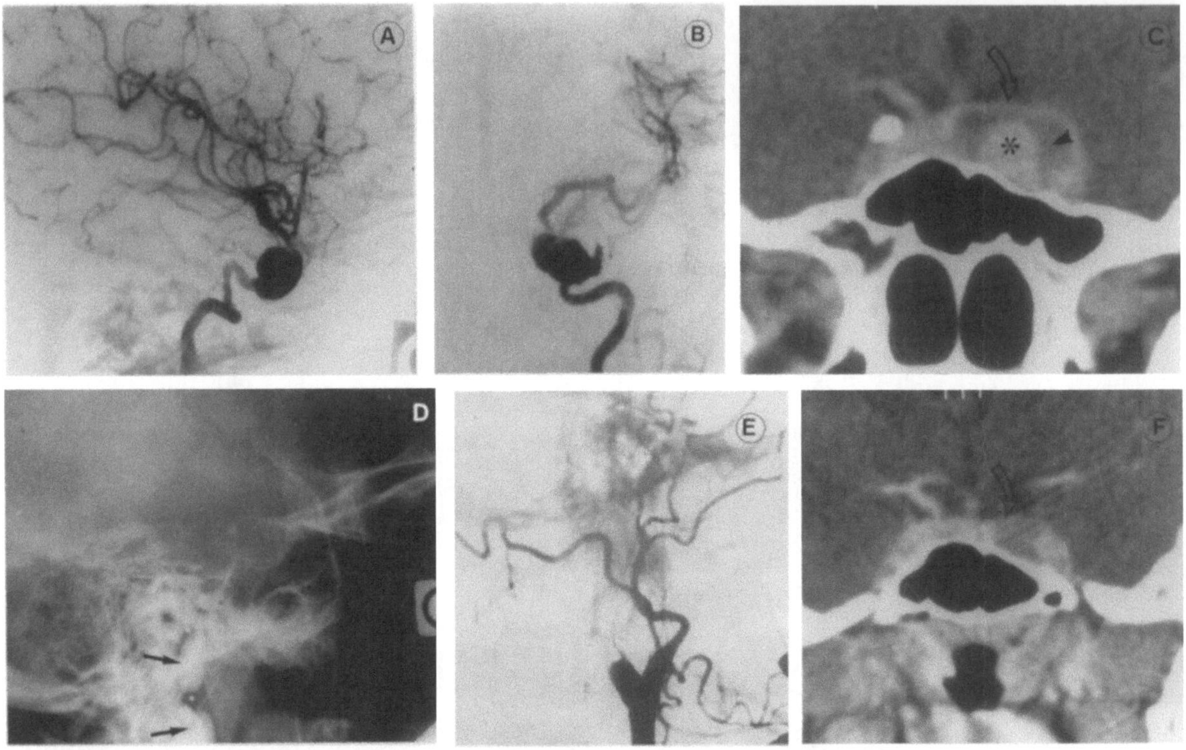

Fig. 115A–F. Left giant intracavernous aneurysm revealed by sudden onset of orbital pain and ophthalmoplegia in a 70-year-old woman. **A, B** Selective left internal carotid artery angiogram: partially thrombosed giant aneurysm inside the cavernous sinus compressing the neighbouring internal carotid artery (**A**, lateral, **B** anteroposterior view). **C** CT scan performed in coronal section with intravenous injection of a bolus of contrast medium. *Arrowhead* partial thrombosis of the aneurysmal sac; *star* circulating channel; *open arrow* limits of the distended left cavernous sinus. **D** Internal carotid artery balloon occlusion (*arrows*) performed after a clinical test of tolerance of internal carotid artery occlusion. **E** Left common carotid artery angiogram. **F** CT scan performed in coronal section 3 months later with intravenous injection of bolus of contrast medium show the thrombosis of the intracavernous internal carotid artery. Note the dramatic decrease in size of the left cavernous sinus (*open arrow*). No neurological deficit was observed

The duration of the test is a subject of controversy. Serbinenko proposes a 10-min test in the internal carotid artery (prolonged, according to the same author, to 15 min if his aim is to study the supply from the ophthalmic artery and measure central retinal pressure). Debrun mentions equivalent figures in the region of 10 min. This duration of occlusion seems sufficient for detecting clinical manifestations of acute ischemia in a conscious patient. However, in the acute phase, the test does not guarantee that there will be no clinical manifestations due to secondary ischemia associated with low blood flow. Nevertheless, these tests cannot be prolonged any further owing to the risk of thrombosis both proximal and distal to the occlusion and of embolic migration following the removal of carotid artery occlusion. Intravenous heparin is given at the beginning of the occlusion for safety whenever the lesion has not manifested itself by subarachnoid hemorrhage, a relatively common occurrence in the case of giant aneurysms.

However, this method is not without its *disadvantages*:

– If performed without due care, it can cause arterial trauma, as evidenced by Dujovny et al. [15] in the common carotid arteries of the rabbit, occluded with Fogarty catheters. Electron scan microscopy revealed crushing type lesions of the endothelia with hemorrhagic platelet deposits. These lesions are most pronounced if the balloon is overinflated or rapidly distended. This necessitates the use of adequately lubricated syringes to avoid sudden overpressure.

– Owing to its short duration, this test cannot guarantee the secondary and long-term consequences of the therapeutic occlusion. Therefore, much interest has been shown in supplementing the clinical evaluation during the occlusion studies of the cerebral flow and intravascular pressure. (See pp. 114–117.)

The intravascular methods make it possible to evaluate the *quality of the collateral supply from the circle of Willis* as explored angiographically

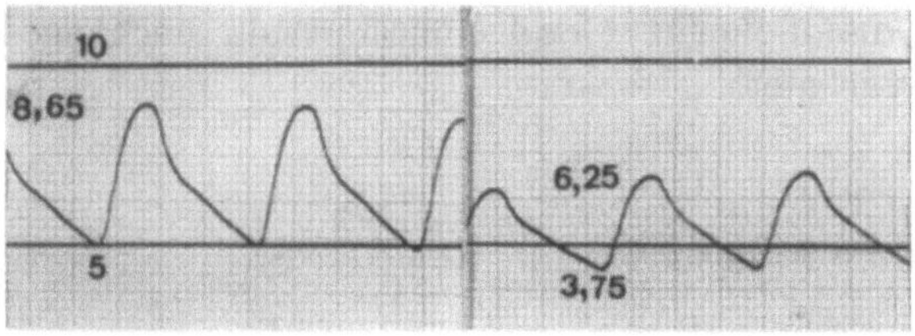

Fig. 116. Occlusion test with the study of distal residual pressure. This test can be combined with cerebral vascular exploration. In the present case, it was performed by positioning a 7F introducer in the common carotid artery (by Seldinger's technique).

Introduction of a double-lumen balloon catheter through the introducer: one lumen allows inflation of the balloon, and the other, recording of the pressure distal to the occlusion. Intravascular pressures measured before occlusion (*left*): maximum 86.5 mmHg, minimum 50 mmHg; dropping – during occlusion (*right*) – to 62.5 mmHg and 37.5 mmHg respectively, i.e. a 25% decrease. The recording shows the pulsatile character of the pressure curve.

This method, coupled with a study of clinical tolerance in the conscious patient, permits an evaluation of the functional capacities of the collateral supply from the circle of Willis

with cervical carotid artery compression. Beatty and Richardson [2] and Jawad et al. [19] stress the increased risk of ischemia in patients who show hypoplasia of the A_1 segment of the anterior cerebral artery and in whom one or two posterior communicating arteries are voluminous, of the fetal type, suggesting the limited character of the supply brought by the vertebrobasilar system to the occluded carotid artery.

The introduction of an intravascular catheter allows direct measurement *of the pressure in the internal carotid artery distal to the occlusion*, reflecting the prevailing pressure in the circle of Willis. This type of exploration is easily accomplished using a double-lumen balloon, as we did in the case in Fig. 116.

Techniques of Permanent Occlusion

Several techniques are possible. Occlusion can either be carried out at the segment located proximally to the aneurysm or, even better, at its neck. When occlusion must be performed at the *segment located proximally to the aneurysm*, the technique is simple and can be carried out by means of a Fogarty catheter or with the aid of two detachable balloons inflated with water-soluble contrast medium, the second balloon ensuring that the flow will not recommence in the event of the first balloon deflating accidentally. This technique has mainly been used in the carotid axis but may prove inadequate if the aneurysm is of the carotid-ophthalmic type. In fact, the countercurrent circulation of the ophthalmic artery may be responsible for keeping the aneurysm patent.

Occlusion of the parent artery can be made *across the aneurysmal neck*. This technique is applicable when the neck has a small orifice. The use of a second balloon is necessary as "insurance", as noted above. In a recently published case [23], secondary displacement of a balloon placed in a carotid-ophthalmic aneurysm would certainly have been prevented if a second balloon had been placed proximally to the lesion, thus ensuring carotid occlusion.

Occlusion can be carried out *on both sides of the aneurysmal neck*, thus forming an intravascular trapping. However, it should be noted that in a wide-neck giant aneurysm, especially of the carotid artery, the tendency of the balloon is to follow the arterial flow and to lodge itself exactly within the aneurysm and not distally. This can make it impossible to apply this technique. Moreover, stagnation and the motion of the balloon within the aneurysmal sac can cause cerebral embolism if the aneurysm is only partly thrombosed.

Complications

Whatever system is used for intravascular management, certain complications are inherent in the procedures. In a recent series of 33 patients treated for carotid-cavernous fistulas, vertebrovertebral fistulas, and aneurysms of the internal carotid artery, Scialfa et al. mention several complications due to the equipment itself [31]: rupture of the balloon (four cases), impossibility of deflating the balloon (one case), intimal lesions of the internal carotid artery related to the detachment procedures without clinical consequences, embolism to cortical arteries (two cases), by clot in one case and by detachment of the radiopaque clip in the other. Both of these mishaps remained asymptomatic. Barrow et al. [1] reported a case of asymptomatic sylvian embolism from a series of eight patients managed by the intravascular approach. In 1983, Chalif et al. [6] and Langford et al. [23] each reported a case of distal displacement of the balloon. The balloons had moved into the internal carotid artery, producing hemiplegia with dysphasia. An emergency operation made it possible to perform balloon embolectomy, with a satisfactory postoperative course and disappearance of the initial signs of neurological deficit.

Clinical Experience and Therapeutic Indications

The clinical experience related in this chapter rests on a total of 21 giant aneurysms with a maximum diameter of at least 25 mm which were managed by Debrun in collaboration with three different surgical teams. This study was over the period from 1975 to November 1983 and involved two patients treated at Créteil with J.P. Caron's team, nine patients treated at London-Ontario with Drake's team, and 10 patients treated at Boston with N. Zervas' team. The clinical summary of each case is given below.

Case Histories

Case 1 (Créteil)

Moribund 45-year-old whose giant supraclinoid aneurysm had hemorrhaged. Glasgow coma score: 3. Carotid angiogram revealed greatly reduced and slowed cerebral flow, with spasm of the internal carotid artery below the aneurysm. Attempted intra-arterial guiding with a balloon made it possible, with great difficulty, to reach the carotid siphon and the terminal portion of the internal carotid artery below the aneurysm.

During inflation of the balloon, the aneurysm ruptured and the patient died on the operating table.

Case 2 (Créteil)

60-year-old female, under cave at another clinic for hypopituitarism with an enlarged and laminated sella turcica. For various reasons, the patient was operated on by the transsphenoidal approach for her "pituitary adenoma," but the neurosurgeon realized that it was an aneurysm and closes the transsphenoidal approach without any difficulty.

The patient was then transferred to Créteil where angiography revealed a cavernous aneurysm, 25 mm in diameter, with a relatively narrow neck. Occlusion of the aneurysmal sac with a balloon partly inflated with silicone (single-lumen catheter at that time) and with preservation of the arterial lumen. Good clinical result, unchanged year later.

Case 3 (London)

12-year-old female. Giant aneurysm of the basilar trunk which had bled with lesions of cranial nerves IX, X and XI. Unsuccessful surgical attempt at clipping the aneurysmal neck.

Owing to good posterior communicating arteries, bilateral occlusion of the vertebral arteries was decided upon. The posterior-inferior cerebellar artery arose from the vertebral artery at C1 which made it possible to clip the vertebral artery above this point. The left vertebral artery was managed by progressive and subsequently total occlusion with a Selverstone clamp in the supraclavicular fossa.

Angiography showed recanalization of the left vertebral artery by a clamp which was bent, but did not occlude the vertebral artery. An attempt to place a tourniquet on the left vertebral artery failed after several tries. Finally, the left vertebral artery was occluded by a detachable balloon. Follow-up angiography spread over a period of several months showed considerable (90%) but not total reduction of the aneurysmal sac, which continued to be opacified by higher branches and across cerebellar-basilar anastomoses. However, excellent clinical recovery 1 year later.

Case 4 (London)

56-year-old female. Isolated palsy of the right sixth nerve. Wide-necked giant cavernous aneurysm; widely patent circle of Willis. The balloon easily penetrated the aneurysm but did not completely obliterate the lumen and stenosed the siphon. Occlusion test of the internal carotid artery for 10 min with the balloon inflated proximally to the neck: good tolerance. Balloon detached. Excellent clinical result. No opacification of the aneurysm on follow-up angiography; stable result at 4 years.

Case 5 (London)

20-year-old male. Progressive right-eye blindness. CT and angiography revealed a carotid bifurcation aneurysm, partly thrombosed. Right extra-intracranial bypass and, 5 days later, occlusion of the right carotid artery proximally to the aneurysm with a detachable balloon. Good clinical tolerance. Aneurysm considered to be thrombosed.

Case 6 (London)

46-year-old female. Left retro-orbital pain and palsy of the left sixth nerve. Asymptomatic right fusiform cavernous aneurysm; left giant cavernous aneurysm. Balloon inflated with silicone added to tantalum powder introduced into the aneurysmal sac. Internal carotid artery preserved, but with stenosis. Upon awakening, right brachial paresis with dysphasia. Excellent recovery, but tantalum powder seen on CT in the region of the head of the caudate nucleus and the left Rolandic operculum.

Regression of the left cavernous syndrome. Follow-up angiography 2 months later revealed severe stenosis of the carotid siphon tending towards complete occlusion. Left hemisphere essentially vascularized by the right.

Case 7 (London)

42-year-old female. Left cavernous syndrome with palsy of nerves III and VI. Wide-neck giant aneurysm. Good circle of Willis. Occlusion of the aneurysmal sac by balloons inflated with iodine; carotid flow preserved. Progressive repermeabilization of the aneurysm which is as voluminous 6 months later.

Fresh attempt at occlusion of the aneurysmal sac with preservation of arterial flow, but maximum inflation of the balloon within the aneurysm does not completely occlude it. Decision to perform permanent occlusion of the internal carotid artery. Good clinical result.

Case 8 (London)

30-year-old male. Left sixth nerve palsy and retro-orbital pain. Left giant cavernous aneurysm over 5 cm in diameter. Complete occlusion of the aneurysmal sac with 12 balloons inflated with iodine during two sessions of 3 h each. Carotid artery preserved 1 month later. Patient returned stuporous with severe headaches and fever. CT showed two abcesses, one frontal and the other temporal, next to the aneurysm. Definitive occlusion of the internal carotid artery, draining of abscess and of the aneurysmal sac. Clinical revovery, though with complete left-eye blindness.

Case 9 (London)

34-year-old female. Transient ischemic attacks in the area of the left carotid artery followed by an internal capsule infarct. Angiography revealed a giant left paraophthalmic aneurysm. Unsuccessful attempt at surgical clipping. Bypass followed by permanent occlusion of the internal carotid artery proximally to the neck, preserving the ophthalmic artery. Angiography 1 year later showed no opacification of the aneurysm, bypass functional. Good clinical result.

Case 10 (London)

30-year-old female. Right carotid artery aneurysm. Bypass, followed 2 days later by permanent occlusion of the internal carotid artery by a balloon detached proximally to the neck. Good clinical tolerance but aneurysm still visible 3 months later. Clipping at the origin of the anterior cerebral artery and of the internal carotid artery above the posterior communicating artery. Thrombosis of the aneurysm.

Case 11 (London)

38-year-old male. Signs of right optochiasmatic compression. Giant aneurysm of the right carotid bifurcation. Unsuccessful surgical clipping. Bypass and clipping of the right anterior cerebral artery at its origin. Permanent occlusion of the internal carotid artery proximally to the aneurysm with a detachable balloon.

Case 12 (Boston)

68-year-old male. Intrapetrous aneurysm of the left internal carotid artery 25 mm in diameter which had bled into the middle ear. Good circle of Willis. Permanent occlusion of the internal carotid artery proximally to the aneurysm. Good immediate clinical tolerance. Two days later, right hemiplegia with dysphasia. Embolism obstructing the sylvian artery before its division. Incomplete recovery with major dysphasic sequelae.

Case 13 (Boston)

46-year-old female. Right cavernous syndrome with sixth nerve palsy. Mistaken diagnosis of a meningioma upon CT, rectified upon angiography. Good circle of Willis. Occlusion of the neck and the internal carotid artery. Good clinical result.

Case 14 (Boston)

52-year-old female. Complete right ophthalmoplegia. Frontal headaches. Visual acuity 20/50 on the right, normal on the left. Voluminous right precavernous aneurysm. Good circle of Willis. Complete occlusion of the aneurysmal sac with two balloons was possible only at the cost of complete stenosis of the carotid siphon. Complete occlusion of the carotid artery proximally. Excellent clinical result.

Case 15 (Boston)

62-year-old female. Recent loss of vision of the right eye. Right ophthalmic aneurysm 25 mm in diameter. Good circle of Willis. Balloon detached proximally to the neck in the horizontal portion of the carotid siphon without occlusion of the ophthalmic artery. Ten-minute occlusion test well tolerated. Right brachial paresis noted after balloon detachment. Excellent clinical result but small left opercular infarct shown by CT. Angiography of the right external carotid artery 3 months later showed that the aneurysm was opacified by the ophthalmic artery, whose diameter had doubled.

Case 16 (Boston)

75-year-old female. Retro-orbital headache with progressive left-eye blindness. Left supraophthalmic aneurysm, 3 cm in diameter, lifting the anterior cerebral artery. Good circle of Willis. Narrow neck (4 mm). Balloon placed easily within the aneurysm, but subsequently wedged in the neck with complete occlusion of the internal carotid artery. Good tolerance test. Balloon detached. Right hemiplegia with dysphasia a little later. Progressive aggravation and death 8 days later. Massive left sylvian infarct shown by CT.

Case 17 (Boston)

34-year-old male with a history of recurrent left otitis media. Left retro-orbital pain with left fifth, sixth, and seventh nerve palsy. Left intrapetrous and intracavernous mass shown by CT diagnosed as an "abscess" and treated with antibiotics. In the absence of clinical improvement, carotid artery angiography disclosed a left paracavernous aneurysm, 4 cm in diameter. Very insufficient circle of Willis. Bypass, followed 2 days later by internal carotid artery occlusion using two balloons detached on both sides of the aneurysmal neck. Excellent result.

Case 18 (Boston)

50-year-old female. Headache and left sixth nerve palsy. Left giant cavernous aneurysm. Good circle of Willis. Permanent occlusion of the internal carotid artery proximally to the neck. Good result.

Case 19 (Boston)

76-year-old female. Signs of right optochiasmatic compression. Voluminous supraophthalmic aneurysm with compression of the anterior cerebral artery and the sylvian artery. Poor circle of Willis. Bypass and then, the following day, permanent internal carotid artery occlusion. Very good tolerance to 10-min occlusion test of the left internal carotid artery. Right hemiplegia with dysphasia a few minutes after balloon detachment. Death 1 week later.

Case 20 (Boston)

46-year-old female. Headache and left sixth nerve palsy. Left paraophthalmic carotid aneurysm 25 mm in diameter. Permanent occlusion of the internal carotid artery with a balloon just proximally to the neck. Recent case.

Case 21 (Boston)

49-year-old female with hypertension. Left sixth nerve palsy. Left giant cavernous aneurysm associated with a trigeminal artery. Good circle of Willis. Permanent occlusion of the internal carotid artery below its neck but above the trigeminal artery.

Another balloon obliterates the carotid artery below the trigeminal artery, which is thus excluded. Excellent result 1 year later.

Comments

The first case, which dates from the very beginning of our study, shows that a patient in deep coma with arterial spasm is not a good candidate for any type of intravascular management. The other 20 cases can be divided into two groups: those in which the aim was to obliterate the aneurysmal sac by means of a detachable balloon and preserve the parent artery, and those in which management consisted of permanent occlusion of the parent artery to produce thrombosis of the aneurysm.

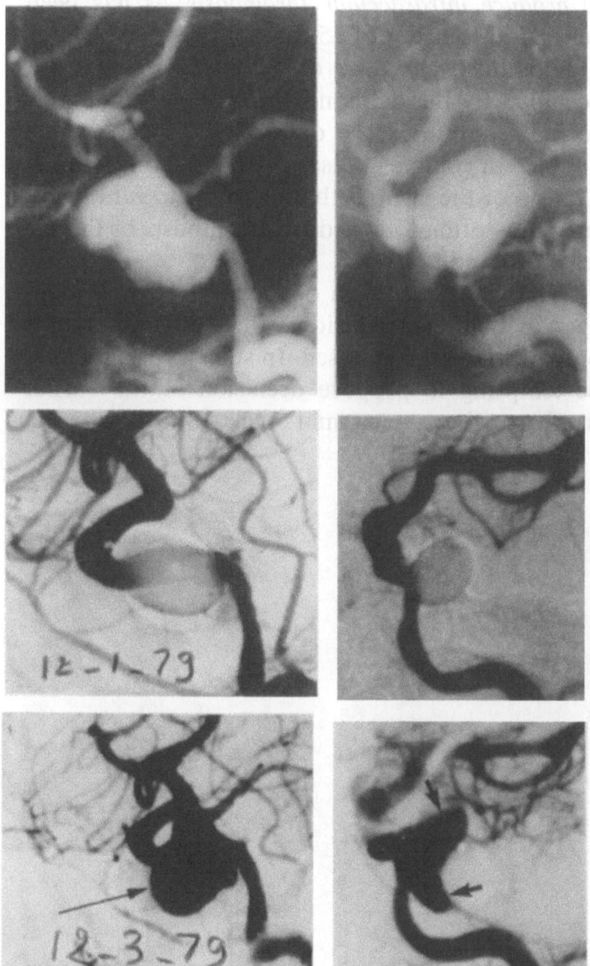

Fig. 117. Left giant intracavernous aneurysm managed by selective occlusion of the sac. *Left* lateral views; *right* frontal views. *Top* preoperative angiogram. *Middle* complete occlusion of the sac with a balloon inflated with iodine, with total preservation of the parent artery. *Bottom* follow-up at 2 months. Improvement of the cavernous syndrome; balloon retraction; partial opacification of the aneurysm (*arrows*). Clinical reaggravation. Subsequent clinical recovery after permanent internal carotid artery occlusion by means of a detachable balloon. (G. Debrun)

Group 1 (Cases 2, 6, 7, 16; Figs. 117, 118)

Case 2 was of an intracavernous aneurysm 25 mm in diameter. It was managed with a good clinical result, because the balloon was largely inflated with silicone and thus kept its volume constant, and also because the aneurysm was not very large.

Case 6 was complicated by sylvian infarct due to secondary occlusion of the internal carotid artery. Clinical recovery has been satisfactory.

Case 7 was managed by a balloon inflated with iodine producing occlusion of the aneurysmal sac for 15 days. There was progressive opacification as the balloons deflated. Contrary to what others have seen in similar cases, there was no intrasaccular thrombosis in spite of complete occlusion for 2 weeks. Six months later, the aneurysm had returned to its original size. After a transient improvement, the clinical condition reverted to its

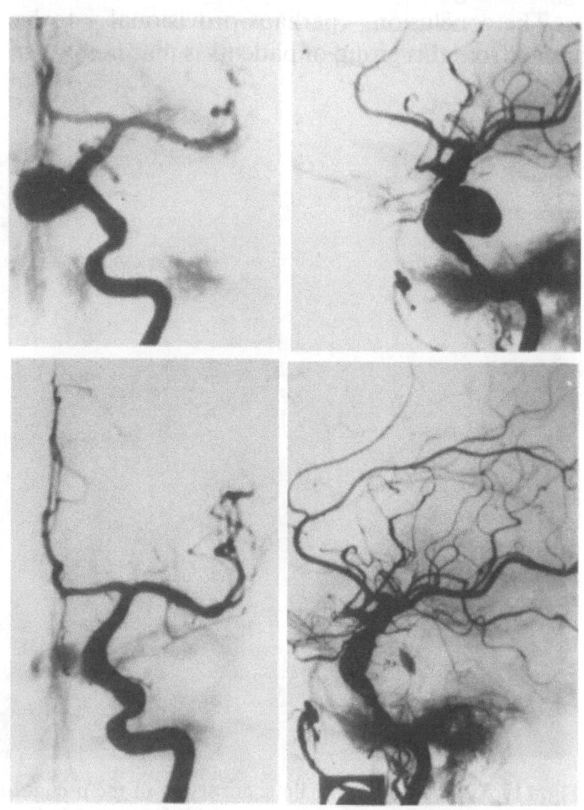

Fig. 118. Left giant intracavernous aneurysm managed by intravascular balloon mainly inflated with silicone. Good clinical and angiographic result. (G. Debrun)

old state. Success was obtained at the cost of permanent occlusion of the carotid artery by another balloon.

Case 8 demonstrates the difficulty in occluding a giant aneurysm with a diameter of more than 5 cm. In fact, the balloons, all inflated by iodine, obstructed the sac but increased the mass effect of the aneurysm. The subsequent cerebral abcess with infection of the aneurysmal content made it necessary to occlude the internal carotid artery in order to drain the contents of the aneurysmal sac.

Case 16 is an attempt at intra-aneurysmal occlusion which ended in a fatal neurological complication for which we have no satisfactory explanation. Contralateral angiography performed 30 min after the onset of right hemiplegia with dysphasia showed good opacification of the left sylvian artery, identical to the preocclusion angiogram. Nor did we find any evidence of vascular obstruction. It is possible that the condition of the circle of Willis was borderline and that left cerebral ischemia was of hemodynamic origin, enhanced by a relative drop in arterial pressure, which we had noted during treatment. In this 75-year-old patient, the absence of bypass might have been an aggravating factor.

The conclusion – perhaps provisional – to be drawn from this group of patients is that *it is better to occlude the parent artery than to attempt occlusion of the aneurysmal sac.*

Group 2

This group, patients whose parent artery was permanently occluded (Fig. 119), makes it possible to define the best way of achieving thrombosis of the aneurysmal sac, and to determine the indication for a bypass prior to occlusion of the parent artery.

Apparently, *occlusion of the parent artery proximal to the aneurysmal neck does not always suffice to produce intrasaccular thrombosis*, as has been verified in four out of 15 cases.

Obviously the neck of the aneurysm was not occluded by the balloon, which allowed countercurrent supply via the ophthalmic artery (which doubled in volume in cases 10 and 11). Intracranial ligation of the arteries that continue to fill the aneurysm is often followed by thrombosis of the sac (cases 10 and 11).

The giant aneurysm of the basilar trunk managed by bilateral occlusion of the vertebral arteries only partially thrombosed. In such a case, it could be tempting to propose occlusion of the basilar trunk at the aneurysmal neck. But if one re-

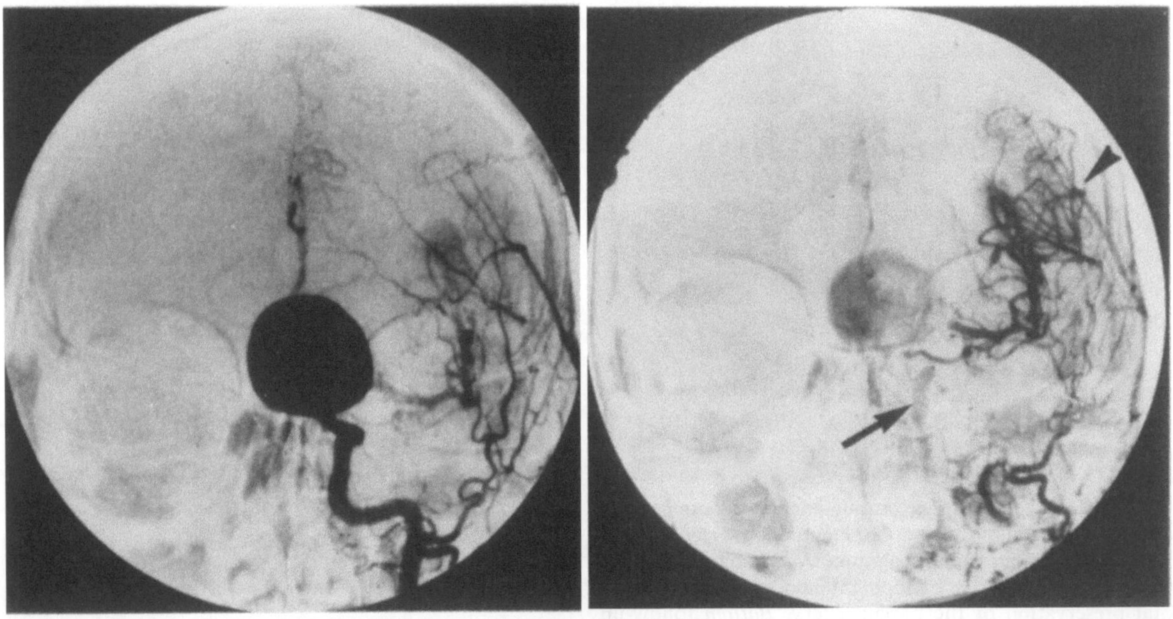

Fig. 119. Left carotid-ophthalmic aneurysm of the pseudotumoral type, managed by proximal occlusion with a detachable balloon, preceded by an extra-intracranial bypass. Left carotid preoperative angiogram shows an inadequate circle of Willis. Extra-intracranial bypass, followed the next day by proximal occlusion of the left internal carotid artery (*arrow*). Excellent tolerance during the 10-min occlusion test. Balloon detachment. Right hemiplegia with dysphasia several minutes later, despite adequate functioning of the bypass (*arrowhead*). (G. Debrun)

members the numerous perforating arteries arising from the basilar trunk supplying the brainstem, it will be realized that any occlusion, however small, is much more hazardous than those obtained by the tournique of Drake. For this reason, we never dared to detach the balloon in the basilar trunk.

The best results in sac thrombosis were obtained when the sac was completely occluded with balloons (case 14) or when the balloon simultaneously occluded the neck and the parent artery (cases 13, 14), or, what amounts to the same thing, when the neck of the aneurysm was isolated by one balloon detached distally and by another detached proximally (case 17).

Cavernous aneurysms whose neck is proximal to the ophthalmic artery generally thrombose readily (cases 4, 18, 21). This does not mean that an ophthalmic aneurysm will not thrombose if the ophthalmic artery remains functional by countercurrent flow (case 9), but nevertheless the latter may be a cause of failure (case 15).

Should supraophthalmic and supraclinoid carotid aneurysms be managed by balloon at the cost of occlusion of the ophthalmic artery? We have always tried to avoid occluding the origin of this artery for fear of producing unilateral blindness. However, in a number of cases where the ophthalmic artery was accidentally occluded, no decrease of visual acuity ensued, no doubt owing to the various anastomoses between the ophthalmic artery and the branches of the external carotid artery. Certainly, in case 15, where the ophthalmic artery doubled in volume during the 3 months after occlusion of the internal carotid artery and had to be approached intracranially, we regretted not having been more daring and occluded its origin.

The *role of extra-intracranial bypass* in relation to permanent occlusion of the parent artery remains to be discussed. Some authors perform a systematic bypass in the days preceding permanent occlusion of the parent artery. Our material proves that a bypass is not necessary when the circle of Willis is largely patent, but it should be done whenever the patency is borderline or in older patients. On the other hand, it is imperative to perform it when the circle of Willis is poorly developed or nonexistent. Moreover, it has been shown that a bypass affords no protection against embolic complications (case 19). In fact, the bypass was largely functional in this patient who developed sylvian embolism 48 h after occlusion of the internal carotid artery.

It is also necessary to discuss the best timing for intravascular occlusion following a bypass. It can be hazardous to perform occlusion just after the bypass in the hope of reducing the risk of its becoming nonfunctional some days later. Undoubtedly the major factor in the flow of a bypass is the actual requirement of blood flow. It seems prudent to wait 24–48 h for the patient to stabilize after the bypass. We routinely checked the bypass before occluding the parent artery. In all cases we found it functional. It is spectacular to find that occlusion of the parent artery leads to an instantaneous doubling in size of the anastomotic arteries.

Should patients be kept on aspirin, dipyridamole, and anticoagulants after occlusion of the parent artery? All the patients treated in this group were fully heparinized during the procedure [13]. At the end of the intravascular management, the heparin was neutralized with protamine sulfate.

Is it preferable to keep patients anticoagulated for a few days? This question arises as we have observed embolic complications in a patient treated with bypass and permanent occlusion of the internal carotid artery by a Selverstone clamp.

Finally, *can occlusion of the parent artery by intravascular balloon be compared with progressive surgical clamping?* Classically it is thought that stepwise clamping of the parent artery favors the development of collateral circulation, minimizing the risk of ischemia, whereas occlusion by balloon leads to acute ischemia that cannot be controlled as easily. Nevertheless, intravascular occlusion can and must be performed with a 10-min occlusion test of the parent artery, during anticoagulation treatment with perfusion of the proximal artery with heparinized serum. Balloon detachment can only be carried out if the patient tolerates occlusion perfectly. It is no doubt hazardous to reestablish blood flow in an artery that has been occluded for more than 10 min, whether by balloon or with a tightening clamp. Neurological complications occurring beyond this period of tolerance, sometimes several hours or several days after permanent occlusion of the artery, are almost always secondary to embolism proven by angiography (case 12).

It is imperative that occlusion by progressive clamp tightening be carried out at a distance from the aneurysmal neck. This increases the risk of revascularization of the aneurysmal sac from collaterals, which normally link the internal carotid artery to its homologue and to the external carotid artery. There is also a long segment of artery which

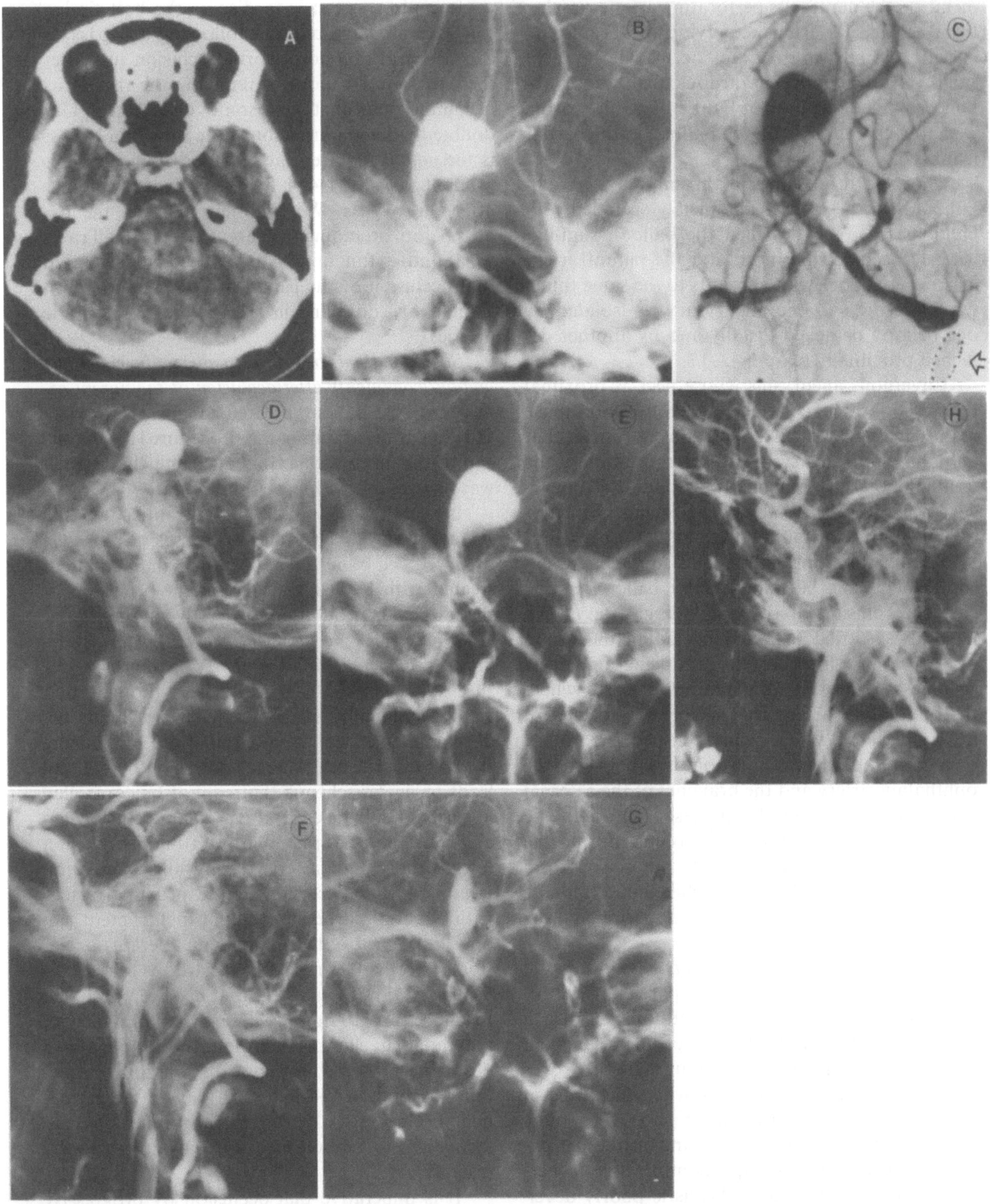

Fig. 120 A–H. Intravascular management of a giant aneurysm of the basilar trunk. A 20-year-old female with a history of several months of progressive symptomatology combining a crippling bilateral cerebellar syndrome of walking and swallowing disturbances with bronchoaspiration. CT and angiography revealed a giant aneurysm of the basilar trunk. CT scan (**A**) shows a voluminous mass filling the entire region of the basilar trunk. Angiogram (**B**) with simultaneous injection of both vertebral arteries demonstrates the large aneurysm arising from the middle third of the basilar trunk. The left vertebral artery is dominant. Management (**C**): occlusion of the left vertebral artery below C1 by detachable

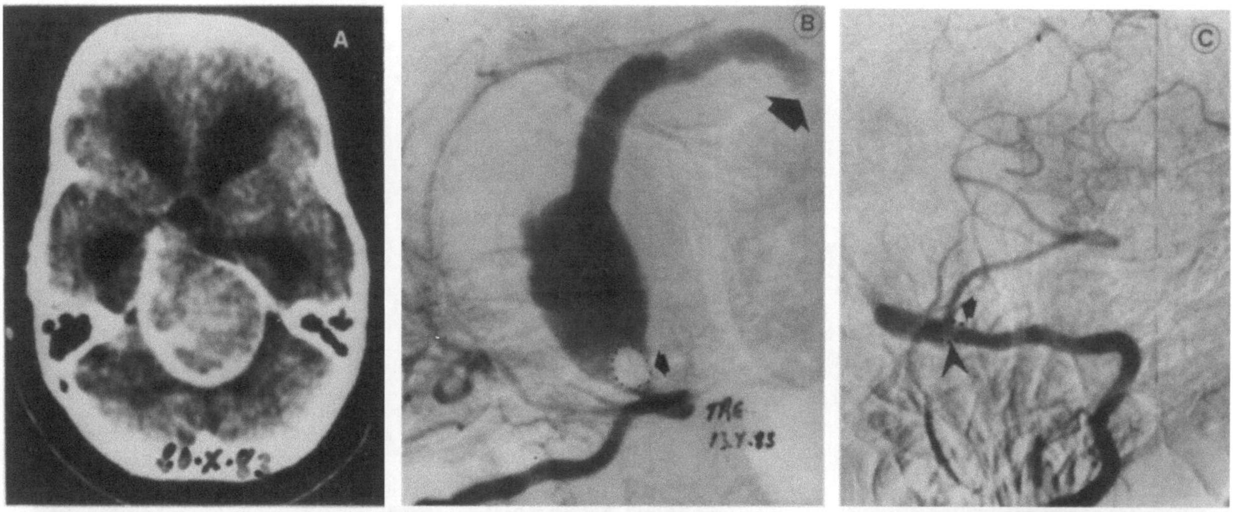

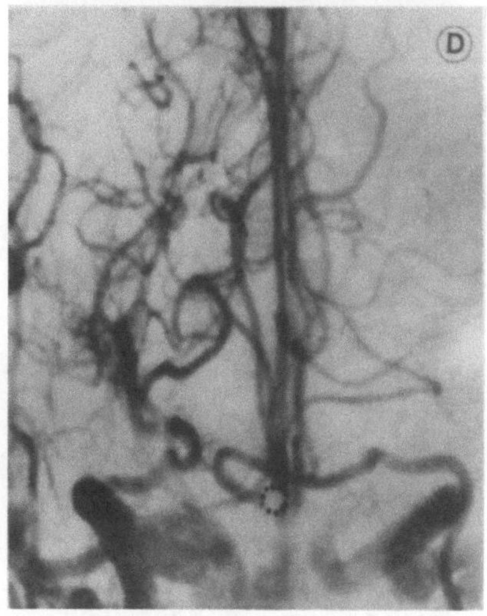

Fig. 121 A–D. Intravascular management of a giant basilar aneurysm. A 13-year-old male presenting in August 1981 a picture of subarachnoid hemorrhage from a partly thrombosed basilar aneurysm, confirmed by angiography. Initially the patient deteriorated, with onset of a left motor deficit, bilateral cerebellar syndrome, and dysphagia. Progressive improvement allows the child to lead a fairly normal life until March 1983. From this date onwards: progressive reappearance of the bilateral cerebellar syndrome, a motor deficit in all four limbs, and facial diplegia leading to a sedentary state.

A CT scan shows a mass with a calcified contour, not enhanced by contrast medium. **B** Angiography by right and left vertebral approach shows a large aneurysmal lumen but with no features in common with the aneurysmal mass seen on CT. The aneurysmal lumen probably represents the basilar trunk itself; its extremity seems obliterated (*upper arrow*). A balloon is guided up to the origin of the aneurysm (*lower arrow*) by the left vertebral approach. Inflated at this level, it is impossible to clamp the aneurysm itself, as the balloon advances distally. **C** The balloon is guided towards the immediate preaneurysmal portion: on this frontal view, there is opacification of the left vertebral artery, which twists itself before giving rise to the inferior cerebellar artery (*arrow*). The balloon is inflated and left in position immediately distal to the inferior cerebellar artery (*arrowhead*). The aneurysm is totally excluded. Angiography of both right and left vertebral arteries shows opacification of the whole cerebellar network starting from both inferior cerebellar arteries. **D** Bilateral injection 8 days later: disappearance of the aneurysmal lumen. Opacification of the inferior cerebellar arteries via the right posterior communicating artery (left carotid artery angiogram showed opacification of the left posterior cerebral artery). In the weeks following this treatment, progressive regression of the symptomatology: progressive disappearance of the cerebellar syndrome, functional recovery, and ability to walk on the 15th day; disappearance of the facial diplegia with recovery of ocular motor activity. (Courtesy of Professor J. Merland, Lariboisière Hospital, Paris)

balloon (*arrow*); injection of the right vertebral artery shows opacification of the basilar trunk, the aneurysm, and the distal segment of left vertebral artery reopacifying the left inferior cerebellar artery by countercurrent. Follow-up: comparative angiograms on the day of treatment (**D**, **E**) and 8 days later (**F**, **G**; frontal and lateral views) show a progressive decrease in the aneurysmal lumen, whereas the vertebrobasilar system remains unchanged (injection by the humeral approach). Clinically, on the 8th day after treatment, spectacular improvement: considerable regression of the cerebellar syndrome; writing, speech, and gait are improved. The vestibular syndrome is gone. Dysphagia of solids has disappeared and dysphagia of liquids has clearly regressed. Angiographic follow-up at 4 months (**H**): right humeral artery injection (left carotid artery not shown); the vertebrobasilar system is clearly visible, although the upper third of the basilar trunk seems narrowed. Nonvisualization of the aneurysm. The patient is asymptomatic. (Courtesy of Professor J. Merland, Lariboisière Hospital, Paris)

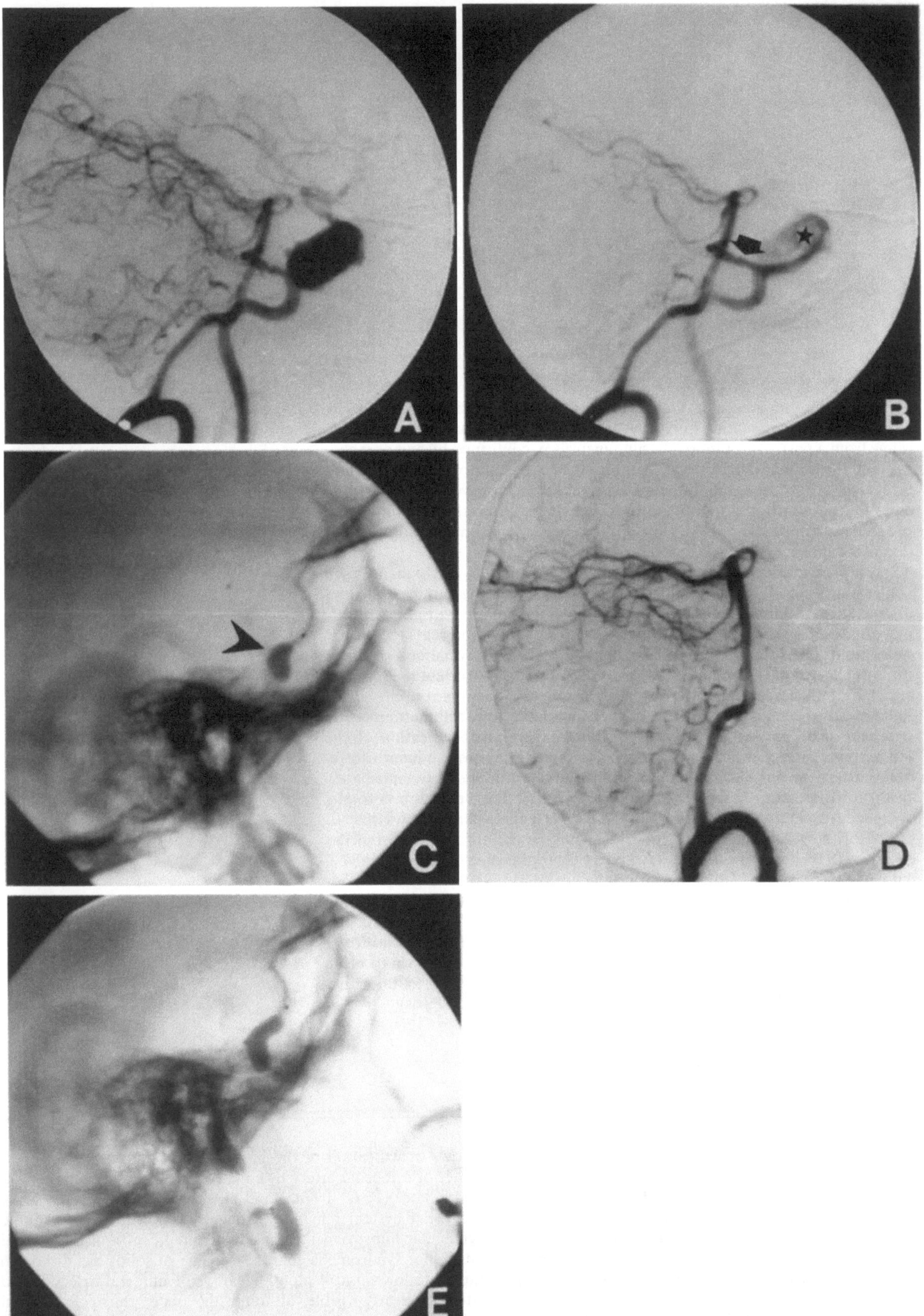
A
B
C
D
E

undergoes thrombosis, producing a greater risk of clot migration.

One of the advantages of intravascular occlusion is that it allows occlusion of the aneurysmal neck in a number of cases and also diminishes the contribution of collaterals which might revascularize the aneurysmal sac.

Conclusion

The management of intracranial giant aneurysms relies on the frequent combination of microsurgical and intravascular techniques.

At present, giant basilar trunk aneurysms apparently cannot be managed any safer by intravascular techniques than the current surgical approach. Intravascular occlusion is probably limited to the vertebral arteries proximal to the basilar trunk (Figs. 120, 121).

Giant internal carotid artery aneurysms most often manifest themselves by their mass effect. The more voluminous the aneurysm, the more reasonable it appears not to attempt obliteration of the sac, but to content oneself with occlusion of the parent artery (Fig. 122) and if possible the aneurysmal neck as well [3, 11, 12].

The need for an extra-intracranial bypass must be considered in each particular case. It does not seem necessary in all cases. It certainly offers protection against hemodynamic ischemia, but not against embolic complications.

Occlusion of the parent artery, even after bypass, may be badly tolerated by older patients and should therefore be contemplated only with great caution.

Fig. 122 A–E. Intravascular management of a right giant intracavernous aneurysm revealed by right ophthalmoplegia in a 65-year-old female. **A** Right vertebral angiogram with manual cervical compression of right carotid artery shows a right giant intracavernous aneurysm. **B** A persistent trigeminal artery (*arrow*) lies between the right carotid and right vertebral arteries. A short segment of internal carotid artery (*star*) can be seen between the origin of the trigeminal artery and the aneurysmal sac. In accordance with this anatomical disposition, it was decided to perform occlusion of both trigeminal and right internal carotid artery and not to try to occlude the internal carotid artery selectively, in order to avoid risks of turbulent flow and clot embolism through the patent trigeminal artery. **C** Temporary occlusion of the internal carotid artery was performed with a no. 16 balloon catheter (Lab. Ingenor, France) inflated with contrast medium (*arrow*). The balloon occluded both the right internal carotid artery and the trigeminal artery. There was good clinical tolerance of occlusion for 15 min under general heparinization. **D** During the test, injection of the right vertebral artery confirmed occlusion of the trigeminal artery and good circulation in the basilar trunk. **E** Secondary permanent occlusion of the internal carotid artery was performed with three balloons. Uneventful postoperative course but ophthalmoplegia persisted 1 month later (photograph by courtesy of Dr. Chiras, la Salpetrière Hospital, Paris)

General Conclusions

In the first part of this report, we have tried to summarize the data concerning the *mechanisms of formation, the anatomical and clinical features, and the neuroradiological characteristics* which may have implications for the management of intracranial giant aneurysms.

The second part was devoted to *therapeutic approaches*, based on the experience of French-speaking neurosurgeons as well as on a review of the literature of the past 12 years. We have outlined as accurately as possible the problems connected with indications and technical difficulties encountered by the various authors. The diversity of the therapeutic methods used by the different surgical teams involved in this field illustrates the difficulty of codifying rules of management.

Moreover, this report reveals the still relatively high rates of mortality and morbidity encountered with these lesions. On the other hand, it highlights a not inconsiderable number of therapeutic successes.

1. This study aims at bringing out the tendencies common to all authors.

Firstly, *reliance must not in general be placed on a favorable spontaneous outcome of these lesions.* Some publications do indeed mention cases of progressive clotting developing spontaneously towards total thrombosis and sac calcification, thus evidencing an arrest of the pathological process and, as a result, offering a guarantee against hemorrhagic rupture. But such favorable courses are rare and leave the patient exposed to possible thromboembolic complications. What is more, the thrombosed aneurysm continues to cause a mass effect, most often leading to incapacitating neurological deficits and decreased cerebral blood flow.

In the great majority of cases, giant aneurysms are complicated by hemorrhagic ruptures and pseudotumoral syndromes which compress the basal structures of the brain, the brainstem, and the surrounding cranial nerves. Moreover, ischemic manifestations can occur by reduction in cerebral blood flow or thromboembolic mechanisms.

Finally, development towards partial thrombosis, with or without parietal calcification, in no way hinders enlargement of the aneurysmal mass; no more does it afford protection against hemorrhagic complications.

These complications justify all the efforts made to conceive a form of *definitive management* for them, even in cases where the risks are far from negligible.

As in the case of small- and medium-sized aneurysms, the treatment of choice is *selective neck occlusion* by surgical or intravascular means. Whenever this can be reasonably attempted, there is no doubt that it is the treatment of choice. Drake and Peerless [1] as well as Sundt and Piepgras [2] concluded the recent review of their huge series of giant aneurysms, published in Kikuchi et al. by advocating that most cases should be explored, since more than one-third are found to have a neck small enough to permit definitive clipping. This holds particularly true with the new generation of clips, like those especially designed by Sugita, Yasargil and Sundt for complex and/or giant aneurysms. The use of microsurgical techniques is mandatory and over the last two decades has helped to decrease the mortality to acceptable rate (around 10%), as shown in Yasargil's recently published series [3]. Microsurgical techniques make it possible to attempt reconstruction of the parent artery in cases of excision of the aneurysmal malformation. But surgical methods can be hazardous and the intravascular ones uncertain. Also, when selective occlusion of the malformation entails too many risks or proves impracticable, even with temporary clamping or with circulatory arrest during extracorporeal circulation, the methods of interruption of the parent artery are a useful aid. These techniques, whether performed by the surgical or the intravascular approach, can be combined in specific cases with an extra-intracranial bypass so as to diminish the potential risks of ischemia.

Direct surgical exploration is for some authors the only way to ascertain whether the neck is suitable for selective occlusion. However, in the view of a large number of surgeons, neuroradiological assessment alone should be used to determine the most efficient and least hazardous method to adopt. These two – apparently contradictory – approaches reflect the complexity of the therapeutic problem and justify our idea that, if not a formulation of rules, then at least a clarification of the indications should be attempted by outlining, when several approaches are possible, two types of therapy: one maximal and the other minimal.

2. The *therapeutic management* to be adopted depends upon the mode of manifestation of the aneurysm, the degree of its mass effect, and, in particular, its anatomical features as evaluated by neuroradiological exploration. Establishment of the surgical treatment must take the greatest account of the topographic localization of the giant aneurysm, the type of implantation of the neck on the parent artery, the relationships of the sac with the surrounding vascular and nervous structures, and, above all, the *degree of thrombosis of the aneurysmal mass:*

a) In *totally thrombosed* aneurysms (rarely encountered), surgery is indicated when the lesion produces a mass effect with clinical manifestations and/or if it is complicated with ischemic manifestations or decrease in cerebral blood flow. When the neck is narrow, decompression can be carried out by complete resection of the aneurysmal mass after neck occlusion. Otherwise, it is safer to leave in situ the basal part of the sac which can be wrapped by plastic coating. When total excision of the aneurysm is felt to be hazardous, owing to its adhesions to the surrounding structures, the mass may be decompressed and pieces of its walls left in situ.

b) In *partly-thrombosed* aneurysms in which a direct surgical approach seems reasonable, neck occlusion, preceded by thrombectomy with temporary clamping, is the most radical method. Decompression of the sac can thus be easily achieved. If selectively occluding the neck seems dangerous or impossible, interruption of the parent artery by surgical or intravascular approach, provided that the anastomotic supply is adequate, can lead to complete thrombosis of the malformation. If postoperative neuroradiological investigation reveals that simple proximal occlusion has failed to produce complete thrombosis of the sac, the initial operation can be supplemented by secondary intracranial trapping. Finally, if mass effect persists despite total thrombosis secondary to initial thrombosis, a subsequent surgical approach may be indicated for the purpose of decompressing the aneurysmal mass. Serpentine aneurysms, which should be considered a distinct group of partially thrombosed giant aneurysms, may sometimes be excised and the parent artery reconstructed. Where this is not done, progressive proximal occlusion may be attempted.

c) *Non-thrombosed* aneurysms are undoubtedly those which lend themselves best to a direct surgical approach for selective occlusion of the neck and decompression of the sac by intraluminal aspiration of blood. In the most difficult types, temporary clamping or trapping (or even circulatory arrest with extracorporeal circulation, in rare circumstances), can afford the surgeon the time required to shrink the sac and reduce the diameter of the neck in order to properly place a clip or a ligature. In cases where the neck, even though narrow, cannot be exposed without danger, because of adhesive collaterals incorporated into the aneurysmal wall (as encountered in the vertebrobasilar system), intraluminal thrombosis of the sac, which only calls for a minimal exposure of a part of it, can be an effective alternative method. As for wrapping of the sac, this must be considered a pis aller, as the method is both hazardous – because it is necessary to expose the whole sac – and not very effective, since it generally fails to prevent the developmental complications of these aneurysms.

When neck occlusion or intraluminal sac thrombosis is found to be impossible or simply too dangerous, proximal occlusion by a progressive occluding system (tourniquet or inflatable clamp) or trapping of the parent artery can be the safest therapeutic method. But these procedures call for prior ascertainment that the anastomotic supply is good; otherwise, an extra-intracranial bypass must be performed and its functionality checked by doppler sonography and/or angiography prior to occlusion of the parent artery. As for the other types, when complete thrombosis of the sac is not accompanied by a sufficient reduction of its mass effect, secondary surgical decompression is justified.

Although direct surgical exploration of the malformation is theoretically the only reliable means of determining the best therapeutic method, its potential risks may in certain cases justify recourse in the first instance to an indirect approach considered to be less dangerous. Indications will be selected on the basis of the anesthesiological risk factors, the anatomical and circulatory data provided by neuroradiological assessments, and the lessons drawn from the neurosurgeon's own experiences.

3. Therapeutic management also varies according to the *topographic localization of the giant aneurysms.*

a) In *giant aneurysms of the internal carotid artery*, which have classically been managed by interruption of the parent artery, the current tendency – encouraged by the possibilities offered by the microsurgical techniques – is to attempt a direct surgical approach first. This is particularly true for the *carotid-ophthalmic type* of aneurysm, which has become relatively accessible to a direct clipping, provided that the possibility of intraoperative temporary clamping of the segment proximal to the internal carotid artery is planned and the operative field is enlarged by resection of the anterior clinoid process to expose the ophthalmic artery and unroofing of the optic canal in order to reroute the optic nerve.

Carotid artery-posterior communicating artery aneurysms can be directly approached for neck clipping or, when this is impracticable, exclusion by trapping the parent segment.

The high rates of mortality and morbidity linked with attempts at selective neck occlusion of *aneurysms of the carotid bifurcation* may justify immediate recourse to proximal occlusion, particularly if the neck is very wide and/or the perforators cannot be safety preserved.

Finally, for *intracavernous aneurysms*, the general tendency is to prefer occlusion of the parent artery, either surgically at the cervical level or by the intravascular approach. However, stress was recently laid on the reasonable possibility of approaching the cavernous sinus directly and dissecting its different structures by current microsurgical techniques.

b) *Giant aneurysms of the middle cerebral artery, the anterior communicating complex, the posterior cerebral artery, and, in general, the distal arteries* (whether of the carotid or the vertebrobasilar system), always require a direct surgical approach to selectively occlude the neck, or when this is not possible, interrupt the parent segment by proximal occlusion or trapping.

c) Management of *giant aneurysms of the vertebral artery and basilar trunk* can be extremely difficult and hazardous. The development of new clips adapted to the surgery of giant aneurysms has made it possible to push back the boundaries of the operability of these aneurysms by direct surgical approach, especially when neuroradiological findings suggest that neck occlusion is practicable. This holds particularly for vertebral artery aneurysms. In certain cases of narrow-necked giant nonthrombosed aneurysms, access and neck dissection of which is felt to be hazardous, intraluminal thrombosis can be performed by a minimal approach of a limited portion of the sac. This technique has been found to be particularly useful in the hands of those trained to manage specific types located in the basilar trunk or at its bifurcation.

When direct occlusion of the aneurysm turns out to be impracticable, progressive proximal occlusion of the parent artery as close to the aneurysm as possible, by either the surgical or the intravascular approach, is the method of choice. Prior creation of an extra-intracranial bypass has proved to increase its tolerance.

This attempt at a synthesis of the indications for surgery, based on common tendencies emerging from the recent literature, form, as it were, no more than a snapshot of current therapeutic options. With the rapid advances being made not only in microsurgical and intravascular but also in neuroanesthesiological techniques, as also in monitoring methods, it is probable that in the next few years the management of giant aneurysms will make considerable headway, becoming safer and more effective.

Bibliography

This review of the literature, which covers 12 years (1973–1985), has been compiled from the Medline system (key-word: "Giant aneurysms"). The bibliography, owing to its abundance (618 references in all), has been grouped under chapters in order to facilitate consultation by the reader. Abundant and recent references can be found in books by Fox and Yasargil ([32, 135] in the reference list for "Direct Surgical Treatment by Neck Occlusion").

Mechanisms of Formation: Pathological Features

1. Aarabi B, Chambers J (1978) Giant thrombosed aneurysm associated with an arteriovenous malformation. J Neurosurg 44:278–282
2. Amacher LA, Drake CG (1975) Cerebral artery aneurysms in infancy, childhood and adolescence. Childs Brain 1:72–80
3. Artmann H, Vonofako D, Muller H, Grau H (1984) Neuroradiologic and neuropathologic findings with growing giant intracranial aneurysm. Review of the literature. Surg Neurol 21:391–401
4. Barabas A (1970) The effect of C.S.F. on blood clotting. Minerva Neurochir 14:314–323
5. Black SP (1963) Experimental saccular aneurysm by an arterio-venous fistula method. Mo Med 60:340–343
6. Black SP, German WJ (1960) Observation on the relation ship between the volume and the size of the orifice of experimental aneurysms. J Neurosurg 17:984–990
7. Bremer JL (1943) Congenital aneurysms of the cerebral arteries. Arch Pathol 35:819–831
8. Brill CB, Peyster RG, Hoover Ed, Keller MS (1985) Giant intracranial aneurysm in a child with tuberous sclerosis: CT demonstration. J Comput Assist Tomogr 9:311–380
9. Cajander S, Hassler O (1976) Enzymatic destruction of the elastic lamella at the mouth of cerebral aneurysm. Acta Neurol Scand 53:171–181
10. Cambria S, Cardia E, Macri E (1976) Anévrysme géant de l'artère sylvienne chez un enfant de quatre ans (exérèse, guérison). Neurochirurgie 22:85–90
11. Carrillo R, Carreira LM, Prada I, Rosas C, Egas G (1984) Giant aneurysms arising from a single arteriovenous fistula in a child. Case report. J Neurosurg 60:1085–1088
12. Carlson DH, Thomson D (1976) Spontaneous thrombosis of a giant cerebral aneurysm in five days. Report of a case. Neurology (Minneap) 26:334–336
13. Carmichael R (1945) Gross defects in the muscular and elastic coats of the larger cerebral arteries. J Pathol Bact 57:345–351
14. Carmichael R (1950) The pathogenesis of non inflammatory cerebral aneurysms. J Pathol Bact 62:1–19
15. Chiappetta F, Vangelista S, Pirroner R (1982) Recurrent massive otorrhagia caused by a petrous carotid aneurysm. J Neurosurg Sci 26:205–207
16. Crawford T (1959) Some observations of the pathogenesis and natural history of intracranial aneurysms. J Neurol Neurosurg Psychiatry 22:259–266
17. Crompton MR (1966) Mechanisms of growth and rupture in cerebral berry aneurysms. Br Med J 1:1138–1142
18. Cuatico W, Cook AW, Tyshchenko V, Khatib R (1967) Massive enlargement of intracranial aneurysm following carotid ligation. Arch Neurol 17:609–613
19. Dharker SR, Chandy MJ, Chandy SM, Abraham J (1975) Giant traumatic aneurysm of the intracranial carotid artery (case report). Neurol India 23:207–209
20. Drennan AM (1921) Aneurysms of the larger cerebral vessels. NZ Med J 324–349
21. Faria MA, Fleischer AS, Spector RH (1980) Bilateral giant intracavernous carotid aneurysms treated by bilateral carotid ligation. Surg Neurol 14:207–210
22. Finney LH, Roberts TS, Anderson RE (1976) Giant intracranial aneurysm associated with Marfan's syndrome. Case report. J Neurosurg 45:342–347
23. Fodstad H, Liliequist B, Wirell S, Nilsson PE, Boquist L, Abdul Rahman A (1978) Giant serpentine intracranial aneurysm after carotid ligation. Case report. J Neurosurg 49:903–909
24. Forbus WD (1930) On the origin of miliary aneurysms of the superficial cerebral arteries. Bull Johns Hopkins Hop 47:239–284
25. Fischer EG, Strand RD, Shapiro F (1984) Congenital hemihypertrophy and abnormalities of the cerebral vasculature. Report of two cases. J Neurosurg 61:163–168
26. Fox JL (1979) Multiple giant aneurysms. Surg Neurol 12:147–151
27. Fukamachi A, Hirato M, Wakao T, Kawafuchi J (1982) Giant serpentine aneurysm of the posterior cerebral artery. Neurosurgery 11:271–276
28. Garcia-Bengochea F, Deland FH (1975) Bilateral giant carotid ophthalmic aneurysms. Case report. J Neurosurg 42:589–592
29. Gautier JC, Morelot D, Gray F, Awada A (1982) Anévrysme géant des deux artères vertébrales, drop attacks. Rev Neurol (Paris) 1:63–67
30. Gerosa M, Licata C, Fiore DL, Iraci G (1980) Intracranial aneurysms in childhood. Childs Brain 6:295–302
31. Glynn LE (1940) Medial defects in the circle of Willis and their relation to aneurysm formation. J Pathol Bacteriol 51:213–222
32. Goetz RH, Weissberg D, Hoppenstein R (1966) Vascular necrosis caused by application of methyl 2, cyanoacrylate (Eastman 910 Monomer): 7 month following in dogs. Ann Surg 163:242–248
33. Gupta SK, Gupta OP, Singh MM, Varma DN, Kesharwani R (1979) Giant aneurysm of the internal carotid artery in the carotid canal. J Laryngol Otol 93:299–305

34. Guttman M, Tanen SM, Lambert CD (1984) Visual loss secondary to a giant aneurysm in a patient with tuberous sclerosis. Can J Neurol Sci 11:472–474
35. Hashimoto N, Handa H, Hazama F (1978) Experimentally induced cerebral aneurysm in rats. Surg Neurol 10:3–8
36. Hashimoto N, Handa H, Hazama F (1979) Experimentally induced cerebral aneurysm in rats II. Surg Neurol 11:243–246
37. Hashimoto N, Handa H, Hazama F (1979) Experimentally induced cerebral aneurysms in rats III. Surg Neurol 11:299–304
38. Hashimoto N, Handa H (1983) The size of cerebral aneurysms in relation to repeated rupture. Surg Neurol 19:107–111
39. Hassler O, Saltzmann GF (1959) Histologic changes in infundibular widening of the posterior communicating artery. Acta Pathol Microbiol Scand [A] 46:305–312
40. Hassler O (1961) Morphological studies on the large cerebral arteries with reference to the aetiology of subarachnoid hemorrhage. Acta Psychiatr Scand [Suppl 154] 1:145
41. Hassler O (1963) Media defects in human arteries. Angiology 14:368–371
42. Hassler O, Saltzman GF (1963) Angiographic and histologic changes in infundibular widening of the posterior communicating artery. Acta Radiol (Stockh) 1:321–327
43. Hassler O (1972) Scanning electron microscopy of saccular intracranial aneurysms. Am J Pathol 68:511–519
44. Hayashi M, Kobayashi H, Kawano H, Handa Y, Kabuto M (1985) Giant aneurysm of an azygos anterior cerebral artery: report of two cases and review of the literature. Neurosurgery 17:341–344
45. Hirsch CS, Roessmann V (1975) Arterial dysplasia with ruptured basilar artery aneurysms. Report of a case. Hum Pathol 6:749–758
46. Howe JF, Harris AB, Sypert QW (1976) Giant aneurysms of the middle cerebral artery. Surg Neurol 6:231–233
47. Iglesias CG, Torres VE, Offord KP, Holley KE, Beard CM, Kurland LT (1983) Epidemiology of adult polycystic kidney disease. Olmsted country Minnesota. Am J Kidney Dis 2:630–639
48. Jackson AC (1983) Association of mitral valve prolapse and intracranial aneurysms. South Med J 76:712–713
49. Johnsen SD, Okamoto G, Kooiker J (1977) Fusiform basilar artery aneurysm in a child. Neurology (Minneap) 27:334–336
50. Kalyanaraman UP, Elwood PW (1980) Fibromuscular dysplasia of intracranial arteries causing multiple intracranial aneurysms. Hum Pathol 11:481–484
51. Katakura R, Yoshimoto T, Suzuki J (1979) A case of giant aneurysm of the basilar artery. Acta Neurochir 49:87–93
52. Kraus H (1952) Ein besonders großes intrakranielles Aneurysma der Arteria carotis interna. Wien Z Nervenheilk 5–23
53. Kuwabara S, Ohta K, Ueda T, Takahashi M (1981) Giant aneurysms of the bilateral vertebral arteries with serpentine vascular channels. A case report. No To Shinkei 33:1227–1234
54. Lang ER, Kidd M (1965) Electron microscopy of human cerebral aneurysms. J Neurosurg 22:554–562
55. Ley Valle A, Vilalta J, Sahuqvillo J, Garcia M, Nogues P (1983) Giant calcified aneurysm on the posterior cerebral artery in a nine year old child. Surg Neurol 20:396–398
56. Lipper S, Morgan D, Krigman MR, Staab EV (1978) Congenital saccular aneurysm in a 19 days old neonate. Case report and review of the literature. Surg Neurol 10:161–165
57. Little JR, St Louis P, Weinstein M, Dohn DF (1981) Giant fusiform aneurysm of the cerebral arteries. Stroke 12:183–188
58. Locksley HB (1966) Report of the cooperative study of intracranial aneurysms and subarachnoid hemorrhage. Section V. Part II. Natural history of subarachnoid hemorrhage, intracranial aneurysms and arteriovenous malformations based on 6368 cases in the cooperative study. J Neurosurg 25:321–368
59. McCormick WF, Acosta Rua GJ (1970) The size of intracranial saccular aneurysms: an autopsy study. J Neurosurg 33:422–427
60. McCune WS, Samadi A, Blades B (1953) Experimental aneurysms. Ann Surg 138:216–218
61. Matsuda M, Matsuda I, Handa H, Okamoto K (1979) Intracavernous giant aneurysm associated with Marfan's syndrome. Surg Neurol 12:119–121
62. Messimy R, Metzger J, Schaison G, Pfister A, Laccourreye H (1975) Elastopathies cutanées et anomalies vasculaires associées à des déficits neurologiques. A propos de deux cas. Rev Neurol (Paris) 131:419–431
63. Meyermann R, Yasargil MG (1978) Ultrastructural studies of cerebral aneurysms and angiomas gained operatively. Adv Neurol 20:557–567
64. Naruse S, Odake G (1979) Primitive trigeminal artery associated with an ipsilateral intracavernous giant aneurysm. A case report. Neuroradiology 17:259–264
65. Neil Dwyer G, Bartlett JR, Nicholls AC, Narcisi P, Pope FM (1983) Collagen deficiency and ruptured cerebral aneurysms, a clinical and biochemical study. J Neurosurg 59:16–20
66. Niemeyer-Filho P, Jahara F, Laterman H (1983) Spontaneous thrombosis of a giant aneurysm after excision of an associated vascular malformation. Report of a case. Arq Neuropsiquiatr 41:274–279
67. Nishikawa M, Smith RD, Yonekawa Y (1977) Experimental intracranial aneurysms. Surg Neurol 7:241–244
68. Nishizaki T, Tamaki N, Matsumoto S, Fujita S (1985) Multiple giant fusiform aneurysms with hydrocephalus. Surg Neurol 24:101–104
69. Nyström SHM (1963) Development of intracranial aneurysms as revealed by electron microscopy. J Neurosurg 20:329–337
70. Nyström SHM (1979) Factors related to growth, rupture and spontaneous healing of cerebral aneurysms. In: Pia HW, Langmaid C, Zierski J (eds) Cerebral aneurysms: Advances in diagnosis and therapy. Springer, Berlin Heidelberg New York, pp 20–27
71. Orozco M, Trigueros F, Quintana F, Dierssen G (1978) Intracranial aneurysms in early childhood. Surg Neurol 9:247–252
72. Ostergaard JR, Voldby B (1983) Intracranial arterial aneurysms in children and adolescents. J Neurosurg 58:832–837
73. Patel DV, Sherman IC, Hemmati M, Ferguson RJL (1981) Giant serpentine intracranial aneurysm. Surg Neurol 16:402–407
74. Pianetti-Filho G, Barros RS, Cabral-Filho G, Carneiro

FD (1978) Giant aneurysms of the middle cerebral artery. Report of a case. J Neurosurg 49:100–102
75. Read D, Esiri MM (1979) Fusiform basilar artery aneurysm in a child. Neurology (Minneap) 29:1045–1049
76. Rebollo M, Quintana F, Combarros O, Berciano J (1983) Giant aneurysm of the intracavernous carotid artery and bilateral carotid fibromuscular dysplasia. J Neurol Neurosurg Psychiatry 46:284–285
77. Reddy SV, Sundi TM (1981) Giant traumatic false aneurysm of the internal carotid artery associated with a carotid cavernous fistula. Case report. J Neurosurg 55:813–818
78. Reid TL, Cornnell B, Murtagh FR, Cahill DW (1985) Port wine nevus associated with ipsilateral saccular aneurysms treatment by intraarterial balloon trapping. Surg Neurol 23:541–544
79. Resende LA, Asseis EA, Costa LS, Gallina RA (1984) Marfan syndrome and giant intracranial aneurysms: report of a case. Arq Neuropsiquatr 42:294–297
80. Reznik M, Mouchette R, Delcour C (1984) Giant fusiform aneurysm of the basilar artery. Clinico-pathological report of 3 cases. Acta Neurol Belg 84:141–150
81. Sadik AR, Budzilovich GN, Shulman K (1965) Giant aneurysm of middle cerebral artery. J Neurosurg 22:177–181
82. Salcman M, Botero E, Bellis E (1985) Giant post-traumatic aneurysm of the intracranial carotid artery: evolution and regression documented by computed tomography. Neurosurgery 16:218–221
83. Scanarini M, Mingrino S, Zuccarello M, Trincia G (1978) Scanning electron microscopy (SEM) of biopsy specimens of ruptured intracranial saccular aneurysms. Acta Neuropathol 44:131–134
84. Scanarini M, Mingrino S, Giordano R, Baroni A (1978) Histological and ultrastructural study of intracranial saccular aneurysmal wall. Acta Neurochir 43:171–182
85. Segal HD, Mc Laurin RL (1977) Giant serpentine aneurysm. Report of two cases. J Neurosurg 46:115–120
86. Sekhar LN, Heros RC (1981) Origin, growth and rupture of saccular aneurysms. A review. Neurosurg 2:248–260
87. Shishido T, Watanabe M, Kuramoto S (1979) A case of giant aneurysm associated with vertebral fenestration. No Shinkei Geka 7:79–83
88. Sonntag VKN, Yuan RH, Stein BM (1977) Giant intracranial aneurysms. A review of 13 cases. Surg Neurol 8:81–84
89. Spallone A (1982) Giant completely thrombosed intracranial aneurysm simulating tumor of the foramen magnum. Surg Neurol 18:372–376
90. Stehbens WE (1954) Intracranial arterial aneurysms. Arch Ann Med 3:214
91. Stehbens WE (1959) Medial defects in the cerebral arteries of man. J Pathol Bacteriol 78:179–185
92. Stehbens WE (1963) Aneurysms and anatomical variation of cerebral arteries. Arch Pathol 75:45–64
93. Stehbens WE (1963) Histopathology of cerebral aneurysms. Arch Neurol 8:272–285
94. Stehbens WE (1972) Intracranial arterial aneurysm. In: Pathology of the cerebral blood vessels. Mosby Co, St Louis, pp 351–470
95. Stehbens WE (1973) Experimental production of aneurysms by microvascular surgery in rabbits. Vasc Surg 7:165–175
96. Stehbens WE (1975) Ultrastructure of aneurysms. Arch Neurol 32:798–807
97. Steimle R, Jacquet G, Cotte Rittaud M, Pageaut G, Bonneville JF, Razzak AA (1977) Volumineux anévrisme pseudotumoral partiellement thrombosé du territoire de la sylvienne. Neurochirurgie 23:73–80
98. Sutherland GR, Drake CG, Kaufmann JC (1985) Extensive organization in a thrombosed giant intracranial aneurysm: case report. Clin Neuropathol 4:19–22
99. Suzuki J, Ohara H (1978) Clinico-pathological study of cerebral aneurysms: origin, rupture, repair and growth. J Neurosurg 48:505–514
100. Suzuki J, Otsuki T, Yoshimoto T (1984) Arteriovenous malformation and a ruptured giant aneurysm cured by emergency operation in a child. Surg Neurol 22:113–177
101. Terao H, Muraoka I (1972) Giant aneurysm of the middle cerebral artery containing an important blood channel. Case report. J Neurosurg 37:353–356
102. Thauvoy C, Vandresse JH, Stroobandt G, Brucher JM (1978) Accroissement progressif et thrombose d'un anévrysme de la communicante antérieure. Etude clinique, radiologique et histologique. Neurochirurgie 24:423–427
103. Tognetti F, Limoni P, Testa C (1983) Aneurysm growth and hemodynamic stress. Surg Neurol 20:74–78
104. Tomasello F, Albanese V, Cioffi FA (1979) Giant serpentine aneurysms: a separate entity. Surg Neurol 12:429–432
105. Troupp H, Rinne T (1964) Methyl 2, cyano-acrylate (Eastman 910) in experimental vascular surgery with a note on experimental arterial aneurysms. J Neurosurg 21:1067–1069
106. Ventureyra EC, Choo SH, Benoit BG (1980) Super giant globoid intracranial aneurysm in an infant. Case report. J Neurosurg 53:411–416
107. Walker AE, Allegre GW (1954) The pathology and pathogenesis of cerebral aneurysms. J Neuropathol Exp Neurol 13:248
108. Whittle IR, Dorsch NW, Besser M (1982) Spontaneous thrombosis in giant intracranial aneurysms. J Neurol Neurosurg Psychiatry 45:1040–1047

Mechanisms of Formation: Hemodynamic Features

1. Black SWP, German WJ (1960) Observation on the relationship between the volume and the size of the orifice of experimental aneurysms. J Neurosurg 17:984–990
2. Botta JM (1976) Bilan angiographique de 65 anévrysmes opérés de la communicante antérieure. MD Thesis, Lyon
3. Coll AM, Del Corral JF, Yazawa S, Falcon M (1976) Intra-aneurysmal pressure difference in human sacular aneurysms. Surg Neurol 2:93–96
4. Crompton MR (1966) Mechanism of growth and rupture in cerebral berry aneurysms. Br Med J 1:1138–1142
5. Early CB, Fink LH (1976) Some fundamental applications of the law of Laplace in neurosurgery. Surg Neurol 16:185–189
6. Ferguson GG (1970) Turbulence in human intracranial saccular aneurysms. J Neurosurg 33:485–497
7. Ferguson GG (1972) Physical factors in the initiation, growth and rupture of human intracranial saccular aneurysm. J Neurosurg 37:666–676

8. Ferguson GG (1972) Direct measurement of mean and pulsatile blood pressure at operation in human intracranial saccular aneurysms. J Neurosurg 36:560–563
9. Ferguson GG, Roach MR (1972) Flow conditions at bifurcations as determined in glass models with reference to the focal distribution of vascular lesions. In: Bergal DH (ed) Cardiovascular fluid mechanics. Chap 14. Academic Press, London, pp 141–156
10. Fodstad H, Liliequist B, Wirell S et al (1978) Giant serpentine intracranial aneurysm after carotid ligation. Case report. J Neurosurg 49:903–909
11. Fry DL (1968) Acute vascular endothelial changes associated with increased blood velocity gradients. Circ Res 22:165–197
12. German WJ, Black SPW (1954) Experimental production of carotid aneurysms. N Engl J Med 250:104–106
13. German WJ, Black SPW (1954) Intraaneurysmal hemodynamic turbulence. Trans Am Neurol Asso 79:163–165
14. Gilsbach JM (1983) Intraoperative doppler sonography in neurosurgery. Springer, Wien New York, pp 68–88
15. Hashimoto N, Handa H, Nagata T, Hazama F (1980) Experimentally induced cerebral aneurysm in rats. Part V. Relation of hemodynamics in the circle of Willis to formation of aneurysms. Surg Neurol 13:41–45
16. Hayashi S, Arimoto T, Itakura T et al (1981) The association of intracranial aneurysms and arteriovenous malformation of the brain. J Neurosurg 55:971–975
17. Kerber CW, Heilman CB (1983) Flow in experimental berry aneurysms: method and model. AJNR 4, May/June, pp 374–377
18. Koulouris S, Rizzoli H (1981) Coexisting intracranial aneurysm and arteriovenous malformation. Neurosurgery 8:219–222
19. Kwa K, Ohi T, Niizuma H, Suzuki J (1980) Affluent artery and the size of neck of anterior communicating aneurysms. Surg Neurol 13:221–223
20. Miyasaka K, Wolpert SM, Prager RJ (1972) The association of cerebral aneurysms, infundibula and intracranial arteriovenous malformations. Stroke 13:196–203
21. Ozdamar N, Celebi G (1978) Pressure distribution on the wall of experimental aneurysms. Acta Neurochir 45:27–34
22. Robinson JL, Roberts A (1972) Operative treatment of aneurysms and Coanda effect: a working hypothesis. J Neurol Neurosurg Psychiatry 35:804–809
23. Sato O, Kamitani H (1975) Giant aneurysm of the middle cerebral artery: angiographic analysis of blood flow. Surg Neurol 4:27–31
24. Shenkin HA, Jenkins F, Kim K (1971) Arteriovenous anomaly of the brain associated with cerebral aneurysm. J Neurosurg 34:225–228
25. Smith RL, Blick EF, Coalson J, Stein PD (1972) Thrombus production by turbulence. J Appl Physiol 32:261–264
26. Stein PD, Sabbah HN (1974) Measured turbulence and its effect on thrombus formation. Circ Res 35:608–613
27. Sutherland GR, King ME, Peerless SJ (1982) Platelet interaction within giant intracranial aneurysms. J Neurosurg 56:53–61
28. Tognetti F, Limoni P, Testa C (1983) Aneurysm growth and hemodynamic stress. Surg Neurol 20:74–78
29. Van Der Ark GD, Kempe LC (1970) Classification of anterior communicating aneurysms as a basis for surgical approach. J Neurosurg 32:300–303
30. Wright RL (1968) Intraaneurysmal pressure reduction with carotid occlusion: observations in three cases of middle cerebral aneurysms. J Neurosurg 29:139–142
31. Yongchareon W, Young DF (1979) Initiation of turbulence in models of arterial stenoses. J Biomech 12:185–196

Clinical Study

1. Aimard G, Confavreux Ch, Devic M, Vighetto A, Bosson D (1980) Les formes non-hémorragiques des anévrysmes artériels intracrâniens. Rev Neurol (Paris) 136:419–429
2. Allegre G, Aimard G, Dechaume JP, Michel D (1966) Une nouvelle observation d'anévrysme intra-pétreux de la carotide interne à sémiologie optique. Rev Neurol (Paris) 115:1052–1055
3. Alliez B, Tranier J, Gueye M, Sainte Rose C (1978) Tumoral form of an intracranial giant aneurysm in a child. Bull Soc Med Afr Noire Lang Fr 23:365–369
4. Amacher LA, Drake CG (1975) Cerebral artery aneurysms in infancy, childhood and adolescence. Childs Brain 1:72–80
5. Assmann H, Basche S, Pothe H, Dietrich J (1983) Simulation of a hypophyseal tumor in carotid-ophthalmic aneurysms. Zentralbl Chir 108:167–171
6. Bhushan C, Hodges FJ, Posey J (1978) Successful surgical treatment of giant aneurysm of the basilar artery. Case report. J Neurosurg 49:124–128
7. Bohl D, Fenske A, Reulen HJ, Schindler E (1977) Giant aneurysm of the vertebral artery causing compression of the lower medulla oblongata. J Neurol 214:289–293
8. Bose B, Northrup B, Österholm J (1983) Giant basilar artery aneurysm presenting as a third ventricular tumor. Neurosurgery 13:699–702
9. Bull J (1969) Massive aneurysms at the base of the brain. Brain 92:535–570
10. Busse O, Grote E (1982) Recurrent cerebral embolization from a carotid bifurcation aneurysm. Acta Neurochir 62:203–206
11. Cambria S, Cardia E, Macri E (1976) Giant aneurysm of the sylvian artery in a 4 year old child. Neurochirurgie 22:85–90
12. Carrillo R, Carreira LM, Prada J, Rosas C, Egas G (1984) Giant aneurysm arising from a single arteriovenous fistula in a child. Case report. J Neurosurg 60:1085–1088
13. Charamis J, Tsamparlakis T, Scouran J, Doris M, Vassilion G (1976) Ophthalmologic manifestations of intracranial arterial aneurysms. Bull Mem Soc Fr Ophtalmol 87:213–218
14. Cohen AR, Aleksic S, Budzilovich GN, Pinto RS, Flamm ES (1983) Giant intracranial aneurysm presenting as a posterior fossa mass. Surg Neurol 20:160–164
15. Cohen MM, Hemalatha CP, D'Adda Rio RT, Goldmann HW (1980) Embolization from a fusiform middle cerebral artery aneurysm. Stroke 11:158–161
16. Constans JP, Visot A, Fredy D, Dorland P (1976) Anévrysme géant du tronc basilaire révélé par une neuralgie faciale essentielle. Neurochirurgie 22:493–502
17. Copetto JR, Hoffman H (1981) Tolosa-hunt syndrome mimicked by giant aneurysm of posterior cerebral artery. Arch Neurol 38:54–55
18. Copetto JR, Lessell S (1983) Dorsal midbrain syndrome from giant aneurysm of the posterior fossa: report of five cases. Neurology (NY) 33:732–736

19. Creissard P (1980) Les anévrysmes géants. Compte rendu de la Table Ronde de la Société Française de Neurochirurgie. Neurochirurgie 26:309–331
20. Danziger J, Bloch S (1975) Intracranial aneurysms presenting as mass lesion. Clin Radiol 26:267–273
21. David M, Pradat P, Doyon D (1968) Anévrysme de l'artère sylvienne chez un enfant de 3 ans. Neurochirurgie 14:822–823
22. Depierreux M, Retif J, Flament-Durand J (1980) Hydrocephalie provoquée par un anévrysme géant de l'artère basilaire. Acta Neurol Belg 80:80–85
23. De Rougemont J, Abada M, Barge M (1966) Les anévrysmes carotidiens intracaverneux à propos de certains aspects particuliers. Neurochirurgie 12:511–519
24. Dolenc V (1983) A tumor-simulating giant aneurysm of the vertebral artery. Case report. Zentralbl Neurochir 44:215–220
25. Drake CG (1979) Giant intracranial aneurysms: experience with surgical treatment in 174 patients. Clin Neurosurg 26:12–95
26. Duff TA, Gossmann HH (1975) Giant aneurysm of the internal carotid artery simulating posterior fossa tumor in a 13 year old girl. Neurochirurgia 18:190–193
27. Duncan AW, Rumbaugh CL, Caplan L (1979) Cerebral embolic disease: a complication of carotid aneurysms. Radiology 133:379–384
28. Faria MA, Fleischer AS, Spector RH (1980) Bilateral giant intracavernous carotid aneurysms treated by bilateral carotid ligation. Surg Neurol 14:207–210
29. Fischer A, Cooper RL (1976) On the visual disturbances associated with massive basal aneurysms. Proc Aust Assoc Neurol 13:97–107
30. Frydl V (1983) Giant brain-base aneurysms manifested by psychotic symptoms. Fortschr Med 101:1815–1918
31. Ganti SR, Steinberger A, Mc Murtry JG, Hilal SK (1981) Computed tomographic demonstration of giant aneurysms of the vertebro-basilar system. Report of eight cases. Neurosurg 9:261–267
32. Gautier JC, Morelot D, Gray F, Abada A (1982) Anévrysme géant des deux artères vertébrales, drop-attacks. Rev Neurol (Paris) 138:63–67
33. Gerosa M, Licata C, Fiore DL, Iraci G (1980) Intracranial aneurysm of childhood. Childs Brain 6:295–302
34. Gruber D, Brasseur G, Charlin JF, Creissard P, Langloid J (1983) Optochiasmatic compression by a giant intracranial aneurysm. Treatment and favorable visual results. Rev Otoneuroophtalmol 55:289–295
35. Heros RC, Kolluri S (1984) Giant intracranial aneurysms presenting with massive cerebral edema. Neurosurgery 15:512–577
36. Hjer-Pedersen E, Haase J (1981) Giant anterior communicating artery aneurysm with bitemporal hemianopsia: case report. Neurosurgery 8:703–706
37. Jane JA (1961) A large aneurysm of the posterior inferior cerebellar artery in a 1 year old child. J Neurosurg 18:122–124
38. Johnston I (1979) Direct surgical treatment of bilateral intracavernous internal carotid artery aneurysms. J Neurosurg 51:98–102
39. Katakura R, Yoshimoto T, Suzuki J (1979) A case of giant aneurysms of the basilar artery. Acta Neurochir 49:87–93
40. Kobayashi N, Nakagawa Y, Sakuragi M, Tashiro K, Abe H, Tsuru M, Nomura M, Ueno K (1985) Two cases of giant fusiform aneurysm presenting ischemic attacks. No Shinkei Geka 13:919–925
41. Koga H, Mori K (1983) Parinaud syndrome in hydrocephalus due to a basilar artery aneurysm. Surg Neurol 19:548–553
42. Koh CS, Inoue K, Kagay A, Yanagisawa N, Tsukagoshi H (1979) A case report of thrombosed giant basilar aneurysm associated with akinetic mutism. Rinsho Shinkeigaku 19:744–750
43. Lapras C, Goutelle A, Dechaume JP, Brunat M (1968) Les anévrysmes intracrâniens chez l'enfant (à propos de 4 observations). Neurochirurgie 14:91
44. Lapresle J, Lasjaunias P, Verret JM (1979) Anévrysme géant de la carotide intracaverneuse compliqué d'hémorragie méningée. Nouv Presse Med 8:3037–3040
45. Laurent B, Trillet M, Cherabieh R, Fischer C, Schott B (1983) Valeur sémiologique des chutes isolées sans modification de vigilance chez l'adulte et les personnes âgées. Lyon Med 249:239–245
46. Lechelle P, Guiot G, Lestradet H, Pecker J (1948) Volumineux anévrysme de la carotide interne développé dans le sinus caverneux. Considérations diagnostiques et thérapeutiques. Sem Hop Paris 24:1096–1101
47. Ley-Valle A, Vivalta J, Sahuquillo J, Garcia M, Nogues P, Rubio E (1983) Giant calcified aneurysm on the posterior cerebral artery in a nine year old child. Surg Neurol 20:396–398
48. Lumenta CB, Lins E, Bock WJ (1984) Bilateral giant aneurysms of the internal carotid artery suspected as hypophyseal tumor in computerized tomography. Neurochirurgia (Stuttg) 27:117–119
49. Lynch JC, Amaral MA (1983) Giant aneurysm of the petrous portion of the carotid artery. J Neurol Neurosurg Psychiatry 46:685–686
50. Massey CE, El Gamma T, Brooks BS (1984) Giant posterior inferior cerebellar artery aneurysm with dysphagia. Surg Neurol 22:467–471
51. Matsko DE, Bogachenko DV (1981) Giant aneurysms of the cerebral vessels (Russian). Arkh Patol 43:29–35
52. Matson DD (1965) Intracranial arterial aneurysms in childhood. J Neurosurg 23:578–583
53. Maxwell RE, Chou SN (1977) Aneurysmal tumors of the basifrontal region. J Neurosurg 46:438–445
54. McKinna AJ (1983) Eye signs in 611 cases of posterior fossa aneurysms: their diagnostic and prognostic value. Can J Ophtalmol 18:3–6
55. Mehdorn HM, Chater NL, Townsend JJ, Darroch JD, Perkins RK, Lagger R (1980) Giant aneurysm and cerebral ischemia. Surg Neurol 13:49–57
56. Michel D, Dechaume JP, Allegre GE, Pheline C, Cabanis EA, Bret P (1970) Les anévrysmes intrapétreux de la carotide interne. A propos de 2 observations. J Med Lyon 1184:867–875
57. Morley TP, Barr HWK (1969) Giant intracranial aneurysms: diagnosis, course and management. Clin Neurosurg 16:73–94
58. Nakamura Matsuda K, Asakura T (1983) Case of hyperprolactinemia as a manifestation of a thrombosed giant aneurysm of the internal carotid artery. Rinsho Shinkeigaku 23:551–555
59. Osenbach RK, Blumenkopf B, McComb B, Huggins MJ (1986) Occular bobbing with ruptured giant distal posterior inferior cerebellar artery aneurysm. Surg Neurol 25:149–152
60. Pecker J, Geets W (1956) Evolution artériographique d'un volumineux anévrysme sylvien opéré avec succès chez un enfant de 7 ans. Neurochirurgie 2:109–114
61. Pecker J, Hoel J, Javalet A, Fournier M (1960) Volumi-

neux anévrysme carotidien intrapétreux révélé par une paralysie isolée du moteur oculaire externe. Bull Soc Ophtalmol Fr 4:286–290
62. Peiris JB, Ross Russel RW (1980) Giant aneurysms of the carotid system presenting as visual field defect. J Neurol Neurosurg Psychiatry 43:1053–1064
63. Pia HW (1978) Classification of aneurysms of the internal carotid system. Acta Neurochir 40:5–31
64. Pia HW (1979) Classification of vertebro-basilar aneurysms. Acta Neurochir 47:3–30
65. Pia HW (1980) Large and giant aneurysms. Neurosurg Rev 3:7–16
66. Piek J, Lim DP, Bock WJ (1983) Obstructive hydrocephalus caused by a growing, giant aneurysm on the upper basilar artery. Surg Neurol 20:288–290
67. Ravon R, Bouquier JJ, Dupuy JP, Bokor J, Feiss P, Vidal J, Dany A (1976) Un cas d'anévrysme géant intrapétreux et intracaverneux de la carotide interne chez l'enfant. Neurochirurgie 22:621–626
68. Raymond LA, Tew J (1978) Large suprasellar aneurysms imitating pituitary tumor. J Neurol Neurosurg Psychiatry 41:83–87
69. Rodriguez-Gomez D, Jimenez-Escrig A, Astarloa-Gomez R, Gobernado-Serrano JM, Gimeno-Alava A (1985) Giant fusiform cerebral aneurysm as a cause of transient cerebral ischemia. Rev Clin Esp 177:136–137
70. Rouzaud M, Gouaze A, Vigneron P, Jezegabel C (1964) Paralysies oculo-motrices et atteinte du trijumeau par volumineux anévrysme carotidien intracaverneux. Rev Neurol (Paris) 110:155–158
71. Rush JA, Bavis GA, Drake CG (1981) Bitemporal hemianopsia in basilar artery aneurysms. J Clin Neuro Ophtalmol 1:129–133
72. Russegger L, Grunert V (1983) A partly thrombosed basilar artery aneurysm simulating a tumor of the 3rd ventricule. Neurochirurgia (Stuttg) 26:59–62
73. Sarwar M (1977) Abducens nerve paralysis due to giant aneurysm in the medial carotid canal. Case report. J Neurosurg 46:121–123
74. Sato T, Kodama N, Suzuki J (1976) Homonymous hemianopsia due to chiasmal compression by intracranial aneurysm. Neurol Surg Tokyo 4:689–697
75. Shibata S, Mori K (1975) Bilateral giant carotid aneurysms in the cavernous sinus with a carotid-cavernous fistula on one side. Case report. Neurol Surg Tokyo 3:347–352
76. Shimizu Y, Namba S, Kinoshita K (1985) Spontaneous angiographical disappearance of an unruptured giant aneurysm of the basilar top demonstrated by a sequential series of angiograms. A case report. No Shinkei Geka 13:1121–1127
77. Sœur M, Brihaye J, Moerman C (1979) Pseudo-tumoural aneurysm in the third ventricle: report of three cases. Acta Neurochir 45:247–258
78. Spallone A (1982) Giant completely thrombosed intracranial aneurysm simulating tumor of the foramen magnum. Surg Neurol 18:372–376
79. Steel JG, Thomas HA, Strollo PJ (1982) Fusiform basilar aneurysm as a cause of embolic stroke. Stroke 13:712–716
80. Steinberger A, Ganti SR, Mc Murtry JG, Hilal SK (1984) Transient neurological deficits secondary to saccular vertebrobasilar aneurysms. Report of two cases. J Neurosurg 60:410–413
81. Suzuki J, Otsuki T, Yoshimoto T (1984) Arteriovenous malformation and a ruptured giant aneurysm cured by emergency operation in a child. Surg Neurol 22:173–177
82. Swearingen B, Heros RC (1985) Fatal rupture of a thrombosed giant basislar artery aneurysm. Surg Neurol 23:299–302
83. Synowitz HJ, Leonhard T, Unger RR, Kloppick E (1985) Giant aneurysm manifestations, diagnosis and therapy. Zentralbl Neurochir 46:11–30
84. Tabarin A, Eresue J (1983) Anévrysmes de la carotide interne simulant une tumeur hypophysaire. Rev Fr Endocrinol Clin 24:5–12
85. Uozumi T, Shima T, Mori S (1979) A case of arterial carotid giant aneurysm with bilateral visual disturbance and panhypopituitarism treated by direct surgery. No Shinkei Geka 7:25–31
86. Van Zandijcke M, Dehaene I (1983) Isolated bilateral oculomotor paralysis due to a ruptured aneurysm. Acta Neurol Belg 83:191–201
87. Ventureyra EC, Choo SH, Benoit BG (1980) Super-giant globoid in an infant. Case report. J Neurosurg 53:411–416
88. Vinuela F, Fox A, Chang JK, Drake CG, Peerless SJ (1984) Clinico-radiological spectrum of giant supraclinoic internal carotid artery aneurysms. Observations in 93 cases. Neuroradiology 26:93–99
89. White JC, Ballantine HT (1961) Intrasellar aneurysms simulating hypophyseal tumors. J Neurosurg 18:34–50
90. Whittle IR, Allsop JL, Halmagyi GM (1985) Focal seizures: an unusual presentation of giant intracranial aneurysms. A report of four cases with comments on the natural history and treatment. Surg Neurol 24:533–540
91. Whittle IR, Dorsch NW, Besser M (1984) Giant intracranial aneurysms: diagnosis, management, and outcome. Surg Neurol 21:218–230
92. Wozniak M, Mazurowski W, Chrzanowski M (1978) Case of giant aneurysm of the basilar artery. Neurol Neurochir Pol 12:345–349
93. Yoshimoto T, Kayama T, Kodama N, Suzuki J (1978) Distribution of intracranial aneurysms. Tohoku J Exp Med 126:125–132
94. Zubkov I, Matsko DE (1980) Certain clinico-anatomic features of large and giant arterial aneurysms of cerebral vessels (Russe). Zh Nevropatol Psikhiatr 80:1809–1813

Neuroradiological Features

1. Ammerman BJ, Smith DR (1977) Giant fusiform middle cerebral aneurysm: successful treatment utilizing microvascular bypass. Surg Neurol 7:255–257
2. Artmann H, Vonofakos D, Muller H, Grau H (1984) Neuroradiologic and neuropathologic findings with growing giant intracranial aneurysm. Surg Neurol 21:391–401
3. Asari S, Satoh T, Sakurai M, Yamamoto Y, Sadamoto K (1982) Delineation of unruptured cerebral aneurysms by computerized angiotomography. J Neurosurg 57:527–534
4. Babu VS, Eisen H (1979) Giant aneurysm of anterior-communicating artery simulating 3rd ventricular tumor. Comput Tomogr 3:159–163
5. Byrd SE, Bentson JR, Winter J, Wilson GH, Joyce PW, O'Connor L (1978) Giant intracranial aneurysms simulating brain neoplasms on CT. J Comput Assist Tomogr 2:303–307
6. Bradley YWC Jr, Waluch V, Lai KS, Fernandez EJ, Spalter C (1984) The appearance of rapidly flowing

blood on magnetic resonance images. AJNR 143:1167–1174
7. Cantu RC, Lemay M (1966) A large middle cerebral aneurysm presenting as a bizarre vascular malformation. Case report. Br J Radiol 39:317–319
8. Carlson DH, Thomson D (1976) Spontaneous thrombosis of a giant cerebral aneurysm in five days. Report of a case. Neurology 26:334–336
9. Davis KR et al (1977) Complementary role of computed tomography and other neuroradiologic procedures. Surg Neurol 8:437–447
10. Dublin AB, French BN (1980) Cerebral aneurysmal rupture during angiography with confirmation by computed tomography: a review of intra-angiographic aneurysmal rupture. Surg Neurol 13:19–26
11. Eggers FM, Price AC, Allen JH, James AE Jr (1983) Neuroradiologic applications of intra-arterial digital subtraction angiography. AJNR 4:854–856
12. Fiore DL, Pardatscher K, Marin G, Galligioni F, Distefano E, Iraci G (1980) The value and limitations of the CT scan in the diagnosis of giant intracranial aneurysms (2 cases). Acta Neurochir 53:19–24
13. Fodstad H, Liliequist B, Wirell S, Nilsson PE, Boquist L, Abdul-Rahman A (1978) Giant serpentine intracranial aneurysm after carotid ligation. J Neurosurg 49:903–909
14. Fujiwara S, Kodama N, Suzuki J (1982) Sequential CT findings on giant aneurysms of the intracranial internal carotid artery after carotid ligation. Neurol Med Chir (Tokyo) 22:267–275
15. Fukamachi A, Mirato M, Wakao T, Kawafuchi J (1982) Giant serpentine aneurysm of the posterior cerebral artery. Neurosurgery 11:271–276
16. Ganti SR, Steinberger A, McMurtry JG, Hilal SK (1981) Computed tomographic demonstration of giant aneurysms of the vertebro-basilar system: report of eight cases. Neurosurgery 9:261–267
17. Golding R, Peatfield RC, Shawdon HH, Rice Edwards JM (1980) Computed tomographic features of giant intracranial aneurysms. Clin Radiol 31:41–48
18. Handa J, Nakano Y, Aii H, Handa H (1978) Computed tomography with giant intracranial aneurysms. Surg Neurol 9:257–263
19. Jones JN, Schwarz HJ (1977) Two cases of giant intracerebral aneurysms simulating neoplasm on CT scan; one with coexistent chronic sub-dural hematomas. J Neurol 215:49–57
20. Kataoka K, Yamada K, Nakao K, Hayakawa T, Ikeda T, Kawai R, Miura T (1983) Digital subtraction angiography and dynamic computed tomography for evaluating the hemodynamics in cases of giant intracranial aneurysm. Surg Neurol 20:355–360
21. Kazner E, Klein W, Stoch Dorph O (1978) Possibilities and significances of computed tomography in non-tumorous space-occupying intracranial lesions. Rontgenblatter 31:181–198
22. Lavyne MH, Kleefield J, Davis KR, Ojemann RG, Crowell RM (1978) Giant intracranial aneurysms of the anterior circulation: clinical characteristics and diagnosis by CT. Neurosurgery 3:356–363
23. Little JR, St Louis P, Weinstein M, Dohn DF (1981) Giant fusiform aneurysm of the cerebral arteries. Stroke 12:183–188
24. Lukin RR, Chambers AA, Mc Laurin R, Tew J Jr (1975) Thrombosed giant middle cerebral aneurysm. Neuroradiology 10:125–129
25. Milles CM, Brandt-Zawadzki M, Crooks LE, Kaufman L, Sheldon P, Norman D, Bank W, Newton TH (1984) Nuclear magnetic resonance: principles of blood flow imaging. AJNR 142:165–170
26. Morley TP, Barr HWK (1969) Giant intracranial aneurysms: diagnosis, course and management. Clin Neurosurg 16:73–94
27. Nadjmi M, Ratzka M, Wodarz M (1978) Giant aneurysms in CT and angiography. Neuroradiology 16:284–286
28. Naheedy MH, Tyler HR, Wolf MA, Hammerschlag SB (1982) Diagnosis of thrombotic giant basilar artery aneurysm on computed tomographic scan. Arch Neurol 39:64–65
29. Nakstad PH, Skalpe IO (1981) Computed tomography in the evaluation of the supraclinoid arteries in suprasellar pituitary gland tumors. Arch Radiologica Diagnosis 22:399–402
30. Obrador S, Dierssen G, Rodriguez-Hernandez J (1967) Giant aneurysm of posterior cerebral artery. Case report. J Neurosurg 26:413–416
31. O'Neill M, Hope T, Thomson G (1980) Giant intracranial aneurysms: diagnosis with special reference to computerized tomography. Clin Radiol 31:27–39
32. Ostrowski K, Bonicki W, Sadowski Z, Wislawski J (1984) Internal carotid artery aneurysm in the sella turcica area simulating pituitary tumor. Neurol Neurochir Pol 18:187–190
33. Pascaud JL, Merland J, Ravon R, Hummel P, Vigneu P, Pascaud-Ged E (1982) Thrombosed carotid aneurysm and CT scan. Report on three cases. J Radiol 63:283–286
34. Patel DV, Sherman IC, Hemmati M, Ferguson RJ (1981) Giant serpentine intracranial aneurysm. Surg Neurol 16:402–407
35. Perrett LV, Sage MR (1977) Computerized tomography and giant intracranial aneurysms. Australas Radiol 21:308–312
36. Petit-Perrin DP, Aubin ML, Vignaud J (1979) C.T. findings in giant intracranial aneurysms. J Neuroradiol 6:317–326
37. Petit-Perrin D, Vignaud J, Aubin ML (1980) Computed tomography in the giant intracranial aneurysms. Ann Radiol 23:641–645
38. Petit-Perrin D, Vignaud J, Aubin ML (1981) Computed tomography in the giant intracranial aneurysms. Sem Hop Paris 57:1301–1305
39. Pinto RS, Cohen WA, Kricheff IF, Redington RW, Berninger WH (1982) Giant intracranial aneurysms: rapid sequential computed tomography. AJR 139:973–977
40. Pinto RS, Kricheff II, Buttler AR, Murali R (1979) Correlation of computed tomographic angiographic and neuropathological changes in giant cerebral aneurysms. Radiology 132:85–92
41. Pozzati E, Nuzzo G, Gaist G (1982) Giant aneurysm of the pericallosal artery. Case report. J Neurosurg 57:566–569
42. Pressman BD, Gilbert GE, Davis DO (1975) Computerized transverse tomography of vascular lesions of the brain. Am J Roentgenol 124:215–219
43. Sadik AR, Budzilovich GN, Shulman K (1965) Giant aneurysm of the middle cerebral artery. A case report. J Neurosurg 22:177–181
44. Sartor K, Nadjmi M (1979) Angiotomography for aneurysms and arterio-venous malformations of the head and neck. Neuroradiology 17:89–100

45. Sarwar M, Batnitzky S, Schechter M (1976) Tumorous aneurysms. Neuroradiology 12:79–97
46. Schubiger O, Valavanis A, Hayek J (1980) Computed tomography in cerebral aneurysms with special emphasis on giant intracranial aneurysms. J Comput Assist Tomogr 4:24–32
47. Scotti G, Ethier R, Melancon D, Terbrugge K, Tchang S (1977) Computed tomography in the evaluation of intracranial aneurysms and subarachnoid hemorrhage. Radiology 123:85–90
48. Segal HD, Mc Laurin RL (1977) Giant serpentine aneurysm. Report of two cases. J Neurosurg 46:115–120
49. Sellem E, Rougier J, Chauplannaz G, Sindou M (1982) Giant supra-clinoid aneurysm with ophthalmologic disclosure: comparative value of tomodensitometry and arteriography. Bull Soc Ophtalmol 12:1507–1510
50. Slosberg PS (1982) Symptomatic unruptured giant aneurysms: medical treatment. Acta Neurochir 62:207–218
51. Spincemaille GH, Slooff JL, Hogenhuis LA, Lodder J (1985) Completely thrombosed giant aneurysm of the basilar artery trunk: 2 case reports. Neurosurgery 17:968–970
52. Steimle R, Jacquet G, Cotte-Rittaud M, Pageaut G, Bonneville JF, Abdul Razzak A (1977) Volumineux anévrysme pseudo-tumoral partiellement thrombosé du territoire de la sylvienne. Neurochirurgie 23:73–80
53. Stevens JL (1950) Central thrombosis in an intracranial aneurysm. Case report. Br J Radiol 23:614–615
54. Terao H, Muraoka I (1972) Giant aneurysm of the middle cerebral artery containing an important blood channel. J Neurosurg 37:353–356
55. Thauvoy C, Vandresse JH, Stroobandt G, Brucher JM (1978) Accroissement progressif et thrombose d'un anévrysme de la communicante antérieure. Etude clinique, radiologique et histologique. Neurochirurgie 24:423–427
56. Thron A, Bockenheimer S (1979) Giant aneurysms of the posterior fossa suspected as neoplasms on CT. Neuroradiology 18:93–97
57. Tomasello F, Albanese V, Cioffi FA (1979) Giant serpentine aneurysm: a separate entity. Surg Neurol 12:429–432
58. Valentin C, Chauplannaz G, Duquesnel J, Sindou M, Trocme Y, Trillet M (1981) Anévrysme géant juxta-clinoïdien à sémiologie akinéto-hypertonique et endocrinienne. Valeur respective des investigations neuroradiologiques. Lyon Med 246:77–80
59. Vonofakos D, Hacker H, Grau H (1983) Direct visualization of intracranial aneurysms by multiplane dynamic CT. AJNR 4:425–428
60. Whittle IR, Dorsch NW, Besser M (1982) Spontaneous thrombosis in giant intracranial aneurysms. J Neurol Neurosurg Psychiatry 45:1040–1047
61. Whittle IR, Williams DB, Halmagyi GM, Besser M (1982) Spontaneous thrombosis of a giant intracranial aneurysm and ipsilateral internal carotid artery. Case report. J Neurosurg 56:287–289
62. Wilmink JT, Vencken LM (1979) Complementary values of static and dynamic scintigraphy, computerized tomography and angiography in the diagnosis of a partially thrombosed giant intracranial aneurysm. Clin Neurol Neurosurg 81:87–96
63. Worthington BS, Kean DM, Hawkes RC, Holland GN, Moore WS, Corston R (1983) NMR imaging in the recognition of giant intracranial aneurysms. AJNR 4:835–836
64. Yamamoto Y, Satoh T, Sakurai M et al (1982) Minimum dose contrast bolus in computed angiotomography of the brain. J Comput Assist Tomogr 6:575–585
65. Yoshida S, Ezuka I, Ohtsuka A (1981) Follow-up study of the giant aneurysm by CT scan after unilateral carotid ligation. No Shinkei Geka 9:1083–1086

Direct Surgical Treatment by Neck Occlusion

1. Abad Rico JM, Rivas Salas JJ, Marin Zarza F, Lamas Greco E (1978) Giant aneurysm of the posterior cerebral artery. Rev Clin Exp 150:201–203
2. Adams CBT, Jamous MA (1983) The operative treatment of giant aneurysms. J Neurol Neurosurg Psychiatr 46:373
3. Allegre G, Vigouroux R (1957) Traitement chirurgical des anévrysmes intracrâniens du système carotidien. Rapport à la Société de Neurochirurgie de Langue Française, Masson, Paris
4. Almeida GM, Shibata MK, Bianco E (1976) Carotid-ophthalmic aneurysms. Surg Neurol 5:41–45
5. Ammerman BJ, Smith DR (1977) Giant fusiform middle cerebral aneurysms. Successful treatment utilizing microvascular by-pass. Surg Neurol 7:255–257
6. Artero JC, Ausman JJ, Dujovny M, Mora EO, Umansky F, Diaz FG, Mirchandani H, Berman K (1985) Middle cerebral artery reconstruction. Surg Neurol 24:5–11
7. Barr HWK, Blackwood W, Meadows SP (1971) Intracavernous carotid aneurysms: a clinical pathological report. Brain 94:607–622
8. Beck DW, Boarini DJ, Kassell NF (1979) Surgical treatment of giant aneurysm of the vertebral-basilar junction. Surg Neurol 12:283–285
9. Benedetti A, Curri D (1977) Direct attack on carotid-ophthalmic and large internal carotid aneurysms. Surg Neurol 8:49–54
10. Bloor BM, Odom GL, Woodhall B (1951) Direct measurement of intravascular pressure in components of the circle of Willis. Arch Surg 63:821–823
11. Bonnal J, Stevenaert A (1969) Thrombosis of intracranial aneurysms of the circle of Willis after incomplete obliteration by clip or ligature across the neck. J Neurosurg 130:158–163
12. Borne G, Arnoud B, Bedou G, Aresu PJ, Garidou JP (1979) Les anévrysmes géants de la carotide interne intra-caverneuse infra-clinoïdienne. Neurochirurgie 25:101–107
13. Botta JM (1966) Bilan angiographique de 65 anévrysmes opérés de la communicante antérieure. MD Thesis, Lyon
14. Cantore GP, Ciappetta P, Vagnozzi R, Bozzao L (1982) Giant aneurysm of the anterior inferior cerebellar artery simulating cerebellar pontine angle tumor. Surg Neurol 18:76–78
15. Constans JP, Dilenge D, De Divitiis E, Aboulker J (1965) Anévrysmes carotidiens infra-clinoïdiens bilatéraux. Neurochirurgie 11:421–440
16. Chou SN, Ortiz-Suarez H (1974) Surgical treatment of arterial aneurysms of the vertebro-basilar circulation. J Neurosurg 41:671–680
17. Cophignon J, Georges B (1984) Personal communication
18. Dawson B (1958) The blood vessels of the human optic

chiasma and their relation to those of the hypophysis and hypothalamus. Brain 81:207–217
19. De Morais JV, Lana-Peixoto MA (1978) Bilateral intracavernous carotid aneurysms. Treatement by bilateral carotid ligation. Surg Neurol 9:379–381
20. Dolenc V (1982) End-to-end suture of the posterior inferior cerebellar artery after the excision of a large aneurysm: case report. Neurosurgery 11:690–693
21. Dolenc V (1983) Direct microsurgical repair of intracavernous vascular lesions. J Neurosurg 58:824–831
22. Dolenc V, Tivada I, Skaric I, Lamovec Z, Cerk M (1983) Direct microsurgical intra-arterial procedures on ICA and MCA. Neurosurg Rev 6:7–12
23. Donzelli R, De Divitiis (1984) Personal communication
24. Drake CG (1968) The surgical treatment of aneurysms of the basilar artery. J Neurosurg 29:436–446
25. Drake CG (1978) Treatment of aneurysms of the posterior cranial fossa. Prog Neurol Surg 9:122–194
26. Drake CG (1979) Giant intracranial aneurysms: experience with surgical treatment in 174 patients. Clin Neurosurg 26:12–95
27. Drake CG (1974) Surgical treatment of vertebral-basilar aneurysms. In: Sano K, Ishii S (eds) Recent progress in neurological surgery. Proceeding of the Vth International progress of neurological surgery. Excerpta Medica, Amsterdam, pp 183–190
28. Drake CG (1979) The treatment of aneurysms of the posterior circulation. Clin Neurosurg 96–114
29. Faria MA, Fleischer AS, Spector RH (1980) Bilateral giant intra-cavernous carotid aneurysms treated by bilateral carotid ligation. Surg Neurol 14:207–210
30. Flamm ES (1981) Suction decompression of aneurysms. Technical note. J Neurosurg 54:275–276
31. Fox JL (1979) Multiple giant aneurysms. Surg Neurol 12:147–151
32. Fox JL (1983) Intracranial aneurysms. Springer, Berlin Heidelberg New York
33. French LA, Chou SN, Story JL et al (1966) Aneurysm of the anterior communicating artery. J Neurosurg 24:1058–1062
34. Fukuoka S, Suematsu K, Fujiwara H, Hashimoto I, Nakamura J (1984) Completely thrombosed giant aneurysm of the angular artery. Surg Neurol 22:145–148
35. Ganti SR, Steinberger A, McMurtry JG, Hilal SK (1981) Computed tomographic demonstration of giant aneurysms of the vertebro-basilar system. Report of eight cases. Neurosurgery 9:261–267
36. Garcia-Bengochea F, Deland FH (1975) Bilateral giant carotid-ophthalmic aneurysms. Case report. J Neurosurg 42:589–592
37. Glasscock ME (1969) Exposure of the intra-petrous portion of the carotid artery. In: Hamberger CA, Wersall J (eds) Disorders of the skull base region; proceedings of the tenth Nobel Symposium, Stockholm, 1968. Almquist and Wiksell, pp 135–143
38. Grand W, Hopkins LN (1977) The microsurgical anatomy of the basilar artery bifurcation. Neurosurgery 1:128–131
39. Guidetti B, Latorre E (1975) Management of carotid-ophthalmic aneurysms. J Neurosurg 42:438–442
40. Hammon WM, Kempe LG (1972) The posterior fossa approach to aneurysms of the vertebral and basilar arteries. J Neurosurg 37:339–347
41. Handa H, Hashimoto N, Yonekawa Y (1982) Surgical treatment of giant aneurysms. Neurosurg Rev 5:169–172
42. Harris FS, Rhoton AL Jr (1976) Anatomy of the cavernous sinus. A microsurgical study. J Neurosurg 46:169–180
43. Hayakawa T, Kamikawa K, Ohnishi T, Yoshimine T (1981) Prevention of post-operative complications after a transoral approach to basilar aneurysms. Technical note. J Neurosurg 54:699–703
44. Heros RC, Nelson PB, Ojeman RG, Crowell RM, Debrun G (1983) Large and giant paraclinoid aneurysms: surgical techniques, complications and results. Neurosurgery 12:153–163
45. Hitchcock E, Cowie RA (1983) Clipping of vertebro-basilar aneurysms. J Neurol Neurosurg Psychiatry 46:373
46. Hook O, Norlen G, Guzman J (1963) Saccular aneurysms of the vertebral basilar arterial system. A report of 28 cases. Acta Neurol Scand 39:271–304
47. Hosobuchi Y (1979) Direct surgical treatment of giant intracranial aneurysms. J Neurosurg 51:743–756
48. Howe JF, Harris AB, Sypert GW (1976) Giant aneurysms of the middle cerebral artery. Surg Neurol 6:231–233
49. Ishii R, Koike T, Takevchi S, Ohsugi S, Tanaka R, Konno K (1983) Anastomosis of the superficial temporal artery to the distal anterior cerebral artery with interposed cephalic vein graft. J Neurosurg 58:425–429
50. Ito Z (1982) The microsurgical anterior interhemispheric approach suitably applied to ruptured aneurysms of the anterior communicating artery in the acute stage. Acta Neurochir 63:85–99
51. Ito H, Shima T, Yamamoto S (1975) Giant anterior communicating artery aneurysm. Neurol Surg Tokyo 3:171–176
52. Ito Z (1985) A new technique of intracranial inter-arterial anastomosis between distal anterior cerebral arteries and its indication (unpublished work)
53. Jamieson KG (1968) Aneurysms of vertebro-basilar system. Further experience with nine cases. J Neurosurg 28:544–555
54. Jane JA (1961) A large aneurysm of the posterior inferior cerebellar artery in a 1 year old child: case report. J Neurol 18:245–247
55. Jefferson G (1938) On the saccular aneurysms of the internal carotid artery in the cavernous sinus. Br J Surg 26:267–302
56. Johnston I (1979) Direct surgical treatment of bilateral intracavernous internal carotid artery aneurysms. J Neurosurg 51:98–102
57. Judice D, Conolly ED (1978) Foramen magnum syndrome caused by a giant aneurysm of the posterior inferior cerebral artery. Case report. J Neurosurg 48:639–641
58. Kempe LG (1979) Aneurysm of the vertebral artery. In: Pia HW, Langmaid C, Zierski J (eds) Cerebral aneurysm: advances in diagnosis and therapy. Springer, Berlin Heidelberg New York, pp 119–120
59. Kothandaram P, Dawson BM, Kruyt RE (1971) Carotid-ophthalmic aneurysms. A study of 19 patients. J Neurosurg 34:544–548
60. Krayenbuhl H, Yasargil MG, Flamm ES et al (1972) Microsurgical treatment of intracranial saccular aneurysms. J Neurosurg 37:678–686
61. Kunc Z (1979) Giant intracranial aneurysm. Cesk Neurol Neurochir 42:297–303

62. Kwa K, Ohi T, Niizuma H, Suzuki J (1980) Afferent artery and the site of neck anterior communicating aneurysms. Surg Neurol 13:221–223
63. Laine E (1968) Arterial vertebro-basilar aneurysms. Prog Brain Res 30:323–346
64. Litvak J, Sumners TC, Barron JL, Fisher LS (1981) A successful approach to vertebro-basilar aneurysms. Technical note. J Neurosurg 55:491–494
65. MacFarlane MR, McAllister VL, Whitby DJ, Sengupta RR (1983) Posterior circulation aneurysms. Results of direct operations. Surg Neurol 20:399–413
66. Matsuda M, Matsuda I, Handa H et al (1979) Intracavernous giant aneurysm associated with Marfan's syndrome. Surg Neurol 12:119–121
67. Maxwell RE, Chou SN (1977) Aneurysmal tumors of the basifrontal region. J Neurosurg 46:438–445
68. Meadows SP (1959) Intracavernous aneurysms of the internal carotid artery: their clinical features and natural history. Arch Ophthalmol 62:566–574
69. Mineura K, Kodama N, Suzuki J (1979) Surgical treatment of the carotid-ophthalmic aneurysms. No Shinkei Geka 7:233–237
70. Morley TP, Barr HWK (1969) Giant intracranial aneurysms: diagnosis, course and management. Clin Neurosurg 16:73–94
71. Nakahara A, Ajakura T, Kawabatake H, Inoue K, Kitamura K (1975) A giant aneurysm of the internal carotid artery treated by intracranial direct surgery with a special reference to the anatomical relationship between the cavernous sinus and the internal carotid artery. Neurol Surg Tokyo 3:783–789
72. Nakao S, Kikuchi H, Takahashi V (1981) Successful clipping of carotid ophthalmic aneurysms through a controlateral pterional approach. Report of two cases. J Neurosurg 54:532–536
73. Nutik S (1978) Carotid paraclinoid aneurysms with intradural origin and intracavernous location. J Neurosurg 48:526–533
74. O'Neill M, Hope T, Thomson G (1980) Giant intracranial aneurysms: diagnosis with special reference to computerized tomography. Clin Radiol 31:27–39
75. Onuma T, Suzuki J (1979) Surgical treatment of giant intracranial aneurysms. J Neurosurg 51:33–36
76. Parkinson D (1965) A surgical approach to the cavernous portion of the carotid artery. Anatomical studies and case report. J Neurosurg 23:474–483
77. Parkinson D (1973) Carotid cavernous fistula: direct repair with preservation of the carotid artery. Technical note. J Neurosurg 38:99–106
78. Parkinson D (1981) Airgun retraction for major bifurcation saccular aneurysms. Technical note. J Neurosurg 54:844
79. Pasqualin A, Daplian R, Colomaria V, Bardin PG (1979) Giant unruptured aneurysm of the middle cerebral artery, manifesting with epilepsy; successful surgical treatment. J Neurosurg Sci 23:303–310
80. Patel DV, Sherman IC, Hemmati M, Perguson RJ (1981) Giant serpentine intracranial aneurysm. Surg Neurol 16:402–407
81. Paullus WS, Pait TG, Rhoton AL (1977) Microsurgical exposure of the petrous portion of the carotid artery. J Neurosurg 47:713–726
82. Peiris JB, Ross Russell RW (1980) Giant aneurysms of the carotid system presenting as visual field defect. J Neurol Neurosurg Psychiatry 43:1053–1064
83. Pertuiset B, Van Effenterre R, Robert G (1978) Chronology of diagnostic and therapeutic activities in the 3 weeks following rupture of an intracranial saccular aneurysm (series of 316 cases). Rev Neurol 134:23–34
84. Pertuiset B, Van Effenterre R, Robert G (1979) Surgery of upper basilar artery aneurysms. Experience with 11 cases. In: Pia HW, Langmaid C, Zierski I (eds) Cerebral aneurysms. Springer, Berlin Heidelberg New York, pp 311–318
85. Pertuiset B, Ancri D, Lienhart A, Goutorbe J, Sichez JP (1980) Electrothermic reduction and clipping of ruptured intracranial saccular aneurysms under deep hypotension (MAP ≤ 50 mm Hg) induced with sodium nitroprusside with reference to vascular autoregulation (series of 377 cases). Neurol Res 2:199–216
86. Pertuiset B, Ancri D, Lienhart A (1981) Profound arterial hypotension (MAP ≤ 50 mm Hg) induced with neurolept-analgesia and sodium nitroprusside (series of 531 cases). Reference to vascular autoregulation mechanism and surgery of vascular malformations of the brain. In: Krayenbuhl H (ed) Advances and technical standards in neurosurgery. Springer, Wien New York 8, pp 75–118
87. Pia HW, Fontana H (1977) Aneurysms of the posterior cerebral artery. Locations and clinical pictures. Acta Neurochir 38:13–35
88. Pia HW (1978) Classification of aneurysms of the internal carotid system. Acta Neurochir 40:5–31
89. Pia HW, Zierski J (1979) Giant cerebral aneurysms: problems in treatment. In: Pia HW, Langmaid C, Zierski J (eds) Advances in diagnosis and therapy. Cerebral aneurysms. Springer, Berlin Heidelberg New York, pp 336–342
90. Pia HW, Langmaid C, Zierski J (1979) Advances in diagnosis and therapy: cerebral aneurysms. Springer, Berlin Heidelberg New York, 468 p
91. Pia HW (1979) Classification of vertebro-basilar aneurysms. Acta Neurochir 47:3–30
92. Pia HW (1980) Large and giant aneurysms. Neurosurg Rev 3:7–16
93. Pianetti Filha G, Barros RS, Cabral Filho G, Carneiro FD, Lauar EH (1978) Giant aneurysms of middle cerebral artery: report of a case. Arq Neuropsiquiatr 36:155–159
94. Pozzati E, Nuzzo G, Gaist G (1982) Giant aneurysm of the pericallosal artery. Case report. J Neurosurg 57:566–569
95. Ravon R (1971) Les anévrysmes artériels du système vertébrobasilaire. MD Thesis, Lyon, 132 p
96. Rhoton AL Jr, Hardy DG, Chambers SM (1979) Microsurgical anatomy and dissection of the sphenoid bone, cavernous sinus and sellar region. Surg Neurol 12:63–104
97. Rout D, Sharma A, Mohan PK, Rao VR (1984) Bacterial aneurysms of the intracavernous carotid artery. J Neurosurg 60:1236–1242
98. Saeki N, Rhoton AL Jr (1977) Microsurgical anatomy of the upper basilar artery and the posterior circle of Willis. J Neurosurg 46:563–578
99. Santini JJ, Gouaze A (1975) L'endo-anévrysmorraphie. A propos de 2 cas d'anévrysme sylvien géant. ONO 47:9–13
100. Sato O, Kamitani H (1975) Giant aneurysm of the middle cerebral artery: angiographic analysis of blood flow. Surg Neurol 4:27–31
101. Sato T, Komatsu S, Sakurai Y, Suzuki J (1980) A case

of giant aneurysm at the anterior communicating artery treated by direct surgery. No Shinkei Geka 8:93–98
102. Schoolman A, Kepes JJ (1967) Bilateral spontaneous carotid-cavernous fistulae in Ehlers-Danlos syndrome. Case Report. J Neurosurg 26:82–86
103. Segal HD, Mc Laurin RL (1977) Giant serpentine aneurysm. Report of 2 cases. J Neurosurg 46:115–120
104. Sekhar LN, Nelson PB (1983) A technique of clipping giant intracranial aneurysms with the preservation of the parent artery. Surg Neurol 20:361–368
105. Seltzer J, Hurteau EF (1957) Bilateral symmetrical aneurysms of internal carotid artery within the cavernous sinus. Case report. J Neurosurg 14:448–451
106. Sengupta RP, Lassman LP, Moraes AA, Garvan N (1975) Treatment of internal carotid bifurcation aneurysms by direct surgery. J Neurosurg 43:343–351
107. Sengupta RP, Gryspeerdt GL, Hankinson J (1976) Carotid-ophthalmic aneurysms. J Neurol Neurosurg Psychiatry 39:837–853
108. Sengupta RP (1982) Management of large and giant aneurysms. Neurosurg Rev 5:173–178
109. Smith RR, Parent AD (1982) End-to-end anastomosis of the anterior cerebral artery after excision of a giant aneurysm. Case report. J Neurosurg 56:577–580
110. Sonntag VKH, Yuan RH, Stein BM (1977) Giant intracranial aneurysms: a review of 13 cases. Surg Neurol 8:81–84
111. Steimle R, Jacquet G, Cotte-Rittaud M, Pageaut G, Bonneville JF, Aboul Razzak A (1977) Volumineux anévrysme pseudo-tumoral partiellement thrombosé du territoire de la sylvienne. Neurochirurgie 23:73–80
112. Sugita K, Shintani A, Mutsuga N et al (1977) Microsurgery for vertebrobasilar aneurysms. Neurol Med Chir 2:351–360
113. Sugita K, Kobayashi S, Shintani A, Mutsuga N (1979) Microneurosurgery for aneurysms of the basilar artery. J Neurosurg 51:615–620
114. Sugita K, Kobayashi S, Inoue T et al (1981) New angled fenestrated clips for fusiform vertebral artery aneurysms. J Neurosurg 54:346–350
115. Sugita K, Kobayashi S, Kyoshima K et al (1982) Fenestrated clips for unusual aneurysms of the carotid artery. J Neurosurg 57:240–246
116. Sundt TM Jr, Pluth JR, Gronert GA (1972) Excision of giant basilar aneurysm under profound hypothermia: report of a case. Mayo Clin Proc 47:631–634
117. Sundt TM Jr, Piepgras DG (1979) Surgical approach to giant intracranial aneurysms. Operative experience with 80 cases. J Neurosurg 51:731–742
118. Suzuki J (1979) Prognosis of 1000 pure saccular aneurysms operated upon, in "Cerebral Aneurysms". In: Pia HW, Langmaid C, Zierski J (eds). Springer, Berlin Heidelberg New York, pp 413–418
119. Suzuki J, Mizoi K, Yoshimo T (1986) Bifrontal interhemispheric approach to aneurysms of the anterior communicating artery. J Neurosurg 64:183–190
120. Suzuki J, Sato T (1980) Direct surgical treatment of giant intracranial aneurysms. Neurol Res 2:305–325
121. Symon L, Vajda J (1984) Surgical experiences with giant intracranial aneurysms. J Neurosurg 61:1009–1028
122. Terao M, Muraoka I (1972) Giant aneurysm of the middle cerebral artery containing an important blood channel. J Neurosurg 37:353–356
123. Thauvoy C, Vandresse JH, Stroobandt G (1978) Accroissement progressif et thrombose d'un anévrysme de la communicante antérieure. Neurochirurgie 24:423–427
124. Thurel C, Rey A, Thiebaut JB et al (1974) Anévrysmes carotido-ophtalmiques. Neurochirurgie 20:25–39
125. Tomasello F, Albanese V, Cioffi FA (1979) Giant serpentine aneurysm: a separate entity. Surg Neurol 12:429–432
126. Tulleken CA (1976) Giant aneurysms of the posterior fossa presenting as space occupying lesions. Clin Neurol Neurosurg 79:161–186
127. Umansky F, Nathan M (1982) The lateral wall of the cavernous sinus. With special reference to the nerves related to it. J Neurosurg 56:228–234
128. Van Der Ark GD, Kempe LC (1970) Classification of anterior communicating aneurysms as a basis for surgical approach. J Neurosurg 32:300–303
129. Verbalis JG, Nelson PB, Robinson AG (1982) Reversible panhypopituitarism caused by a suprasellar aneurysm: the contribution of mass effect to pituitary dysfunction. Neurosurgery 10:604–611
130. White JC, Ballantine HT (1961) Intra-sellar aneurysms simulating hypophyseal tumors. J Neurosurg 18:34–50
131. Wilson CB, Myers FK (1963) Bilateral saccular aneurysms of the internal carotid artery in the cavernous sinus. J Neurol Neurosurg Psychiatry 26:174–177
132. Wilson CB, U HS (1976) Surgical treatment for aneurysms of the upper basilar artery. J Neurosurg 44:537–543
133. Wilson CB, Spetzler RF (1979) Operative approaches to aneurysms. Clin Neurosurg 26:232–247
134. Yasargil MG (1969) Microsurgery applied to neurosurgery. Thieme, Stuttgart
135. Yasargil MG (1984) Microneurosurgery II: clinical considerations, surgery of the intracranial aneurysm and results. Thieme, Stuttgart
136. Yasargil MG, Fox JL (1975) The microsurgical approach to intracranial aneurysms. Surg Neurol 3:7–14
137. Yasargil MG, Fox JL, Ray MW (1975) The operative approach to aneurysms of the anterior communicating artery. In: Krayenbuhl H (ed) Advances and technical standards in neurosurgery. Springer, Wien New York, pp 113–170
138. Yasargil MG, Antic J, Laciga R, Jain KK, Hodosh RM, Smith RD (1976) Microsurgical pterional approach to aneurysms of the basilar bifurcation. Surg Neurol 6:83–91
139. Yasargil MG, Smith RD (1977) Surgery on the carotid system in the treatment of hemorrhage stroke. Adv Neurol 16:181–209
140. Yasargil MG, Gasser JC, Hodosh RM et al (1977) Carotid-ophthalmic aneurysms: direct microsurgical approach. Surg Neurol 8:155–165
141. Yasargil MG, Smith RD, Gasser C (1978) Microsurgery of the aneurysms of the internal carotid artery and its branches. Prog Neurol Surg 9:58–121
142. Yeh HS, Tew JM (1985) Anterior interhemispheric approach to aneurysms of the anterior communicating artery. Surg Neurol 23:98–100
143. Yoshi Y, Maki Y, Egashira T (1979) Giant aneurysms of the distal portion of the posterior inferior cerebellar artery. Eur Neurol 18:382–386
144. Yoshimoto T, Uchida K, Kanekou et al (1979) An analysis of follow-up results of 1000 intracranial saccular aneurysms with definitive surgical treatment. J Neurosurg 50:152–157

Clips and Giant Aneurysms

1. Bradford DW (1977) A simple method of measuring aneurysm clip tension. J Neurosurg 47:788–789
2. Bradford OW, Ray R (1978) Metallurgical analysis of aneurysm and microvascular clips. J Neurosurg 48:614–621
3. Colombo F, Curri D, Benedetti A (1980) The broken clip. Neurochirurgia 23:126–129
4. Drake CG, Allcock JM (1973) Post-operative angiography and the "slipped" clip. J Neurosurg 39:683–689
5. Drake CG (1978) Treatment of aneurysms of the posterior cranial fossa. Prog Neurol Surg 9:122–194
6. Dujovny M, Kossovsky N, Kossovsky R et al Magnetic fields and metal implants: study of aneurysm clips (personal communication)
7. Dujovny M, Wakenhut N, Kossowsky N et al (1979) Minimum vascular occlusive force. J Neurosurg 51:662–668
8. Edner GF, Ericson K, Forster DMC et al (1978) The broken clip. Acta Neurochir 40:145–149
9. Fox JL (1976) Vascular clips for the microsurgical treatment of stroke. Stroke 5:489–499
10. Heifetz MD (1969) A new intra-cranial aneurysm clip. J Neurosurg 30:753
11. Heifetz MD (1982) Failure of aneurysm clip. J Neurosurg 57:866–867
12. Kossowsky R, Dujovny M, Kossowsky N, Keravel Y (1982) Failure of a Heifetz aneurysm clip. J Neurosurg 57:233–239
13. Mayfield FH, Kess G Jr (1971) A brief history of the development of the Mayfield clip. Technical note. J Neurosurg 35:97–100
14. McFadden JT (1972) Tissue reaction to standard neurosurgical metallic implants. J Neurosurg 36:598–603
15. Quest DO, Countee RW (1977) Fractured aneurysm clip. J Neurosurg 47:466–468
16. Rosenbaum TJ, Sundt TM (1978) Inter-relationship of aneurysm clips and vascular tissue. J Neurosurg 48:929–934
17. Servo A, Puranen M (1977) Delayed breaking of a Heifetz aneurysm clip. J Neurosurg 47:463–465
18. Shahababian S, Mayfield FH (1978) Modification of intracranial aneurysm clip. J Neurosurg 49:935–936
19. Sugita K, Hirota T, Iguchi I (1976) Comparative study of the pressure of various aneurysm clips. J Neurosurg 44:723–727
20. Sugita K, Kobayashi S, Inoue T et al (1981) New angled fenestrated clips for fusiform vertebral artery aneurysms. J Neurosurg 54:346–350
21. Sugita K, Kobayashi S, Shintani A et al (1979) Microneurosurgery for aneurysms of the basilar artery. J Neurosurg 51:615–620
22. Sugita K, Kobayashi S, Kyoshima K et al (1982) Fenestrated clips for unusual aneurysms of the carotid artery. J Neurosurg 57:240–246
23. Sugita K, Kobayashi S, Inoue T, Takemae T (1984) Characteristics and use of ultra-long aneurysm clips. J Neurosurg 60:145–150
24. Sundt TM Jr, Piepgras DG, Marsh WR (1984) Booster clips for giant and thick based aneurysms. J Neurosurg 60:151–162
25. Yasargil MG (1978) Microsurgery of the aneurysm of the internal carotid artery and its branches. Prog Neurol Surg 9:55–121

Direct Surgical Treatment by Wrapping and Intravascular Thrombosis

1. Alksne JF, Rand RW (1962) Current status of metallic thrombosis intracranial aneurysms. Prog Neurol Surg 3:212–229
2. Alksne JF, Smith RW (1977) Iron-acrylic compound for stereotaxic aneurysm thrombosis. J Neurosurg 44:137–141
3. Alksne JF, Smith RW (1980) Stereotaxic occlusion of 22 consecutive anterior communicating artery aneurysms. J Neurosurg 52:790–793
4. Carney PG, Oatey PE (1983) Muslin wrapping of aneurysms and delayed visual failure. A report of three cases. J Clin Neuro Ophthalmol 3:91–96
5. Dott NM (1983) Intracranial aneurysms: cerebral arteriography: surgical treatment. Edinb Med J 40:219–234
6. Drake CG (1979) Giant intracranial aneurysms: experience with surgical treatment in 174 patients. Clin Neurosurg 26:12–95
7. Dutton J (1969) Acrylic investment of intracranial aneurysms. A report of 12 years experience. J Neurosurg 31:652–657
8. Gallagher JP (1964) Pilojection for intracranial aneurysms. Report of progress. J Neurosurg 21:129–134
9. Ganti SR, Steinberger A, Mc Murty JG, Hilal SK (1981) Computed tomographic demonstration of giant aneurysms of the vertebro-vascular system. Report of eight cases. Neurosurg 9:261–267
10. Gillingham FJ (1958) The management of ruptured intracranial aneurysm. Ann R Coll Surg 23:78–177
11. Hosobuchi Y (1975) Electrothrombosis of carotid cavernous fistula. J Neurosurg 42:76–85
12. Hosobuchi Y (1979) Direct surgical treatment of giant intracranial aneurysms. J Neurosurg 51:743–756
13. Mazars G (1956) Communication à la Société Française de Neurologie
14. McMurtry JG, Housepian EM, Bowman FO, Mateo RS (1974) Surgical treatment of basilar artery aneurysms. Elective circulatory arrest with thoracotomy in 12 cases. J Neurosurg 40:486–494
15. Mount LA, Antunes JI (1975) Results of treatment of intracranial aneurysms by wrapping and coating. J Neurosurg 42:189–193
16. Mullan S (1974) Experiences with surgical thrombosis of intracranial berry aneurysms and carotid cavernous fistulas. J Neurosurg 41:657–670
17. Mullan S (1979) Treatment of carotid cavernous fistulas by cavernous sinus occlusion. J Neurosurg 50:131–144
18. Northfield DWC (1952) Comment on Norlen G: The pathology, diagnosis and treatment of intracranial saccular aneurysms. Proc R Soc Med 45:302
19. Selverstone B (1963) Treatment of intracranial aneurysms with adherent plastics. Clin Neurosurg 9:201–213
20. Smith RW, Alksne JF (1977) Stereotaxic thrombosis of inaccessible intracranial aneurysms. J Neurosurg 47:833–839
21. Sonntag VKH, Yuan RH, Stein BM (1979) Giant intracranial aneurysms: a review of 13 cases. Surg Neurol 8:81–84
22. Velpeau A (1831) Mémoire sur la piqûre ou l'acupuncture des artères dans le traitement des anévrysmes. Gaz Med Paris 2:1–4
23. Werner SC, Blakemore AH, King BG (1941) Aneurysm

of internal carotid artery within the skull: wiring and electrothermic coagulation. JAMA 116:578–582
24. Wilson CB, U HS (1976) Surgical treatment for aneurysms of the upper basilar artery. J Neurosurg 44:537–543

Extracorporeal Circulation

1. Chalnot P, Lepoire J avec la collaboration de Grosdidier J, Frisch R, Montaut J, Bouchot M, Picard JM, Meyer (1963) L'arrêt circulatoire sous hypothermie profonde et CEC dans le traitement des anévrysmes intra-crâniens. Neurochirurgie 9:129–146
2. Davison Ph, Mc Ilveen DJS, Small JM et al (1968) Elective circulatory arrest with continuous coronary perfusion during neurosurgical operation. Br Heart J 30:705–712
3. Drake CG, Barr HWK, Coles JC, Gergely NF (1964) The use of extra-corporeal circulation and profound hypothermia in the treatment of ruptured intracranial aneurysm. J Neurosurg 21:575–581
4. Gissen AJ, Matteo RS, Housepian EM et al (1969) Elective circulatory arrest during neurosurgery for basilar artery aneurysms. JAMA 207:1315–1318
5. Gonski A, Johnston JB (1966) Profound hypothermia as an adjunct in the surgical management of intracranial aneurysms. Report of eight cases. Pac Med Surg 74:259–263
6. Guegan Y, Scarabin JM, Le Guilcher C, Guillou L, Logeais Y, Pecker J (1985) Extracorporeal circulation with deep hypothermia and circulatory arrest in the treatment of intracranial arterial aneurysms. Surg Neurol 24:441–448
7. Guiot G, Rougerie J, Arfel G, Dubost C, Blondeau P (1960) Le "Grand Froid" en neurochirurgie. Possibilités et perspectives d'avenir. Neurochirurgie 6:332–346
8. Housepian EM, Bowman FO, Gissen AJ (1967) Elective circulatory arrest in intracranial surgery. J Neurosurg 26:594–597
9. McMurtry JG III, Housepian EM, Bowman FO (1974) Surgical treatment of basilar artery aneurysms. Elective circulatory arrest with thoracotomy in 12 cases. J Neurosurg 40:486–494
10. Michenfelder JD, Kirklin JW, Uihlein A et al (1964) Clinical experience with a closed-chest method of producing profound hypothermia and total circulatory arrest in neurosurgery. Ann Surg 159:125–131
11. Patterson RH Jr, Ray BS (1962) Profound hypothermia for intracranial surgery: laboratory and clinical experience with extra-corporeal circulation by peripheral cannulation. Ann Surg 156:377–393
12. Rey A (1973) L'arrêt circulatoire encéphalique en neurochirurgie. Neurochirurgie 19:251–252
13. Riemens V, Baudet E, Chauve A, Roques X (1982) Intérêt de l'arrêt circulatoire en hypothermie profonde par canulation périphérique et circulation extra-corporelle sans ouverture du thorax pour le traitement chirurgical des lésions anévrysmales intracraniennes géantes. Communication à la SNCLF, Paris
14. Silverberg GD, Reitz BA, Ream AK, Taylor G, Enzmann DR (1980) Operative treatment of a giant cerebral artery aneurysm with hypothermia and circulatory arrest report of case. Neurosurgery 6:301–305
15. Silverberg GD, Reitz BA, Ream AK (1981) Hypothermia and cardiac arrest in the treatment of giant aneurysms of the cerebral circulation and hemangioblastoma of the medulla. J Neurosurg 55:337–346
16. Silverberg GD (1984) Giant aneurysms: surgical treatment. Neurol Res 6:57–63
17. Small JM, Stevenson SC (1966) Circulatory arrest in neurosurgery. Lancet 1:569–570
18. Sundt TM, Pluth JR, Gronert GA (1972) Excision of a giant basilar aneurysm under profound hypothermia. Report of a case. Mayo Clin Proc 47:631–634
19. Uihlein A, MacCarty CS, Michenfelder JD et al (1966) Deep hypothermia and surgical treatment of intracranial aneurysms. A five-year surgery. JAMA 195:639–641
20. Woodhall B, Sealy WC, Hall KD et al (1960) Craniotomy under conditions of guinidine-protected cardioplegia and profound hypothermia. Ann Surg 152:37–44

Surgical Occlusion of the Parent Artery

1. Ausman JI, Lee MC, Chater N et al (1979) Superficial temporal artery to superior cerebellar artery anastomosis for distal basilar artery stenosis. Surg Neurol 12:277–282
2. Bakay L, Sweet WH (1952) Cervical and intracranial intraarterial pressures with and without vascular occlusion. Surg Gynecol Obstet 95:67–75
3. Bakay L, Sweet WH (1958) Intra-arterial pressures in the neck and brain. J Neurosurg 10:353–359
4. Bhushan C, Hodges FJ, Posey J (1978) Successful surgical treatment of giant aneurysm of the basilar artery. Case report. J Neurosurg 49:124–128
5. Black SPW, German WJ (1953) The treatment of internal carotid artery aneurysms by proximal arterial ligation. A follow-up study. J Neurosurg 10:590–601
6. Bloor BM, Glista GG (1977) Observations on simultaneous internal carotid artery and total cerebral blood flow measurements in man. Neurosurgery 1:249–255
7. Bloor BM, Odom GL, Woodhall B (1951) Direct measurement of intravascular pressure in components of the circle of Willis. Arch Surg 63:821–823
8. Brunon J (1973) Les possibilités chirurgicales dans la pathologie vertébro-basilaire ischémique. MD Thesis, Lyon, 320 p
9. Brunon J, Goutelle A (1974) L'ischémie cérébrale dans le territoire vertébro-basilaire. Fabre, 157 p
10. Christiansson J (1962) On the late effect of carotid ligation upon the humain eye. Acta Ophthalmol 40:271–280
11. Drake CG (1975) Ligation of the vertebral (unilateral or bilateral) or basilar artery in the treatment of large intracranial aneurysms. J Neurosurg 43:255–274
12. Drake CG (1979) Giant intracranial aneurysms: experience with surgical treatment in 174 patients. Clin Neurosurg 26:12–95
13. Drake CG (1979) The treatment of aneurysms of the posterior circulation. Clin Neurosurg 26:96–144
14. Ferguson GG (1972) Direct measurement of mean and pulsatile blood pressure at operation in human intracranial saccular aneurysms. J Neurosurg 36:560–563
15. Fodstad H, Lillequist B, Wirell S, Nilsson PE, Boquist L, Abdul-Rahman A (1978) Giant serpentine intracranial aneurysm after carotid ligation. Case report. J Neurosurg 49:903–909
16. German WJ, Black SPW (1954) Experimental production of carotid aneurysms. N Engl J Med 250:104–106
17. Gratzl O, Schmiedek P, Steinhoff H (1975) Extracranial-intracranial arterial bypass in patients with occlusion

of cerebral arteries due to trauma and tumor. In: Handa H (ed) Microneurosurgery. University Park Press, Baltimore, pp 68–80
18. Hashimoto N, Handa H, Hazama F (1978) Experimentally induced cerebral aneurysms in rats. Surg Neurol 18:3–8
19. Hassler O (1963) Experimental carotid ligation followed by aneurysmal formation and other morphological changes in the circle of Willis. J Neurosurg 20:1–7
20. Heyman A, Tindall GT, Finney WHM, Woodhall B (1960) Measurement of retinal artery, intra-carotid pressures following carotid artery occlusion with the Crutchfield clamp. J Neurosurg 17:297–305
21. Hirato M, Fukamachi A, Toyoda O, Kaneko M, Wakao T, Nukui H (1983) A newly-developed aneurysm after controlateral common carotid ligation for arteriovenous malformation with porencephalia. Case report. Neurol Med Chir (Tokyo) 23:163–166
22. Hockley AD (1975) Proximal occlusion of the anterior cerebral artery for anterior communicating artery. J Neurosurg 43:426–431
23. Hosobuchi Y (1979) Direct surgical treatment of giant intracranial aneurysms. J Neurosurg 51:743–746
24. Ishii R, Koike T, Takeuchi S, Ohsugi S, Tanaka R, Konno K (1983) Anastomosis of the superficial temporal artery on the distal anterior cerebral artery with interposed cephalic vein graft. J Neurosurg 58:425–429
25. Ishii R, Tanaka R, Koike T, Takeda N, Takeuchi S, Sasaki O, Okada K (1983) Computed tomographic demonstration of the effect of proximal parent artery ligation for giant intracranial aneurysms. Surg Neurol 19:532–540
26. Kak VK, Taylor AR, Gordon DS (1973) Proximal carotid ligation for internal carotid aneurysms. A long term follow-up study. J Neurosurg 39:503–513
27. Karvounis PC, Singounas EG (1983) Proximal ligation of the anterior cerebral artery for the treatment of the anterior communicating aneurysms. Neurochirurgia 26:118–119
28. Kondo T, Higashi H, Murakami T, Goto T, Sugawara T, Tsubokawa T, Moriyasu N (1978) A case of giant aneurysm at the posterior cerebral artery. No Shinkei Geka 6:907–911
29. Landolt AM, Millikan CH (1970) Pathogenesis of cerebral infarction secondary to mechanical carotid artery occlusion. Stroke 1:52–62
30. Love IG, Dart LH (1967) Results of carotid ligation with particular reference to intracranial aneurysms. J Neurosurg 27:89–93
31. Matsuda M, Shiino A, Handa J (1985) Rupture of previously unruptured giant carotid aneurysm after superficial temporal middle cerebral artery bypass and internal carotid occlusion. Neurosurgery 16:177–184
32. Morris L (1963) Arteriographic studies in aneurysms of the internal carotid artery treated by carotid occlusion. Acta Radiol 1:367–372
33. Mount LA (1959) Results of treatment of intracranial aneurysms using the Selverstone clamp. J Neurosurg 16:611–618
34. Mount LA, Taveras JM (1956) The results of surgical treatment of intracranial aneurysms as demonstrated by progress arteriography. J Neurosurg 13:618–626
35. Mount LA, Taveras JM (1962) Ligation of the basilar artery in the treatment of an aneurysm at the basilar bifurcation. J Neurosurg 19:167–170
36. Murphey F (1965) Extracranial carotid ligation: technical aspects. In: Fields WS, Sahs AL (eds) Intracranial aneurysms and subarachnoid haemorrhage, Thomas, Springfield (Ill) pp 315–323
37. Nakao S, Fukumitsu T, Ogata M (1982) Transient total ophthalmoplegia following internal carotid artery ligation for treatment of intracavernous giant aneurysm. Surg Neurol 17:458–463
38. Nishioka H (1966) Results of the treatment of intracranial aneurysm by occlusion of the carotid artery in the neck. J Neurosurg 25:660–682
39. Odom GL, Tindall GT (1968) Carotid ligation in the treatment of certain intracranial aneurysms. Clin Neurosurg 15:101–116
40. Oldershaw JB, Voris HC (1966) Internal carotid artery ligation. A follow-up study. Neurology 16:937–938
41. Pelz DM, Vinuela F, Fox AJ, Drake CG (1984) Vertebrobasilar occlusion therapy of giant aneurysms. Significance of angiographic morphology of the posterior communicating arteries. J Neurosurg 60:560–565
42. Pool JL, Potts DG (1965) Aneurysms and arterio-venous anomalies of the brain. Harper & Row, New York
43. Poppen JL, Fager CA (1960) Intracranial aneurysms: results of surgical treatment. J Neurosurg 17:283–296
44. Pozzati E, Fagioli L, Servadei F, Gaist G (1981) Effect of common carotid ligation on giant aneurysms of the internal carotid artery: computerized tomography study. J Neurosurg 55:527–531
45. Roski RA, Spetzler RF, Nulsen FE (1980) Late ischemic complications of carotid ligation in the treatment of intracranial aneurysms. Presented at American Association of Neurological Surgeons Annual Meeting, April 21, New York
46. Rozario RA, Stein BM (1980) Ligation of the basilar artery as the definitive treatment for a giant aneurysm of the basilar artery apex: case report. Neurosurgery 6:87–91
47. Schott B, Bourrat C, Trillet M, Goutelle A (1965) Pathologie du système vertébro-basilaire. Rapport de Neurologie présenté au Congrès de Neurologie et de Psychiatrie de Langue Française, Masson, Paris
48. Scott M, Skwarok E (1961) The treatment of cerebral aneurysms by ligation of the common carotid artery. Surg Gynecol Obstet 113:54–61
49. Sengupta D, Harper M, Jennett B (1973) Effect of carotid ligation on cerebral blood flow in baboons. Response to altered pCO2. J Neurol Neurosurg Psychiatry 36:736–741
50. Shibata T, Ito A, Enomoto H, Harada J (1982) Proximal ligation of the vertebral artery for treatment of vertebral aneurysms. No Shinkei Geka 10:1327–1332
51. Sindou M, Brunon J, Fischer G, Goutelle A, Mansuy L (1977) L'anastomose extra-intracrânienne préalable à la ligature de la carotide. Neurochirurgie 23:205–213
52. Somak FM, Shenkin HA (1966) Angiographic end-results of carotid ligation in treatment of carotid aneurysms. J Neurosurg 24:966–974
53. Sonntag VKH, Yuan RH, Stein BH (1977) Giant intracranial aneurysms: a review of 13 cases. Surg Neurol 8:81–84
54. Sundt TM Jr, Campbell JK, Houser OW (1981) Transpositions and anastomoses between the posterior cerebral and superior cerebellar arteries. Report of two cases. J Neurosurg 55:967–970
55. Sundt TM Jr, Piepgras DG (1979) Surgical approach to giant intracranial aneurysms. Operative experience with 80 cases. J Neurosurg 51:731–742

56. Sundt TM Jr, Piepgras DG, Houser OW, Campbell JK (1982) Interposition saphenous vein grafts for advanced occlusive disease and large aneurysms in the posterior circulation. J Neurosurg 56:205–215
57. Sweet WH, Bennett HS (1948) Changes in internal carotid pressure during carotid and jugular occlusion and their significance. J Neurosurg 5:178–195
58. Sweet WH, Sarnoff SJ, Bakay L (1950) A clinical method for recording internal carotid pressure. Surg Gynecol Obstet 90:327–334
59. Tindall GT, Goree JA, Lee JF, Odom GL (1966) Effect of common carotid ligation on size of internal carotid aneurysms and distal intracarotid and retinal artery pressures. J Neurosurg 25:503–511
60. Tindall GT, Odom GL (1969) Treatment of intracranial aneurysms by proximal carotid ligation. Prog Neurol Surg 3:66–114
61. Tindall GT, Odom GL, Cupp HB Jr, Dillon ML (1962) Studies on carotid artery flow and pressure. Observations in 18 patients during graded occlusion of proximal carotid artery. J Neurosurg 19:917–923
62. Tindall GT, Odom GL, Dillon ML, Cupp HB Jr, Mahaley MS Jr, Greenfield JC Jr (1963) Direction of blood flow in the internal and external carotid arteries following occlusion of the ipsilateral common carotid artery. J Neurosurg 20:985–994
63. Tytus JS, Ward AA (1970) The effect of cervical carotid ligation on giant intracranial aneurysms. J Neurosurg 33:184–190
64. Vlahovitch B, Fuentes JM, Reynaud C, Benbouzid T, Mazariegos R (1985) Série de 17 cas d'anévrysmes géants intra-crâniens, suites chirurgicales éloignées et effets hémodynamiques des occlusions artérielles. Neurochirurgie 31:255–263
65. Voris HC (1951) Complications of ligation of the internal carotid artery. J Neurosurg 8:119–131
66. Winn HR, Richardson AE, Jane JA (1977) Late morbidity and mortality of common carotid ligation for posterior communicating aneurysms. J Neurosurg 47:727–736
67. Woodhall B, Odom GL, Bloor BM, Golden J (1952) Direct measurement of intravascular pressure in components of circle of Willis. A contribution to the surgery of congenital cerebral aneurysms and vascular anomalies of the brain. Ann Surg 135:911
68. Woodhall B, Odom GL, Bloor BM, Golden J (1953) Studies on cerebral intravascular pressure: Further data concerning residual pressure in components of the circle of Willis and in blind arterial segments. J Neurosurg 10:28–34
69. Wright RL (1968) Intra-aneurysmal pressure reduction with carotid occlusion. Observations in three cases of middle cerebral aneurysms. J Neurosurg 29:139–142
70. Wright RL, Sweet WH (1963) Carotid or vertebral occlusion in the treatment of intracranial aneurysms. Value of early and late readings of carotid and retinal pressures. Clin Neurosurg 13:163–192
71. Wright RL, Sweet WH (1965) Intra-arterial pressure determinations at the time of carotid occlusion. Correlation with clinical tolerance of occlusion and subsequent subarachnoid hemorrhage. In: Fields WS, Sahs AL (eds) Intracranial aneurysms and subarachnoid hemorrhage. Thomas, Springfield (Ill), pp 324–347
72. Yasargil MG, Antic J, Laciga R, Jain KK, Hodosh RM, Smith RD (1976) Microsurgical pterional approach to aneurysms of the basilar bifurcation. Surg Neurol 6:83–91
73. Yonekawa Y, Yasargil MG (1976) Extra-intracranial anastomosis: clinical and technical aspects. Results. In: Krayenbühl H (ed) Advances and technical standards in neurosurgery. Springer, Wien New York, pp 45–78
74. Youmans JR, Kindt GW, Mitchell OC (1967) Extended studies of direction of flow and pressure in the internal carotid artery following common carotid artery ligation. J Neurosurg 27:250–254

Extra-intracranial Bypass

1. Albanese W, Tomasello F, Cioffi FA (1980) Combined extra-intracranial arterial bypass and trapping procedure for giant intracavernous carotid aneurysms. Acta Neurochir 53:129 (abstract)
2. Ammerman BJ, Smith DR (1977) Giant fusiform middle cerebral aneurysm: successful treatment utilizing microvascular bypass. Surg Neurol 7:255–257
3. Ausman JI, Diaz FG, De Los Reyes RA et al (1981) Anastomosis of occipital artery to anterior inferior cerebellar artery for basilar artery stenosis. Neurosurgery 9:56–60
4. Ausman JI, Diaz FG, De Los Reyes FA, Pak H, Patel S, Metha B, Boulos R (1982) Posterior circulation revascularization. Superficial temporal artery to superior cerebellar artery anastomosis. J Neurosurg 56:766–776
5. Ausman JI, Lee MC, Chater N et al (1979) Superficial temporal artery to superior cerebellar artery anastomosis for distal basilar artery stenosis. Surg Neurol 12:277–282
6. Barnett HJM (1978) Delayed cerebral ischemic episodes distal to occlusion of major cerebral arteries. Neurology 28:769–774
7. Brambilla G, Paoletti P, Rodriguez Y, Baena R (1982) Extracranial-intracranial arterial bypass in the treatment of inoperable giant aneurysms of the internal carotid artery. Report of a case. Acta Neurochir 60:63–69
8. Bushe KA, Bockhorn J (1980) Extracranial-intracranial arterial bypass for giant aneurysms. Acta Neurochir 54:107–115
9. Cesari JB, Fuentes JM, Prince P, Castan P, Vlahovitch B (1980) Ultrasonic surveillance of an extra-intracranial anastomosis in the process of ligature of the homolateral internal carotid. Ultrasons 1:399–407
10. Debrun G (1984) Personal communication
11. Diaz FG, Ausman JI, Pearce JE (1982) Ischemic complications after combined internal carotid artery occlusion and extracranial intracranial anastomosis. Neurosurgery 10:563–570
11a. Diaz FG, Pearce J, Ausman JI (1985) Complications of cerebral revascularization with autogenous vein grafts. Neurosurgery 17:271–276
12. Diaz FG, Umansky F, Mehta B, Montoya S, Dujovny M, Ausman JI, Cabezudo J (1985) Cerebral revascularization to a main limb of the middle cerebral artery in the sylvian fissure. An alternative approach to conventional anastomosis. J Neurosurg 63:21–29
13. Donaghy RMP (1967) Patch and bypass in microsurgical surgery. In: Donaghy RMP, Yasargil MG (eds) Microvascular surgery. Mosby Co, St Louis, pp 75–86
14. Drake CG (1979) Giant intracranial aneurysms: experience with surgical treatment in 174 patients. Clin Neurosurg 26:12–95
15. Eguchi T, Mayanagi Y, Takakura K (1983) Extra-intracranial bypass and internal carotid artery ligation in one

stage operation for intracavernous and giant carotid aneurysm. No Shinkei Geka 11:1037–1046
16. Ferguson GG, Drake CG, Peerless SJ (1980) Extra-intracranial arterial bypass in the treatment of giant intracranial aneurysms. Stroke 8:11 (abstract)
17. Fischer CM (1975) Clinical syndromes in cerebral thrombosis, hypertensive hemorrhage, and ruptured saccular aneurysm. Clin Neurosurg 22:117–147
18. Gelber BR, Sundt TM Jr (1980) Treatment of intracavernous and giant carotid aneurysms by combined internal carotid ligation and extra to intracranial bypass. J Neurosurg 52:1–10
19. German WJ, Black SPW (1965) Cervical ligation for internal carotid aneurysms. An extended follow-up. J Neurosurg 23:572–577
20. Grote E, Schönmayr R (1982) Extracranial-intracranial bypass in giant aneurysms. Neurosurg Rev 5:83–85
21. Gurdjian ES, Lindner DW, Thomas LW (1965) Experiences with ligation of the common carotid artery for treatment of aneurysms of the internal carotid artery, with particular reference to complications. J Neurosurg 23:311–318
22. Hassler O (1963) Experimental carotid ligation followed by aneurysmal formation and other morphological changes in the circle of willis. J Neurosurg 20:1–7
23. Heros RC (1984) Thromboembolic complications after combined internal carotid ligation and extra to intracranial bypass. Surg Neurol 21:75–79
24. Heros RC, Ameri AM (1984) Rupture of a giant basilar aneurysm after saphenous vein interposition graft to the posterior cerebral artery. Case report. J Neurosurg 61:381–390
25. Heros RC, Nelson PB (1980) Intracerebral hemorrhage after microsurgical cerebral revascularization Neurosurgery 6:371–375
26. Heros RC, Nelson PB, Ojemann RG, Crowell RM, Debrun G (1983) Large and giant paraclinoid aneurysms: surgical techniques, complications and results. Neurosurgery 12:153–163
27. Hirato M, Fukamachi A, Toyoda O, Kaneko M, Wakao T, Nukui H (1983) A newly-developed aneurysm after controlateral common carotid ligation for arteriovenous malformation with porencephalia. Case report. Neurol Med Chir (Tokyo) 23:163–166
28. Hopkins LN, Budny JL, Castellani D (1983) Extra-intracranial arterial bypass and basislar artery ligation in the treatment of giant basilar artery aneurysms. Neurosurgery 13:189–194
29. Hopkins LN, Fein JM, Flamm ES, Spetzler RF (1982) The role of cerebral bypass in the treatment of aneurysms. In: Hopkins LN, Long DM (eds) Clinical management of intracranial aneurysm. Raven, New York, pp 287–293
30. Hopkins LN, Grand W (1979) Extracranial-intracranial arterial bypass in the treatment of aneurysms of the carotid and middle cerebral arteries. Neurosurgery 5:21–31
31. Hosobuchi Y (1979) Direct surgical treatment of giant intracranial aneurysms. J Neurosurg 51:743–756
32. Ishii R, Koike T, Takeuchi S, Ohsugi S, Tanaka R, Konno K (1983) Anastomosis of the superficial temporal artery to the distal anterior cerebral with interposed cephalic vein graft. J Neurosurg 58:425–429
33. Iwabuchi T, Kudo T, Hatanaka M, Oda N, Maeda S (1979) Vein graft bypass in treatment of giant aneurysm. Surg Neurol 12:463–466
34. Kak VK, Taylor AR, Gordon DS (1973) Proximal carotid ligation for internal carotid aneurysms. A long term follow-up study. J Neurosurg 39:503–513
35. Khodadad G, Singh RS, Olinger CP (1977) Possible prevention of brain stem stroke by microvascular anastomosis in the vertebro-basilar system. Stroke 8:316–321
36. Leclercq TA, Ambler MW (1980) Fatal subdural bleeding following superficial temporal-middle cerebral artery anastomosis. Case report. J Neurosurg 52:392–394
37. Lougheed WM, Marshall BM, Hunter M, Michel ER, Sandwith-Smyth H (1971) Common carotid to intracranial internal carotid bypass venous graft: technical note. J Neurosurg 34:114–118
38. Love JG, Dart LH (1967) Results of carotid ligation with particular reference to intracranial aneurysms. J Neurosurg 27:89–93
39. Miller JD, Jawad K, Jennett B (1977) Safety of carotid ligation and its role in the management of intracranial aneurysms. J Neurol Neurosurg Psychiatry 40:64–72
40. Odom GL, Tindall GT (1968) Carotid ligation in the treatment of certain intracranial aneurysms. Clin Neurosurg 15:101–116
41. Oldershaw JB, Voris HC (1966) Internal carotid artery ligation. A follow-up study. Neurology 16:937–938
42. Ouaknine GE (1984) Pontage temporo-sylvien et ligature carotidienne dans les anévrysmes intracraniens géants. Union Med Can 113:246–250
43. Peerless SJ (1976) Techniques of cerebral revascularization. Clin Neurosurg 23:258–269
44. Peerless SJ, Fergusson GG, Drake CG (1982) Extracranial-intracranial bypass in the treatment of giant intracranial aneurysms. Neurosurg Rev 5:77–81
45. Pouyanne H, Banayan A, Guérin J, Riemens V (1973) Les anévrysmes sacculaires multiples du système carotidien supra-clinoïdien. Rapport à la société de neurochirurgie de langue française, vol 19. Masson, Paris [Suppl 1] 96 p
46. Reichman OH (1976) Complications of cerebral revascularization. Clin Neurosurg 23:318–335
47. Robbins J, Fein JM, Lantos G, Hooshangi N (1984) Reflow into a thrombosed giant middle cerebral artery aneurysm after extracranial-intracranial bypass. Neurosurgery 15:120–124
48. Samson DS, Boone S (1978) Extracranial-intracranial (EC-IC) arterial bypass: past performance and current concepts. Neurosurgery 3:79–86
49. Scott RM, Liu HC, Yuan R, Adelman L (1982) Rupture of a previously unruptured gaint middle cerebral artery aneurysm after extra-intracranial bypass surgery. Neurosurgery 10:600–603
50. Sindou M, Grunewald P, Guegan Y, Redondo A, Rey A (1979) Cerebral revascularization with extra-intracranial anastomoses for vascular lesions of traumatic, malformative and tumorous origin. Acta Neurochir 28:282–286
51. Sindou M, Guegan Y, Grunewald P, Redondo A, Rey A (1978) Revascularisation cérébrale par anastomoses extra-intracrâniennes en pathologie vasculaire: traumatique, malformative et tumorale. In: Rey A (ed) Revascularisation cérébrale par anastomoses extra-intracrâniennes, Table Ronde de la société française de Neurochirurgie de langue française. Favre, Paris, pp 178–192
52. Spetzler RF, Rhodes RS, Roski RA, Likavec MJ (1980) Subclavian to middle cerebral artery saphenous vein bypass graft. J Neurosurgery 53:465–469
53. Spetzler RF, Roski RA, Schuster H, Takaoda Y (1980)

The role of EC-IC in the treatment of giant intracranial aneurysms. Neurol Res 2:345–359
54. Spetzler RF, Schuster H, Roski RA (1980) Elective extracranial-intracranial arterial bypass in the treatment of inoperable giant aneurysms of the internal carotid artery. J Neurosurg 53:22–77
55. Spetzler RF, Selman W, Carter LP (1984) Elective EC-IC bypass for unclippable intracranial aneurysms. Neurol Res 6:64–68
56. Story JL, Brown WE Jr, Eidelberg E, Arom KV, Stewart JR (1978) Cerebral revascularization: common carotid to distal middle cerebral artery bypass. Neurosurgery 2:131–134
57. Sundt TM, Piepgras DG (1978) Occipital to posterior inferior cerebellar artery bypass surgery. J Neurosurg 48:916–928
58. Sundt TM, Piepgras DG (1979) Surgical approach to giant intracranial aneurysms. Operative experience with 80 cases. J Neurosurg 51:731–742
59. Sundt TM, Piepgras DG, Houser OW, Campbell JK (1982) Interposition saphenous vein grafts for advanced occlusive discase and large aneurysms in the posterior circulation. J Neurosurg 56:205–215
60. Tew JM Jr (1975) Reconstructive intracranial vascular surgery for prevention of stroke. Clin Neurosurg 22:264–280
61. Tew JM Jr (1979) Techniques of supratentorial cerebral revascularisation. Clin Neurosurg 26:330–345
62. Tognetti F, Andreoli A, Testa C (1984) Giant fusiform aneurysm of the middle cerebral artery treated with extracranial intracranial arterial bypass and Drake tourniquet. Surg Neurol 22:33–35
63. Winn HR, Richardon AE, Jane JA (1977) Late morbidity and mortality of common carotid ligation for posterior communicating aneurysms. A comparison to conservative treatment. J Neurosurg 47:727–736
64. Yasargil MG (1969) Anastomosis between the superficial temporal artery and a branch of the middle cerebral artery. In: Yasargil MG (ed) Microsurgery applied to neurosurgery. Thieme, Stuttgart, pp 105–115
65. Yonekawa Y, Yasargil MG (1976) Extra-intracranial anastomosis: clinical and technical aspects. Results. In: Krayenbühl H (ed) Advances and technical standards in neurosurgery, vol 3. Springer, Wien New York, pp 45–78
66. Ausman JI, Pearce J, De los Reyes RA, Scharz G (1983) Treatment of high extracranial carotid aneurysm with CCA-MCA bypass and carotid ligation. J Neurosurg 58:421–424
67. Diaz FG, Pearce J, Ausman JI (1985) Complications of cerebral revascularization with autogenous vein grafts. Neurosurgery 17:271–276
68. Little J, Farlan A, Bryerton B (1983) Short vein grafts for cerebral revascularization. J Neurosurg 59:384–388

Tests for Tolerance to Therapeutic Occlusion

1. Cathignol D, Chapelon JY, Fourcade C (1978) Vélocimètre doppler à l'usage des petits vaisseaux: "le Microflo". Biosigma (Paris) 426–429
2. Cathignol D, Chapelon JY, Mestas JL et al (1983) Description et application d'un vélocimètre ultrasonore doppler pour les petits vaisseaux. Med Biol Eng Comput 21:358–364
3. Chacornac R, Poussel JF, Perrin G, Goutelle A (1982) Modifications des pressions intracrâniennes au cours du clampage de la carotide. Agressologie 23:77–81
4. Chater N (1976) Surgical results and measurements of intraoperative flow in micro-neurosurgical anastomoses. In: Austin GM (ed) Micro-neurosurgical anastomoses for cerebral ischemia. Thomas, Springfield (Ill), pp 295–304
5. Espagno J (1969) La circulation cérébrale: du morphologique au fonctionnel normal ou pathologique. Neurochirurgie [Suppl 2] 15:178
6. Fuentes JM, Cesari JB, Prince P (1980) Place du "doppler" dans le bilan pré et postopératoire des anastomoses extra-intracrâniennes (à propos de 40 cas). Ultrasons 1:301–308
7. Gelber BR, Sundt TM Jr (1980) Treatment of intracavernous and giant carotid aneurysms by combined internal carotid ligation and extra-intracranial bypass. J Neurosurg 52:1–10
8. Gilsbach JM (1983) Intra-operative doppler sonography in neurosurgery. Springer, Wien New York, 104 p
9. Heilbrun MP, Reichman OH, Anderson RE et al (1975) Regional cerebral blood flow studies following superficial temporal-middle cerebral artery anastomosis. J Neurosurg 43:706–716
10. Hosobuchi Y (1976) Direct surgical treatment of giant intracranial aneurysms. J Neurosurg 51:743–756
11. Jennett B, Miller JD, Harper AM (1976) Effect of carotid artery surgery on cerebral blood flow. Excerpta Medica, Amsterdam, 170 pp
12. Little JR, Yamamoto YL, Feindel W et al (1979) Superficial temporal artery to middle cerebral artery anastomosis. Intra-operative evaluation by fluoresceine angiography and xenon-133 clearance. J Neurosurg 50:560–569
13. Lye CR, Summer DS, Strandness DE (1976) The accuracy of the supra-orbital doppler examination in the diagnosis of hemodynamically significant carotid occlusive disease. Surgery 79:12–15
14. Miller JD, Jawad K, Jennett B (1977) Safety of carotid ligation and its role in the management of intracranial aneurysms. J Neurosurg Neurol Psychiatry 40:64–72
15. Moritake K, Handa H, Yonekawa Y, Takebe Y, Kishimoto S, Makimoto K (1981) Ultrasonic doppler assessment of hemodynamics in gradual carotid ligation. Stroke 12:177–182
16. Nornes H, Wickeby P (1977) Cerebral arterial blood flow and aneurysm surgery. J Neurosurg 47:810–827
17. Ouaknine GE (1984) Pontage temporo-sylvian et ligature carotidienne dans les anévrysmes intracrâniens géants. Union Med Can 113 (4):246–250, 292
18. Perrin G, Chacornac R, Goutelle A (1984) Corrélation entre pression intra-crânienne et pression artérielle carotidienne résiduelle au cours du clampage carotidien. Agressologie 25 [6]:691–696
19. Poussel JF, Chacornac R, Perrin G, Goutelle A (1982) Incidences du clampage carotidien sur la pression intracrânienne. Lyon Chir 78:361–364
20. Roski RA, Spetzler RF (1982) Carotid ligation in the treatment of cerebral aneurysms. In: Hopkins LN, Long DM (eds) Clinical management of intracranial aneurysms. Raven Press, New York, pp 11–19
21. Schmiedek P, Gratzl O, Spetzler R (1976) Selection of patients for extra-intracranial arterial bypass surgery based on R-CBF measurements. J Neurosurg 44:303–312
22. Sindou M, Peronnet F, Fischer G, Gérin P, Mansuy

L (1972) Exploration du cortex chez l'homme, par les méthodes transcorticographiques et straticorticographiques. Neurochirurgie 18:213–234
23. Sundt TM Jr, Piepgras DG (1979) Surgical approach to giant intracranial aneurysms. Operative experience with 80 cases. J Neurosurg 51:731–742
24. Sundt TM Jr, Sharbrough FW, Anderson RE et al (1974) Cerebral blood flow measurements and electroencephalogram during carotid endarterectomy. J Neurosurg 41:310–320
25. Symon L, Wang AD, Costa e Silva IE, Gentili F (1984) Peri-operative use of somatosensory evoked responses in aneurysm surgery. J Neurosurg 60:269–275
26. Wilkins RH (1982) Partial carotid artery ligation in the treatment of intracranial aneurysms. In: Hopkins LN, Long DM (eds) Clinical management of intracranial aneurysms. Raven Press, New York, pp 39–47
27. Yoneda S, Nukada T, Kimura K, Tanaka K, Ashida K, Asai T, Etani H, Imaizumi M, Abe H (1981) Evaluation of cross-circulation through circle of Willis using an ultrasonic doppler technique. Stroke 12:478–488

Management by the Intravascular Approach

1. Barrow OL, Fleischer AS, Hoffman JC (1982) Complications of detachable balloon catheter technique in the treatment of traumatic intra-cranial arterio-venous fistulae. J Neurosurg 56:396–403
2. Beatty RA, Richardson AE (1968) Predicting intolerance to common carotid artery ligation by carotid angiography. J Neurosurg 28:9–13
3. Berenstein A, Ransohoff J, Kupersmith M, Flamm E, Graed D (1984) Transvascular treatment of giant aneurysms of the cavernous carotid and vertebral arteries. Functional investigation and embolization. Surg Neurol 21:3–12
4. Brooks B (1930) The treatment of traumatic arteriovenous fistulae. South Med J 23:100–106
5. Carlens E, Hanson HE, Nordenstrom BEW (1951) Temporary unilateral occlusion of the pulmonary artery. J Thorac Surg 22:527
6. Chalif DJ, Flamm ES, Berenstein A, In Sup Choi (1983) Microsurgical removal of a balloon embolus to the internal carotid artery. J Neurosurg 58:112–116
7. Debrun G, Lacour P, Caron JP et al (1975) Experimental approach to the treatment of carotid cavernous fistulas with inflatable and isolated balloon. Neuroradiology 9:9–12
8. Debrun G, Lacour P, Caron JP et al (1975) Traitement de fistules artério-veineuses et d'anévrysmes par ballon gonflable et largable. Bases expérimentales et application à l'homme. Nouv Presse Méd 4:2315–2318
9. Debrun G, Lacour P, Caron JP et al (1975) Inflatable and released balloon. Technique experimentation in dog. Application in man. Neuroradiology 9:267–271
10. Debrun G, Lacour P, Caron JP et al (1979) Detachable balloon and calibrated-leak balloon techniques in the treatment of cerebral vascular lesions. J Neurosurg 49:635–649
11. Debrun G, Fox AJ, Drake CG, Peerless S, Girvin J, Ferguson G (1981) Giant unclippable aneurysm: treatment with detachable balloons. AJNR 2:167–173
12. Debrun G, Fox AJ (1982) Interventional neuroradiology in the treatment of cerebral aneurysms. In: Hopkins LN, Long DM (eds) Clinical management of intracranial aneurysms. Raven, New York, pp 273–285
13. Debrun G, Vinuela FV, Fox AJ (1982) Aspirin and systemic heparinization in diagnostic and interventional neuroradiology. AJNR 3:337–340
14. Di Tullio MV Jr, Rand RW, Frisch E (1978) Detachable balloon catheter. Its application in experimental arteriovenous fistulae. J Neurosurg 48:717–723
15. Dujovny M, Laha RK, Barrionuevo P (1977) Endothelial changes secondary to use of a Fogarty catheter. Surg Neurol 7:39–41
16. Fogarty TJ, Cranley JJ, Krause RJ et al (1963) A method for extraction of arterial emboli and thrombi. Surg Gynecol Obstet 110:241–244
17. Heifetz MD, Hieshima GB, Mehringer CM (1980) Preliminary report of a hollow-centered balloon for intravascular occlusion of intracranial aneurysms or arteriovenous fistulas. Technical note. J Neurosurg 53:262–265
18. Hieshima GB, Grinnell VS, Mehringer CM (1981) A detachable balloon for therapeutic transcatheter occlusions. Radiology 138:227–228
19. Jawad K, Miller DCh, Wyper DJ, Rowan JO (1977) Measurement of CBF and carotid artery presure compared with cerebral angiography in assessing collateral blood supply after carotid ligation. J Neurosurg 46:185–196
20. Keravel Y, Debrun G, Rottman N (1980) Treatment of experimental aneurysms and carotid jugular fistulas by inflated and detachable balloons. Int J Microsurg 2:33–38
21. Keravel Y, Gaston A, Nguyen JP, Lacaze A, Benabid AL, Marsault C, Debrun C et al (1981) Cathétérisme intra-vasculaire super-sélectif: apport du guidage par aimant supra-conducteur. Résultats préliminaires. Communication Société de Neurochirurgie de Langue Française, December, Paris
22. Laitinen L, Servo A (1978) Embolization of cerebral vessels with inflatable and detachable balloons. J Neurosurg 48:307–308
23. Langford KH, Vitek JJ, Zeiger E (1983) Migration of detachable mini balloon from the ICA causing occlusion of the MCA. Case report. J Neurosurg 58:430–434
24. Luessenhop AJ, Velasquez AC (1964) Observation of the tolerance of intracranial arteries to catheterization. J Neurosurg 21:85–91
25. Marsault C, Gaston A, Nguyen JP, Keravel Y, Benabid A, Lacaze A, Debrun G (1982) Intra-vascular navigation of catheter aided by superconducting magnet. Symposium Neuroradiologicum. Washington DC, October
26. Pevsner PH (1977) Microballoon catheter for superselective angiography and therapeutic occlusion. AJR 128:225–230
27. Picard L, Lepoire J, Montant H et al (1974) Endarterial occlusion of carotid cavernous sinus fistulas using a balloon tipped catheter. Neuroradiology 8:5–10
28. Prolo DJ, Hanbery JN (1971) Intraluminal occlusion of a carotid cavernous sinus fistula with a balloon catheter. (Technical note). J Neurosurg 35:237–242
29. Rodomanov AP, Shcheglov VI (1983) Intravascular occlusion of saccular aneurysm. Adv Neurosurgery 9:25–49
30. Rougerie J, Guilmet D, Bamberger-Bozo (1973) Anévrysme carotido-caverneux. A propos d'une orientation thérapeutique nouvelle. Neurochirurgie 19:649–654
31. Scialfa G, Vaghi A, Valsecchi F et al (1982) Neuroradiological treatment of carotid and vertebral fistulas and

intracavernous aneurysms. Technical problems and results. Neuroradiology 24:13–25

32. Serbinenko FA (1974) Balloon catheterization and occlusion of major cerebral vessels. J Neurosurg 41:125–145
33. Straube K, Dotter CH (1963) Single lumen balloon catheter for percutaneous insertion. AJR 90:650
34. Swan MJL, Ganz W, Forrester F et al (1970) Catheterization of the heart in man with use of a flow directed balloon-tipped catheter. N Engl J Med 283:447–451
35. Taki W, Handa H, Yamagata S, Matsuda I, Yonekawa Y, Ikada Y, Iwata H (1979) Balloon embolization of a giant aneurysm using a newly developped catheter. Surg Neurol 12:363–365
36. Theron J (1980) Cas inhabituels de lésions vasculaires du siphon carotidien intra-caverneux traité par sonde de Fogarty. J Neuroradiol 7:183–191
37. White RI, Kaufman SL, Barth KH et al (1979) Embolotherapy with detachable silicone balloons. Radiology 131:619–627
38. Wholey MH, Kessler L, Boenke M (1972) A percutaneous balloon catheter technique for the treatment of intracranial aneurysms. Acta Radiol 13:286–292
39. Yodh SB, Pierce NT, Weggel JR et al (1968) A new magnetic system for intra-cranial vascular navigation. Med Biol Eng 6:143–147
40. Zanetti PH, Sherman FE (1972) Experimental evaluation of a tissue adhesive as an agent for the treatment of aneurysms and arterio-venous anomalies. J Neurosurg 36:72–79

General Conclusions

1. Drake CG, Peerless SJ (1986) Posterior circulation aneurysms. In: Kikuchi H, Fukushima T, Watanabe K (eds) Intracranial aneurysms: surgical timing and techniques. Nishimura, Japan
2. Sundt TM, Piepgras DG (1986) Surgical management of giant intracranial aneurysms. In: Kikuchi H, Fukushima T, Watanabe K (eds) Intracranial aneurysms: surgical timing and techniques. Nishimura, Japan
3. Yasargil MG (1984) Microneurosurgery II: clinical considerations, surgery of the intracranial aneurysm and results. Thieme, Stuttgart

Subject Index

MIX
Papier aus verantwortungsvollen Quellen
Paper from responsible sources
FSC® C105338

If you have any concerns about our products,
you can contact us on
ProductSafety@springernature.com

In case Publisher is established outside the EU,
the EU authorized representative is:
Springer Nature Customer Service Center GmbH
Europaplatz 3, 69115 Heidelberg, Germany

Printed by Libri Plureos GmbH
in Hamburg, Germany